The Diplegic Child
Evaluation and Management

Shriners Hospitals for Crippled Children Symposium

Published by the
American Academy of Orthopaedic Surgeons

Library of Congress Cataloging-in-Publication Data

The diplegic child: evaluation and management/edited by Michael D.
 Sussman.
  512 p. cm.
  "Symposium, Charlottesville, Virginia, Nov. 21–24, 1991."
  Includes bibliographical references and index.
  ISBN 0-89203-068-2: $75.00
   1. Cerebral palsy—Treatment—Congresses.   2. Cerebral palsy—
Congresses.   3. Cerebral palsied children—Congresses.
I. Sussman, Michael D.
  [DNLM: 1. Cerebral Palsy—diagnosis—congresses.   2. Cerebral
Palsy—in infancy & childhood—congresses.   3. Cerebral Palsy—
therapy—congresses.   4. Movement Disorders—therapy—congresses.
5. Muscle Spasticity—therapy—congresses.   WS 342 D596]
RJ496.C4D58   1992
618.92'836—dc20
DNLM/DLC
for Library of Congress   92-49903
                                                                       CIP

The Diplegic Child: Evaluation and Management/edited by Michael D. Sussman,
MD; supported by the Shriners Hospitals for Crippled Children and published by the
American Academy of Orthopaedic Surgeons.

ISBN 0-89203-068-2

The Diplegic Child
Evaluation and Management

Edited by
Michael D. Sussman, MD
Chief of Staff
Shriners Hospital for Crippled Children
Portland, Oregon

with 150 illustrations

Symposium
Charlottesville, Virginia
Nov. 21–24, 1991

Supported by the
Shriners Hospitals for Crippled Children

in collaboration with the
Pediatric Orthopaedic Society of North America

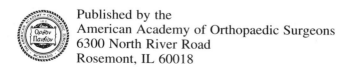

Published by the
American Academy of Orthopaedic Surgeons
6300 North River Road
Rosemont, IL 60018

Contributors

Bennett I. Bertenthal, PhD*†
Professor, Department of Psychology
University of Virginia
Charlottesville, Virginia

James A. Blackman, MD, MPH*†
Professor of Pediatrics
University of Virginia Health Sciences
   Center
Children's Medical Center
Kluge Children's Rehabilitation Center and
   Research Institute
Charlottesville, Virginia

Peter A. Blasco, MD*†
Associate Professor of Pediatrics
University of Minnesota Medical School
Minneapolis, Minnesota

Kristen A. Bowsher, MS†
Doctoral Fellow, Biomedical Engineering
University of Virginia
Charlottesville, Virginia

Patricia A. Burtner, MOT, OTR†
Occupational Therapist
CDRC
Eugene, Oregon

Tom Bylander, PhD†
Assistant Professor
Department of Computer and Information
   Science
The Ohio State University
Columbus, Ohio

Suzann K. Campbell, PhD, PT*†
Professor of Physical Therapy
University of Illinois at Chicago
Chicago, Illinois

S. Terry Canale, MD*
Professor
University of Tennessee Campbell Clinic
Department of Orthopaedic Surgery
Memphis, Tennessee

R. Jay Cummings, MD†
Chairman, Department of Orthopaedics
Nemours Children's Clinic
Jacksonville, Florida

Luciano S. Dias, MD*†
Associate Professor, Orthopaedic Surgery
Northwestern University
Chicago, Illinois

Lisa Federico, PT†
Nemours Children's Clinic
Jacksonville, Florida

Robert L. Freedland, PhD†
Research Fellow, Department of Psychology
University of Virginia
Charlottesville, Virginia

James R. Gage, MD*†
Professor of Orthopaedics
University of Minnesota
St. Paul, Minnesota

Melinda Goins, PT†
Nemours Children's Clinic
Jacksonville, Florida

Michael J. Goldberg, MD*†
Professor and Chairman
Department of Orthopaedic Surgery
Tufts University School of Medicine
Boston, Massachusetts

Neil E. Green, MD*†
Department of Orthopaedics
Vanderbilt University School of Medicine
Nashville, Tennessee

Walter B. Greene, MD*†
Professor of Orthopaedic Surgery and
   Pediatrics
University of North Carolina School of
   Medicine
Chapel Hill, North Carolina

Linda Hanlin, OTR†
Pediatric Occupational Therapist
Henry Ford Hospital
Detroit, Michigan

Susan E. Harryman, MS, RPT*†
Director, Physical Therapy
Kennedy Krieger Institute
Baltimore, Maryland

Eric T. Jones, MD*
Clinical Professor of Pediatric Orthopaedic
  Surgery
West Virginia University
Morgantown, West Virginia

Andre J. Kaelin, MD, Privat-Docent*†
Chief of the Pediatric Orthopaedics Unit
Children's Hospital
Geneva, Switzerland

Susan E. Kirsch, MD, FRCPC, FAAP†
Associate Director
Magee Clinic
Toronto, Ontario, Canada

Boris M. Kogan, PhD†
Institute of General and Forensic Psychiatry
Neurochemistry Laboratory
Moscow, Russia

E. Dennis Lyne, MD*†
Professor of Surgery and Pediatrics
Michigan State University College of Human
  Medicine
Program Director Orthopaedic Surgery
Kalamazoo Center for Medical Studies
Kalamazoo, Michigan

Gerard R. Marty, MD†
Clinical Instructor
Department of Orthopaedics
Northwestern University
Chicago, Illinois

Cirill V. Mashilov, PhD*†
Institute of General and Forensic Psychiatry
Neurochemistry Laboratory
Moscow, Russia

John M. Mazur, MD*†
Nemours Children's Clinic
Jacksonville, Florida

William P. McCluskey, MD†
Nemours Children's Clinic
Jacksonville, Florida

Newton C. McCollough III, MD*†
Director of Medical Affairs
Shriners Hospitals for Crippled Children
Tampa, Florida

Colin F. Moseley, MD*†
Chief Surgeon
Shriners Hospital for Crippled Children
Los Angeles, California

M. Susan Murr, RPT†
Pediatric Physical Therapist
Gillette Children's Hospital
St. Paul, Minnesota

Jodi H. Nashman, BS†
Research Assistant in Biomedical
  Engineering
University of Virginia
Charlottesville, Virginia

Craig Newsam, MPT†
Research Physical Therapist
Rancho Los Amigos Medical Center
Downey, California

William L. Oppenheim, MD*†
Associate Professor
Division of Orthopaedic Surgery
UCLA Medical Center
Los Angeles, California

Karen E. Pape, MD, FRCPC, FAAP*†
Medical Director
Magee Clinic
Toronto, Ontario, Canada

Warwick J. Peacock, MD†
Professor, Division of Neurosurgery
UCLA Center for the Health Sciences
Los Angeles, California

Jacquelin Perry, MD*†
Chief, Pathokinesiology Service
Rancho Los Amigos Medical Center
Downey, California

George T. Rab, MD*†
Professor of Orthopaedic Surgery
Head, Children's Orthopaedic Service
University of California, Davis
Sacramento, California

Michael D. Reed, PharmD, FCCP, FCP†
Associate Professor of Pediatrics
School of Medicine
Case Western Reserve University
Cleveland, Ohio

Jørgen Reimers, MD*†
Chief Surgeon
Orthopaedic Department
Rigshospitalet
Copenhagen, Denmark

Theresa Ricketts, PT†
Pediatric Physical Therapist
Henry Ford Hospital
Detroit, Michigan

Cathleen D. Roberts, DO†
Developmental Fellow
University of Virginia
Charlottesville, Virginia

Bernard Roehr, MD†
Chief Orthopaedic Surgery Resident
Michigan State University
Kalamazoo Center for Medical Studies
Kalamazoo, Michigan

Leon Root, MD*†
Chief, Pediatric Orthopaedics
The Hospital for Special Surgery
New York, New York

Peter L. Rosenbaum, MD, FRCP(C)*†
Professor of Pediatrics, Faculty of Health
  Sciences
McMaster University
Hamilton, Ontario, Canada

Robert K. Rosenthal, MD*†
Assistant Clinical Professor of Orthopaedic
  Surgery
Harvard Medical School and Children's
  Hospital
Boston, Massachusetts

Andrew W. Ryan, MD†
Resident in Orthopaedic Surgery
The Ohio State University
Columbus, Ohio

William Z. Rymer, MD, PhD*†
Director of Research
Rehabilitation Institute of Chicago
Chicago, Illinois

Edward L. Schor, MD†
Associate Professor, Department of Pediatrics
Tufts University School of Medicine
Boston, Massachusetts

Daniel E. Shanks, MD†
Nemours Children's Clinic
Jacksonville, Florida

Sheldon R. Simon, MD*†
Professor and Chief, Orthopaedic Surgery
The Ohio State University
Columbus, Ohio

Stephen R. Skinner, MD*†
Chief of Staff
Shriners Hospital for Crippled Children
San Francisco, California

Evgeny G. Sologubov, MD*†
Head Physician
Children's Psychoneurological Clinical
  Hospital No. 18
Moscow, Russia

Loretta A. Staudt, MS, PT†
Clinical/Research Physical Therapist
UCLA Division of Neurosurgery
Los Angeles, California

J. Andy Sullivan, MD*
Professor and Chair
The University of Oklahoma Health Sciences
  Center
Department of Orthopaedic Surgery and
  Rehabilitation
Section on Children's Orthopaedics
Oklahoma City, Oklahoma

Michael D. Sussman, MD*†
Chief of Staff
Shriners Hospital for Crippled Children
Portland, Oregon

David H. Sutherland, MD*†
Professor
Medical Director, Children's Hospital Motion
  Analysis Laboratory
University of California, San Diego
San Diego, California

Vernon T. Tolo, MD*
John C. Wilson, Jr. Professor of Orthopaedics
Head, Divison of Orthopaedic Surgery
Childrens Hospital Los Angeles
Los Angeles, California

James C. Torner, PhD*†
Associate Professor of Epidemiology
Department of Preventive Medicine and
  Environmental Health
University of Iowa
Iowa City, Iowa

Chester M. Tylkowski, MD*†
Medical Director, The Motion Laboratory
Miami Children's Hospital
Miami, Florida

Christopher L. Vaughan, PhD*†
Director of Motion Analysis Laboratory
Associate Professor of Orthopaedics &
  Biomedical Engineering
University of Virginia
Charlottesville, Virginia

Hugh G. Watts, MD*
Shriners Hospital for Crippled Children
Los Angeles, California

Michael Weintraub, PhD†
Technical Staff
GTE Laboratories, Inc.
Waltham, Massachussetts

Marjorie H. Woollacott, PhD*†
Professor, University of Oregon
Eugene, Oregon

---

* Workshop Participant
† Contributor to Volume

Contents

Contents

Foreword

This volume is the first in a series of pediatric orthopaedic symposia published by the American Academy of Orthopaedic Surgeons and made possible through sponsorship by Shriners Hospitals for Crippled Children. Since 1922, Shriners Hospitals have expended over $2.3 billion, providing free care to nearly half a million children in its 19 orthopaedic hospitals and three burn institutes. During this time, nearly 3,000 residents in orthopaedic surgery have been educated in pediatric orthopaedics at Shriners Hospitals and over $140 million has been expended in support of basic research programs.

During the Opening Ceremony of its 1989 Annual Meeting, the Academy officially recognized Shriners Hospitals for its major contributions to patient care, education, and research in pediatric orthopaedics. In response, Mr. Gene Bracewell, Chairman of the Board of Trustees of Shriners Hospitals, announced that Shriners Hospitals would provide the Academy with the necessary funds to support triennial symposia on important topics in pediatric orthopaedics. The symposia, to be developed in collaboration with the Pediatric Orthopaedic Society of North America, are to define the current status of patient care and to develop consensus on controversial issues. For these symposia to have maximal impact on patient care, it was determined that the proceedings of the symposia should be published and be made widely available to the health-care professions.

Dr. Eric Jones, Chairman of the Academy's Committee on Pediatric Orthopaedics, and Dr. S. Terry Canale, then President of the Pediatric Orthopaedic Society of North America, co-chaired the Steering Committee that led to this first symposium. The Committee selected the topic, determined the format, and chose Dr. Michael Sussman to chair the symposium and to serve as the editor of this publication.

It is hoped that the product of this new and ongoing collaboration between Shriners Hospitals for Crippled Children, the American Academy of Orthopaedic Surgeons, and the Pediatric Orthopaedic Society of North America will assist in improving the care of children throughout the world who have orthopaedic disabilities.

NEWTON C. McCollough III, MD

Preface

This volume is the product of a symposium held in Charlottesville, Virginia, November 21–24, 1991. The symposium was organized by a joint steering committee composed of members from the Academy's Committee on Pediatric Orthopaedics and the Pediatric Orthopaedic Society of North America: S. Terry Canale, MD; Vernon T. Tolo, MD; Colin F. Moseley, MD; Walter B. Greene, MD; J. Andy Sullivan, MD; Eric T. Jones, MD; and Newton C. McCollough III, MD. The final format of this meeting was developed in order to provide a forum in which experts in the field of cerebral palsy could present data to their peers and then use the shared information to develop consensus regarding current practice, as well as critical questions that must be answered in the future. The summary statements at the end of each chapter were compiled by small discussion groups and then were discussed by all participants at the meeting. These statements reflect the current practice of a group of experts and should be used in this context as general guidelines to patient management; they are not meant to be used as rules to be applied in a cookbook fashion.

Making treatment decisions for patients with cerebral palsy is challenging for a variety of reasons. The condition is heterogeneous in degree, as well as type of involvement, and a multitude of factors affect motor function, including (but not limited to) spasticity, dysphasic muscle activity, poor motor planning, balance problems, impaired spatial perception, and poor proprioception. General factors, such as environment, motivation, obesity, intelligence, and age, also affect treatment outcome. Accurate assessment of the outcome of treatment has been limited by lack of objective measurement tools, as well as by the long periods of time required to assess ultimate outcome. In addition, because the children under treatment are in the process of developing motor skills, comparison with the pretreatment state does not provide a valid control for the influence of treatment. Most studies published to date are descriptive and retrospective and do not provide sufficient information to help in the choice between alternative surgical procedures.

Some limitations of outcome assessment in cerebral palsy have been partially overcome in the past decade through the availability of computer-based gait analysis, which is an excellent, objective, functional assessment tool, although it also has limitations. In addition, other clinically based validated measures have recently become available, such as the Gross Motor Performance Measure and Gross Motor Function Measure described by Rosenbaum, in Chapter 10.

Making valid recommendations regarding treatment requires the use of these tools in the format of a controlled clinical trial, wherein two similar groups of patients are compared, with the only difference between them being the intervention strategy (dependent variable) under study. In practice, this type of study is exceedingly difficult to perform. Finding large groups of patients willing to participate requires a large patient population and committed clinical investigators with adequate funding to carry out the studies. Studies have shown that surgeons have a particularly difficult time participating in such clinical trials.[1] Alternative study design may allow patients to make a choice and still provide statistically relevant data that can be analyzed.[2]

An additional problem is that financial support of clinical investigations is severely limited. Most clinicians cannot dedicate the time to the development of such studies, much less their implementation. The American Academy of Orthopaedic Surgeons has recognized the need for clinical studies and has actively promoted the development of outcome studies. It is particularly important that such studies be initiated. A variety of therapeutic techniques, including neurodevelopmental, Peto, and Vojta; a variety of orthotics such as UCBL inserts, SMOs, and articulated and ''dynamic'' ankle-foot orthoses; and a variety of surgical techniques, including selective dorsal rhizotomy, have been introduced as treatments in the past decade with little or no objective evidence of efficacy. Use of these treatments may be associated with significant financial costs, as well as time commitments by patients and families, and may ultimately be deleterious to the child's functional outcome. It is, therefore, imperative that the means be found for competent investigators to carry out valid clinical trials of all of the intervention strategies that we use in treatment of patients with cerebral palsy. Only then will our treatment decisions become as sophisticated and technologically soundly based as the treatment and assessment tools themselves.

MICHAEL D. SUSSMAN, MD

1. Angell M: Patients' preferences in randomized clinical trials, editorial. *New Engl J Med* 1984;310:1385–1387.
2. Rudicel S, Esdaile J: The randomized clinical trial in orthopaedics: Obligation or option? *J Bone Joint Surg* 1985;67A:1284–1293.

Acknowledgments

This symposium and publication would not have occurred without the strong support and help from a variety of people. Dr. Newton C. McCollough III, Medical Director of Shriners Hospitals for Crippled Children, was instrumental in developing this concept. Mr. Gene Bracewell, Chairman of the Joint Board of Shriners Hospitals, led the Board in the decision to provide the funding that supported this entire endeavor. Mr. Thomas Nelson, Executive Director, and the Board of Directors of the American Academy of Orthopaedic Surgeons also provided significant support and are fully responsible for funding the publication itself. Dr. Marilyn Fox and Ms. Joan Abern have been instrumental in managing the publication process, including editing and preparing the manuscripts and the final volume for publication. The Steering Committee, under the direction of Eric Jones and S. Terry Canale, played a significant role in the development of the final format of the symposium. Becky Parks played a large role in organizing the symposium in Charlottesville and saw to it that everything occurred without problems. Karen Schneider also aided me in organizing this event and in preparing the budget.

Finally, I want to thank my wife, Nancy, for helping with the local arrangements and supporting me throughout this process.

MICHAEL D. SUSSMAN, MD

Section One
Spasticity: Pathology and Pathophysiology

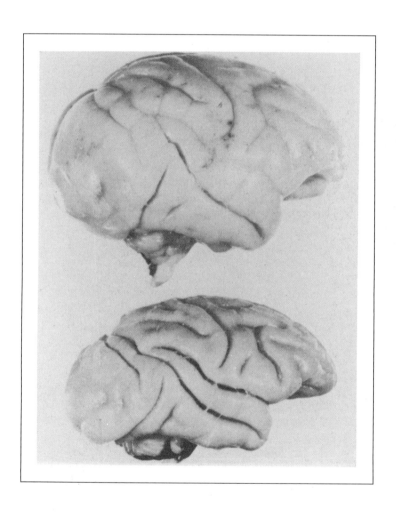

Chapter 1

Pathology of Cerebral Palsy

Peter A. Blasco, MD

Introduction

Cerebral palsy is a disorder of movement and posture (a motor disability) resulting from a nonprogressive central nervous system insult.[1,2] The disorder may stem either from an insult to a normally developing brain or from a central nervous system that developed in an anomalous fashion from an early stage. The exact timing of the insult is important to the epidemiologic description of this disorder but often is difficult to determine, especially during the perinatal period. Furthermore, when considering postnatally acquired cerebral palsy, some favor limiting the time frame of the description to cases present from birth, while others favor later ages. Two to 3 years of age is frequently mentioned as an arbitrary time limit; 6 to 8 years of age is a logical point because of the apparent change in motor plasticity or degree of motor developmental potential around that time; and 16 to 18 years of age is another logical cut point because of the analogy with the developmental plateau in cognitive processing at that time. There is no consensus of opinion on this issue.[3,4] Cerebral palsy is a relatively common disorder (Table 1), affecting approximately one in 200 children, with a prevalence range of 0.1% to 0.7%.[5,6] The higher number probably takes into better account the full spectrum of the disorder by including milder cases,[4] a broader definition of age of insult, and more complete case ascertainment.[7]

The fundamental question underlying the topic of this chapter is: Why do children have cerebral palsy? In addition to understanding the gross and microscopic anatomy of the disorder, what is the pathophysiology linking the disturbed neuroanatomy to the clinical picture (the clinicopathological correlation)? The question also can be addressed by seeking the "why" for the lesion that produces the motor dysfunction. Studies of the etiology and the pathology of this disorder are closely intertwined, with each providing information about the other. Etiologic studies suggest that anywhere from 33% to 65% of cerebral palsy cases are related to perinatal events.[6,8–11] Included are mainly infants born prematurely without an obvious prenatal defect or syndrome and those

Table 1 Prevalence of cerebral palsy relative to other childhood problems

Problem	Prevalence
Cerebral palsy	0.5% (range 0.1% to 0.7%)
Seizure disorders	0.2% to 0.5%
Diabetes mellitus	0.2% to 0.3%
Spina bifida	0.1%
Cystic fibrosis	0.05%

born at any gestational age experiencing significant birth asphyxia or traumatic cranial injury. The variability in reported frequency seems mostly to be a result of arbitrary assumptions about what is considered prenatal and what is perinatal. Postnatally-acquired cerebral palsy is consistently quoted around 10%.[7,8]

Twenty years ago, informal clinical discourse and the literature supported the concept that cerebral palsy usually was a consequence of birth-related injury to the brain. Obstetricians often took blame for causing it. More recently, there has been a major shift in emphasis to unknown prenatal events as the causative factors producing defective babies and precipitating preterm birth and/or difficult deliveries.[4,12] Anatomy such as that seen in Figure 1, for example, indicates that maldevelopment of the nervous system has been present since early prenatal life, dating from the fourth month or before in this particular case. Such a child may have had a difficult birth and would be severely and multiply disabled, but the neuroanatomy shows conclusively that little or none of the developmental dysfunction is a consequence of birth insult. On the other hand, for a child with hemiplegia who had a normal birth history and a sequence of acute clinical events postnatally associated with a cerebrovascular accident, the neuroanatomy defined by imaging studies would support a postnatal insult to a previously normal nervous system. This scenario has been well documented in pathologic studies including confirmation that the rest of the nervous system is normal.[13] Such clean correlations of the etiology and pathology of cerebral palsy are the exception rather than the rule. It is possible to argue (as many defense lawyers will) that every baby born prematurely or with distress of any type was abnormal before labor, and that this undefined abnormality provided the stimulus for premature birth. Anything that happens during delivery is then coincidental to the primary defect.

How much cerebral palsy is related to perinatal insult (prematurity and birth asphyxia) versus prenatal central nervous system abnormality?[14] In this context, the contribution of birth asphyxia to causation[15–19] is a heavily debated issue. Insights in this area come from an understanding of the neuropathology associated with cerebral palsy and from the epidemiologic correlation between certain antecedent events, such as preterm birth, and the ultimate development of cerebral palsy.[20,21] This chapter is an attempt to analyze the information on the pathology of cerebral palsy in order to provide not only a better understanding of

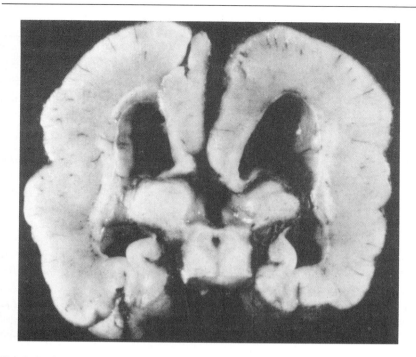

Fig. 1 *Pathology specimen of infant brain, cut in the coronal plane, with lissencephaly. The surface of the cortex is smooth (agyria) as a result of arrested neuronal migration at about the fourth month of gestation. Decreased cerebral volume and increased ventricular size are additional features.*

the nature of the central nervous system insult but also some understanding of how to prevent or limit the multiple causes of these insults.

Historical Background

William John Little (1810–1894), an English orthopaedist, first described cerebral palsy and associated it with difficult birth.[22,23] His name was applied to this disorder (Little's disease) for decades. His hypothesis that orthopaedic deformity was a consequence of neonatal brain injury represented a remarkably novel viewpoint at a time when teething was considered the primary cause of most paralytic syndromes. Sigmund Freud (1856–1939), in his treatises on the classification of cerebral palsy, recognized spastic diplegia and the close association between the spastic diplegic type of cerebral palsy and premature birth.[24,25] However, a decade of work on these childhood motor syndromes failed to elucidate a clear correlation between neuropathology and clinical classification.

In 1888, Sir William Osler[13] popularized use of the term "cerebral palsy" with his review of the clinical details of 151 cases of the "cerebral palsies of children,'' most of whom had spastic hemiplegia. He divided etiologies into seven categories: congenital syphilis, alcohol-related (maternal), difficult labor, forceps (traumatic) delivery, post-natal head trauma, complications of various infectious diseases of infancy (such as pertussis or meningitis), convulsions (the teething hypothesis), and embolism (from bacterial endocarditis). Osler's meticulous review of the pathology literature existing at that time emphasized the varied nature of the lesions encountered and the unsatisfactory state of knowledge. He classified the lesions as primarily vascular/hemorrhagic, atrophic/sclerotic, or porencephalic, and he reported pyramidal tract degeneration descending into the spinal cord. Children with the clinical picture of ''spastic paraplegia'' had much less associated cerebral morbidity and a marked correlation with difficult parturition and prematurity, which he notes quoting Little's work. These cases appear to represent what we would call spastic diplegia today.

Crothers and Paine,[1] in their classic treatise *The Natural History of Cerebral Palsy*, carefully reviewed and contrasted the literature on pathology available from the time of Little and Osler to 1955. The major point of contention through much of this period was whether the insult was primarily vascular/hemorrhagic caused by trauma during delivery or was a primary infectious process involving the motor cortex (polioencephalitis), analogous to poliomyelitis involving the spinal cord. Another approach to the question was to analyze the morbid anatomy of infants who died in the newborn period after suffering abnormal births and who, presumably, would have been at high risk for cerebral palsy had they survived. In this situation, hemorrhage and cerebral tears produced by the tentorium or falx were prominent in otherwise normal brains. Anoxia was included in this analysis as a possible cause of hemorrhage, independent from direct trauma, but was not accorded great importance.

Understanding the Origins of Cerebral Palsy

Four approaches can be used to untangle and elucidate the etiopathology of cerebral palsy: (1) Retrospective studies of children who have cerebral palsy consistently show an increased incidence of birth problems. However, the range of problems and their frequency vary tremendously, as can be seen in the work of Holm,[8] O'Reilly and Walentynowicz,[9] Stanley,[26] and Nelson and Ellenberg.[27] (2) Prospective studies of high-risk newborns show an increased incidence of cerebral palsy as an outcome among survivors. These studies also vary tremendously depending on the risk factor(s) chosen for investigation. Brann,[28] reviewing 16 studies on birth asphyxia in full-term babies, reported neonatal mortality rates ranging from 4% to 61% and neurological sequelae rates ranging from 3.6% to 57% of survivors (Table 2). The variable causing most of this discrepancy was the definition of asphyxia. Both of these approaches led to identification of many, overlapping risk factors that vary widely in degree or severity, making it

Table 2 Incidence of moderate or severe long-term neurologic sequelae in full-term infants surviving birth asphyxia

Investigator	Definition of Asphyxia	Percent Morbidity in Survivors	Percent Mortality
Ergander, 1983	0-3 Apgar at 5 min	22.0	21.0
Finer, 1983	0-5 Apgar at 5 min or IPPV	16.3	0
Storz, 1982	0-5 Apgar at 5 min or IPPV	22.0	—
Finer, 1981	0-3 Apgar at 5 min	28.0	7.0
Fitzhardinge, 1981	0-5 Apgar at 5 min or IPPV more than 2 min	47.0	—
Mulligan, 1980	IPPV more than 1 min	27.0	19.0
Nelson, 1981	0-3 at 15 min	36.0	52.5
	0-3 at 20 min	57.1	59.0
Nelson, 1979	0-3 at 10 min	16.7	34.4
Nelson, 1977	0-3 Apgar at 5 min	4.7	15.5
DeSouza, 1978	0 Apgar at 1 min or onset of breathing after 5 min	8.0	4
Thomson, 1977	0 Apgar at 1 min or 0-3 at 5 min	10.3	50
Scott, 1976	0 Apgar at 1 min or 1-2 at 20 min IPPV	25.0	52
Sarnat, 1976	0-4 Apgar at 1 or 5 min	31.0	10
Steiner, 1975	0-1 Apgar at 15 min	28.0	44
Brown, 1974	0-2 Apgar at 1 min or 0-4 at 5 min or IPPV	26.0	22
Dweck, 1974	0-3 Apgar at 1 min	33.0	61
Drage, 1966	0-3 Apgar at 1 min	3.6	23
	0-3 at 5 min	7.4	50
Robertson, unpublished	0-5 Apgar at 1 or 5 min IPPV	14.7	3.5
Overall		23.4	29.0

IPPV: Intermittent Positive Pressure Ventilation
(Adapted from Brann.)

almost impossible to pinpoint precise causative processes. (3) Pathologic studies of mortally affected human neonates show discrete neuropathology and provide some insights about the origins of cerebral palsy, but correlation between clinical findings and neuroanatomy is possible only to a limited degree. Some examples are detailed in the following section. Specific syndromes of motor and cognitive deficit can be recognized in older children and adults, but material for careful autopsy study at these later ages is infrequently available. (4) Animal models of birth asphyxia have been developed to show the neuropathology resulting from specific insults. Limited clinical follow-through and correlation is available in these models, one of which is reviewed in the final section of this chapter.

Neuropathology Encountered in Autopsy Studies

The term ''birth trauma'' has traditionally been used to include both mechanical traumatic injury and asphyxial injury. From the days of Osler, probably until the 1940s, there was a high prevalence of genuine traumatic cerebral injury at birth. This type of injury is rare today because of the increased use of Caesarean section and the virtual abandonment of high and mid forcep delivery. Physical trauma is more likely to be seen in the spinal cord and peripheral nervous system (facial nerve, brachial plexus) than in the brain.[29,30] As mechanical brain injury has become more rare, birth asphyxia, its antecedents, and its physiologic concomitants have ascended as causative processes in cerebral palsy.

Recognition of the great importance of asphyxia in newborn mortality and morbidity began to appear in the literature during the 1940s.[31,32] Courville and Friedman first described in detail asphyxial central nervous system pathology in babies who died as neonates or in early infancy.[32,33] Asphyxial perinatal brain injury lies along a spectrum of insults that are primarily hypoxic or primarily ischemic in nature.[28,34] The sites of lesions are quite distinct. Hypoxic injury produces necrosis of neuronal groups most sensitive to oxygen deprivation. Scattered neuronal necrosis occurs within the cerebral or cerebellar cortex or in the deep nuclei of the basal ganglia, thalamus, or brain stem. Ischemic lesions represent watershed (arterial border zone) infarcts that appear in the cortical zones between the major cerebral arteries (parasagittal central necrosis)[34,35] or deep in the periventricular white matter (periventricular leukomalacia). The specific lesions seen will vary with the gestational age of the neonate and with the acuteness or severity of the hypoxic and/or ischemic insult. Thus, in the full term baby, cortical and deep gray matter lesions predominate. In the premature newborn, hemorrhage into the germinal matrix and ventricles predominates. Periventricular leukomalacia, though seen at all gestational ages, is much more typical of the preterm infant. Focal brain infarction due to ischemia within the distribution of specific cerebral vessels, is relatively unrelated to gestational age or to parturition. The pathogenesis is highly variable: vascular anomalies, embolism, thrombosis, systemic vascular collapse, etc. Kernicterus—the chronic sequela of bilirubin encephalophy in the newborn—produces a unique pattern of brain damage focused in the basal ganglia, tectum, thalamus, and cochlea.[1] The various pathological entities encountered in cerebral palsy are summarized in Outline 1.

Ellis and associates reviewed the pathological findings in infants who died before reaching 7 days of age in an attempt to distinguish prenatal from later brain damage. Of 25 term and 64 preterm infants studied, only 22 (24.5%) had prenatal damage, mostly minor anomalies. Prenatal pathology was much more common among infants carried to term (12 of 25, or 48%) than among those who were premature (10 of 64, or 16%). Thus, Ellis' data suggest that fetal brain abnormalities are an infrequent contributor to the process causing premature birth. Thus, the question remains whether minor anomalies or prenatal insults represent a set-up for major asphyxial damage during parturition or postnatally. Paneth[14] emphasizes the difficulty analyzing such a sequence of variables and the potential for obscuring the causal role of birth asphyxia. Major congenital anomalies were seen in ten preterm babies, with only one involving the central nervous system. Thus, if anything, it is somatic malformation, not nervous system anomaly, that predisposes

Outline 1 Neuropathology of cerebral palsy

Developmental CNS Anomalies

Encephaloclastic Processes
1. Selective neuronal necrosis (lobar sclerosis)
2. Status marmaratus
3. Parasagittal central necrosis
4. Periventricular leukomalacia (PVL)
5. Germinal matrix/intraventricular hemorrhage (GMH-IVH)
6. Focal infarction
   • Mechanical injury
   • Vascular
   • Infectious
7. Kernicterus

to preterm birth. Going a step further, somatic malformations are not associated with significant central nervous system damage acquired before birth. Nine full-term infants with anomalies not involving the central nervous system were among those without evidence of prenatal central nervous system damage.[36] In summary, the notion that most premature babies already had significant nervous system impairment before the onset of labor is not supported by these autopsy data. Indeed, only a small minority were so affected.

Towbin[37] has emphasized the traumatic nature of the birth process. He reviewed the pathologic findings of over 600 cases of death in early infancy or childhood noting the presence of four general categories of pathology: (1) subdural hemorrhage resulting from traumatic dural venous tears, (2) spinal cord and brain stem damage resulting from mechanical injury, (3) hypoxic damage to the deep cerebral structures, and (4) hypoxic damage to the cerebral cortex. He points out that minor insults in an immature nervous system may or may not be associated with any acute symptomatology and yet have the potential for lasting damage and associated dysfunction. The precise timing of perinatal cerebral damage, which may have occurred just prepartum, during parturition, or soon afterwards, cannot be determined from these studies.[37]

Prematurity and Intraventricular Hemorrhage

Intraventricular hemorrhage originates in the germinal matrix, a richly vascularized but poorly supported zone immediately adjacent to the ventricular wall.[38,39] Germinal matrix hemorrhage, which is localized to the subependymal region, represents the mildest bleeding (grade I) (Fig. 2). More commonly, the blood will rupture into the ventricular space. Grades II and III severity refer to increasing quantities of blood in the ventricular system (Fig. 2), and grade IV includes parenchymal blood.[40] Whether or not the parenchymal blood represents extension of the intraventricular hemorrhage into the periventricular white matter is debated and is probably not the case.[41]

It is well accepted that hypoxia and its effect on the fragile vascular endothelium of the subependymal vascular bed is at least one predisposing factor for intraventricular hemorrhage.[42] Though these hemor-

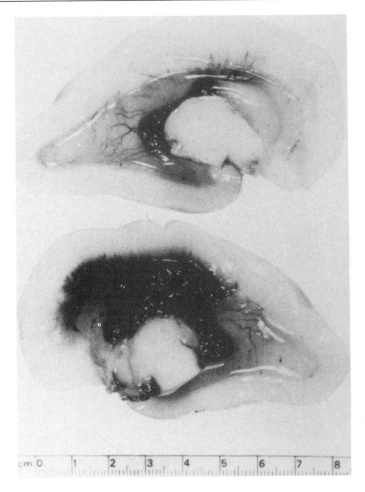

Fig. 2 *Sagittal section of 27 week premature infant's brain with bilateral hemorrhage. The top specimen (left hemisphere) shows germinal matrix hemorrhage localized to the body of the caudate nucleus. The lower portion (right hemisphere) shows rupture into the ventricular space (grade III intraventricular hemorrhage). (Reproduced with permission from Pape et al.[38])*

rhages typically occur following birth, predisposing events precede them by hours to days.[38] When the first prospective studies of intra-ventricular hemorrhage in premature infants were reported, bleeding was found in an unexpectedly high percentage.[40,43] Papile and associates[40] reported a 40% incidence in all premature infants weighing less than 1,250 g. The most striking finding, however, was that neurologic injury was suspected in only half of those babies with documented bleeding; in the other half, the intracranial hemorrhage was silent, unaccompanied by recognizable clinical symptoms.

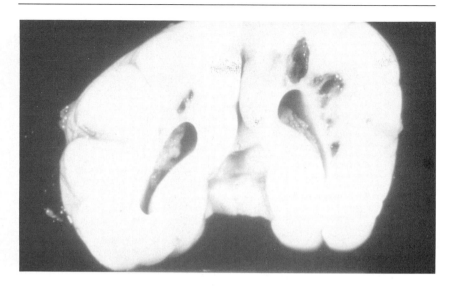

Fig. 3 *Pathology specimen of a premature infant's brain, cut in the coronal plane, with cystic periventricular leukomalacia. The lesion is markedly asymmetric. (Courtesy of T.S. Park, MD.)*

Periventricular Leukomalacia

Periventricular leukomalacia refers to a pathologic diagnosis consisting of patchy areas of necrosis in the periventricular white matter adjacent to the external angles of the lateral ventricles.[34,44-47] Necrotic areas can evolve into periventricular cavities of varying size surrounded by gliosis, with calcified fibers often present in this glial scar tissue (Fig. 3). Associated thinning of the white matter in the centrum semiovale and corpus callosum and mild expansion of the lateral ventricles occur as secondary phenomena. These lesions are seen primarily in premature infants and are a consequence of ischemia in arterial watershed zones close to the ventricular wall (Fig. 4).[44,46] This region would be most vulnerable to a fall in perfusion pressure. The same process that causes periventricular leukomalacia may also result in extensive hemorrhagic infarction in the same region.[41]

The clinicopathologic correlation between spastic diplegic cerebral palsy and periventricular leukomalacia is widely acknowledged,[6,34,48-50] though Gilles[51] disputes this. The pathologic picture predicts the typical clinical picture. The motor syndrome of spastic diplegia consists of spasticity involving all four extremities, with the legs much more impaired than the arms. Pyramidal tract fibers from the lower extremities and trunk sweep most closely past the lateral ventricles before turning down into the internal capsule. The arms and face are relatively spared unless the lesion is exceptionally extensive. Strabismus and occasional cognitive deficits in the form of learning disabilities are

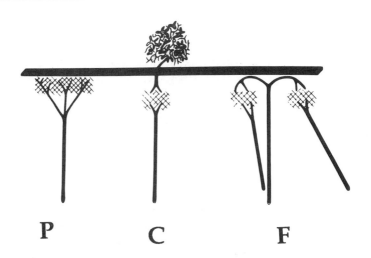

P   C   F

Fig. 4 *Diagram of border zones of arterial blood supply to the periventricular region. Three types of end zones (cross-hatched) are postulated between ventriculopetal (P), ventriculofugal (F), and choroidal (C) arteries. (Reproduced with permission from DeReuck et al.[44])*

fairly common, but mental retardation, articulation deficit, persistent seizure disorders, and hearing loss or peripheral sensory impairment are rare.[52] In the worst cases, spastic quadriplegia plus mental deficiency may be seen as a consequence of extensive pyramidal tract destruction plus destruction of intercortical connections. Autopsy studies tend to overrepresent this severe end of the spectrum.[44] Though the association of this pathological entity with the spastic diplegia syndrome is logical, the neuropathology of older children or adults with the syndrome has not been reported.

Shuman and Selednick[53] make the point that periventricular leukomalacia is a nonlethal lesion. Of the 17 infants in their autopsy study, all probably died from other causes, mainly cardiopulmonary or septic in nature. Spastic diplegia can be viewed as a mild cerebral palsy syndrome that is associated with longevity well into adult life.[34,52] They also point out that periventricular leukomalacia is not necessarily an isolated nervous system insult. Fifty-nine percent (10 of 17) of their cases had other lesions including intraventricular hemorrhage, germinal matrix hemorrhage, status marmaratus (see below), and necrosis of brain stem nuclei.

In the live infant, periventricular leukomalacia can be demonstrated by head ultrasonography, the preferred imaging technique,[54] and appears as periventricular echodensities. In their serial examination of 86 consecutive premature babies by ultrasonography, Weindling and associates[49] identified periventricular hemorrhage and leukomalacia in 40%. Seven (8%) later developed periventricular cysts. Cranial com-

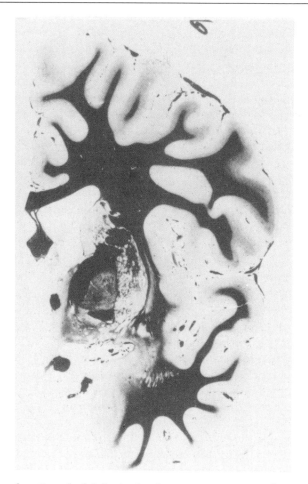

Fig. 5 *Coronal section of adult brain showing status marmaratus due to neonatal asphyxia. The white matter has been stained highlighting the typical marbled appearance seen in the caudate nucleus and putamen of this specimen. (Reproduced with permission from Volpe.[34])*

puted tomography (CT) and magnetic resonance imaging (MRI) are both more sensitive than ultrasonography, but are highly impractical when compared to ultrasound because of transport, time factors, radiation risks, and other factors. The relative insensitivity of head ultrasonography in detecting small lesions or residual scarring[55] becomes a major issue when trying to interpret clinical outcome studies. Hope and associates[56] report only 40% of periventricular lesions seen at autopsy were detected by head ultrasonography.

Status Marmaratus

Status marmaratus refers to the pathologic picture of scarring in the basal ganglia resulting in a marbled appearance (Fig. 5).[34,57] The lesions are typically bilateral and symmetrical with the caudate, putamen, and thalamus most affected. The glial scarring is a consequence of a unique hypermyelination response to anoxic injury.[58] The cortex is usually completely spared. Premortem recognition of the lesion is rare, but at least one case has been reported.[59]

Clinically, one would expect extrapyramidal motor features and little in the way of cognitive deficit or seizure problems. This is the classic syndrome of choreoathetoid cerebral palsy whereby, in some cases of severe motor impairment, intelligence can be normal or superior and epilepsy is uncommon.[1,34,60] More diffuse neuronal injury accompanying status marmaratus can, of course, produce greater functional impairment, including cognitive disability. The typical insult associated with this lesion is a sudden anoxic catastrophe at the time of birth such as maternal cardiac arrest, cord prolapse, abruptio placentae, and others. It closely resembles the events described by Brann and Myers in their model of total anoxia.[61]

What About the Spinal Cord?

The spinal cord receives scant attention in discussions of cerebral palsy pathology. Courville makes no reference to it at all in his comprehensive work on neonatal brain damage.[33] Most references involve traumatic injury to the cord directly[40,57,62] or indirectly via local vascular compromise.[29] Additional findings, attributed to anoxia and/or kernicterus, include focal and petecchial hemorrhage, anterior horn cell loss, edema, atrophy, and long tract degenerative changes.[13,31,57,62] Christensen and Melchior[62] cite one case of anterior horn cell dysplasia on the basis of malformation.

There are insufficient data available to know whether asphyxia causes spinal cord lesions in children surviving the neonatal period. In these children, the motor consequence of asphyxia is typically a picture of hyperreflexia with increased or variable tone and not the hypotonic, hypoflexic state of a dominant lower motoneuron lesion.

Experimental Birth Anoxia

In contrast to the ischemic events causing periventricular leukomalacia, Brann and Myers developed a model of almost pure neonatal hypoxia.[61,63] In the 1950s, their perinatal research laboratory at the National Institutes of Health was the site of elegant studies of asphyxia and resuscitation in the newborn Rhesus monkey. They described two distinct clinical conditions of perinatal oxygen deprivation that resulted in two distinct pathologic outcomes. The first was termed total anoxia and consisted of an acute, complete deprivation of oxygen to the fetus by virtue of abrupt ligation of the umbilical cord in utero. These infants were then immediately delivered and resuscitated. When later sacrificed, their brains showed no edema and a paucity of cortical findings. The neuropathology was localized to the basal ganglia, brain stem, and thalamus in the form of neuronal loss. Their other model was one of prolonged and partial asphyxia whereby maternal hypoxemia was

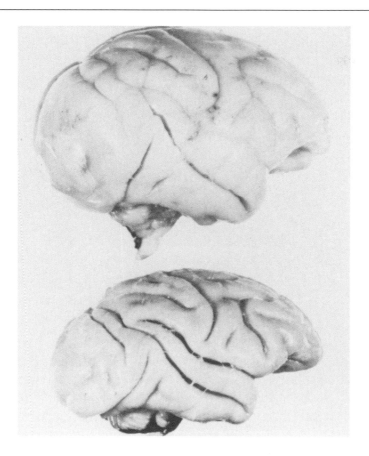

Fig. 6 *Whole brain specimens of experimental term monkey fetus (**top**) exposed to prolonged partial asphyxia and control (**bottom**). There is severe, generalized edema and small superficial hemorrhage visible in the cortex of the experimental animal. (Reproduced with permission from Brann et al.[63])*

induced for extended periods of time. In this situation, markedly different neuropathologic lesions developed, consisting of diffuse cerebral swelling and hemorrhagic and nonhemorrhagic necrosis of parenchyma deep within the sulci (Figs. 6 and 7).

One interesting theme that runs through all of Brann and Myers' work is the observation that creating a brain-damaged newborn was remarkably difficult.[61,63] Even under carefully controlled laboratory-induced asphyxia, most of the newborn animals were either easy to resuscitate and healthy, surviving with no neuropathologic findings, or were difficult to resuscitate and nonsurvivors. It was the exception to produce a newborn who could be successfully resuscitated and would survive with permanent brain damage. This experience is, in fact, quite consistent with the clinical experience of the most severely asphyxiated human newborns.[27,64,65] Severe asphyxia is most often a fatal insult.

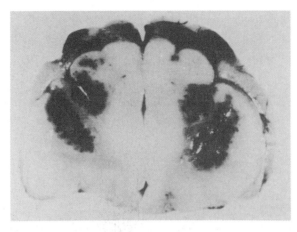

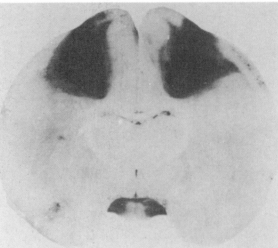

Fig. 7 *Coronal sections through two specimens from experimental term monkey fetuses with prolonged, partial asphyxia. Note the greater extent of hemorrhagic necrosis in the depths of the sulci. (Reproduced with permission from Brann et al.[63])*

However, there is something of an "all-or-none" phenomenon at work. The majority of the survivors do quite well with little or no long-term disability and only a small percentage show neurologic impairment.

Conclusions

The neuropathologic findings associated with perinatal insults and with cerebral palsy have been summarized. Nelson and Ellenberg[21] concluded in 1986 that "we probably do not know what causes most cases of cerebral palsy." Although this applies to individual case histories, we have gained tremendous insight into the general mechanisms involved based on the many contributions to the study of etiology and pathology of cerebral palsy from the time of William John Little to present-day basic science research into cellular events accompanying hypoxia.[66,67] The contribution of birth asphyxia as a definitive cause of cerebral palsy is small,[15,16] but emphatically real.[68] Obstetrical changes that took place decades ago have resulted in unequivocal changes in the types of pathology seen in neonatal deaths, specifically a decrease in traumatic (mechanical) brain insults. Though "close to birth" is still probably the time when asphyxial brain injury occurs, detailed understanding of this process and its antecedents is still lacking. Further decreases in the incidence and morbidity of cerebral palsy are dependent on three conditions. First, decreasing the incidence of preterm births should be possible by changing social and public policy[69,70] in the areas of prepregnancy counseling and prenatal care and education.[71,72] Second, identifying those fetal-placental units that are biophysically marginal in their ability to respond to hypoxic stress can allow for earlier and more definitive obstetrical interventions before asphyxia occurs.[73,74] Third, identifying and successfully intervening in those perinatal and early neonatal circumstances that are hostile to the brain should result in better outcomes.[66,67,75,76]

References

1. Crothers B, Paine RS: *The Natural History of Cerebral Palsy.* Cambridge, Harvard University Press, 1959, pp 54–60.
2. Bax M: Terminology and classification of cerebral palsy. *Dev Med Child Neurol* 1964;6:295–297.
3. Kurland LT: Definitions of cerebral palsy and their role in epidemiologic research. *Neurology* 1957;7:641–654.
4. Capute AJ, Accardo PJ: Cerebral palsy: The spectrum of motor dysfunction, in Capute AJ, Accardo PJ (eds): *Developmental Disabilities in Infancy and Childhood.* Baltimore, Paul Brookes, 1991, pp 335–348.
5. Lipkin PH: Epidemiology of the developmental disabilities, in Capute AJ, Accardo PJ (eds): *Developmental Disabilities in Infancy and Childhood.* Baltimore, Paul Brookes, 1991, pp 43–67.
6. Hagberg B, Hagberg G, Zetterstrom R: Decreasing perinatal mortality: Increase in cerebral palsy morbidity. *Acta Paediatr Scand* 1989;78:664–670.
7. Paneth N, Kiely J: The frequency of cerebral palsy: A review of population studies in industrialized nations since 1950, in Stanley F, Alberman E (eds): *The Epidemiology of the Cerebral Palsies,* Clinics in Developmental Medicine. Oxford, Blackwell Scientific, 1984, no 87, pp 46–56.
8. Holm VA: The causes of cerebral palsy: A contemporary perspective. *JAMA* 1982;247:1473–1477.
9. O'Reilly DE, Walentynowicz JE: Etiological factors in cerebral palsy: An historical review. *Dev Med Child Neurol* 1981;23:633–642.
10. Stanley F, Alberman E: Birthweight, gestational age and the cerebral palsies, in Stanley F, Alberman E (eds): *The Epidemiology of the Cerebral Palsies,* Clinics in Developmental Medicine. Oxford, Blackwell Scientific, 1984, no 87, pp 57–68.
11. Ellenberg JH, Nelson KB: Birth weight and gestational age in children with cerebral palsy or seizure disorders. *Am J Dis Child* 1979;133:1044–1048.
12. Freeman JM: Introduction, in Freeman JM (ed): *Prenatal and Perinatal Factors Associated with Brain Disorders.* Washington, DC, U.S. Department of Health and Human Services (NIH Publication No. 85–1149), 1985, pp 263–358.

13. Osler W: *The Cerebral Palsies of Children: Classics in Developmental Medicine.* Philadelphia, JB Lippincott, 1987, pp 36–43.

14. Paneth N: Birth and the origins of cerebral palsy, editorial. *N Eng J Med* 1986; 315:124–126.

15. Blair E, Stanley FJ: Intrapartum asphyxia: A rare cause of cerebral palsy. *J Pediatr* 1988;112:515–519.

16. Nelson KB: What proportion of cerebral palsy is related to birth asphyxia?, editorial. *J Pediatr* 1988;112:572–574.

17. Freeman JM, Nelson KB: Intrapartum asphyxia and cerebral palsy. *Pediatrics* 1988;82:240–249.

18. Naeye RL, Peters EC, Bartholomew M, et al: Origins of cerebral palsy. *Am J Dis Child* 1989;143:1154–1161.

19. Tobin A: Obstetric malpractice litigation: The pathologist's view. *Am J Obstet Gynecol* 1986;155:927–935.

20. Nelson KB, Ellenberg JH: Antecedents of cerebral palsy: I. Univariate analysis of risks. *Am J Dis Child* 1985;139:1031–1038.

21. Nelson KB, Ellenberg JH: Antecedents of cerebral palsy: Multivariate analysis of risk. *N Eng J Med* 1986;315:81–86.

22. Little WJ: On the influence of abnormal parturition, difficult labours, premature birth and asphyxia neonatorum on the mental and physical condition of the child, especially in relation to deformities. *Trans Obstet Soc London* 1861–1862;3:293–344.

23. Accardo PJ: William John Little and cerebral palsy in the nineteenth century. *J Hist Med Allied Sci* 1989;44:56–71.

24. Freud S: Les diplegies cerebrales infantiles. *Revue Neurologique* 1893;1:177–183.

25. Accardo PJ: Freud on diplegia: Commentary and translation. *Am J Dis Child* 1982;136:452–456.

26. Stanley F: Perinatal risk factors in the cerebral palsies, in Stanley F, Alberman E (eds): *The Epidemiology of the Cerebral Palsies*, Clinics in Developmental Medicine. Oxford, Blackwell Scientfic, 1984, no 87, pp 98–115.

27. Nelson KB, Ellenberg JH: Apgar scores as predictors of chronic neurologic disability. *Pediatrics* 1981;68:36–44.

28. Brann AW: Factors during neonatal life that influence brain disorders, in Freeman JM (ed): *Prenatal and Perinatal Factors Associated With Brain Disorders.* Washington, DC, U.S. Department of Health and Human Services (NIH Publication No. 85–1149), 1985, pp 263–358.

29. Painter MJ, Bergman I: Obstetrical trauma to the neonatal central and peripheral nervous system. *Semin Perinatol* 1982;6:89–104.

30. Freeman JM: Summary, in Freeman JM (ed): *Prenatal and Perinatal Factors Associated with Brain Disorders.* Washington, DC, U.S. Department of Health and Human Services (NIH Publication No. 85–1149), 1985, pp 13–32.

31. Clifford SH: The effects of asphyxia on the newborn infant. *J Pediatr* 1941;18: 567–578.

32. Friedman AP, Courville CB: Atrophic lobar sclerosis of early childhood (ulegyria): Report of two verified cases with particular reference to their asphyxial etiology. *Bull Los Angeles Neurol Soc* 1941;6:32–45.

33. Courville CB: *Birth and Brain Damage.* Pasadena, MF Courville, 1971.

34. Volpe JJ: Perinatal hypoxic-ischemic brain injury. *Pediatr Clin North Am* 1976;23:383–397.

35. Volpe JJ, Pasternak JF: Parasagittal cerebral injury in neonatal hypoxic-ischemic encephalopathy: Clinical and neuroradiologic features. *J Pediatr* 1977;91:472–476.

36. Ellis WG, Goetzman BW, Lindenberg JA: Neuropathologic documentation of prenatal brain damage. *Am J Dis Child* 1988;142:858–866.

37. Towbin A: Organic causes of minimal brain dysfunction: Perinatal origin of minimal cerebral lesions. *JAMA* 1971;217:1207–1214.
38. Pape KE, Wigglesworth JS: *Haemorrhage, Ischaemia and the Perinatal Brain,* Clinics in Developmental Medicine. Oxford, Blackwell Scientific, 1979, no 69/70.
39. Volpe JJ: Intraventricular hemorrhage in the premature infant: Current concepts: Part I. *Ann Neurol* 1989;25:3–11.
40. Papile LA, Burstein J, Burstein R, et al: Incidence and evolutation of subependymal and intraventricular hemorrhage: A study of infants with birth weights less than 1,500 gm. *J Pediatr* 1978;92:529–534.
41. Volpe JJ: Brain injury in the premature: Is it preventable? *Pediatr Res* 1990;27(suppl 6):S28-S33.
42. Weindling AM, Wilkinson AR, Cook J, et al: Perinatal events which precede periventricular hemorrhage and leukomalacia in the newborn. *Br J Obstet Gynec* 1985;92:1218–1223.
43. Ahmann PA, Lazzara A, Dykes FD, et al: Intraventricular hemorrhage in the high-risk preterm infant: Incidence and outcome. *Ann Neurol* 1980;7:118–124.
44. DeReuck J, Chattha AS, Richardson EP Jr: Pathogenesis and evolution of periventricular leukomalacia in infancy. *Arch Neurol* 1972;27:229–236.
45. Banker BQ, Larroche JC: Periventricular leukomalacia of infancy: A form of neonatal anoxic encephalopathy. *Arch Neurol* 1962;7:386–410.
46. Abramowicz A: The pathogenesis of experimental periventricular cerebral necrosis and its possible relation to the periventricular leucomalacia of birth trauma. *J Neurol Neurosurg Psychiatry* 1964;27:85–95.
47. Armstrong D, Norman MG: Periventricular leukomalacia in neonates: Complications and sequelae. *Arch Dis Child* 1974;49:367–375.
48. Bowerman RA, Donn SM, DiPietro MA, et al: Periventricular leukomalacia in the pre-term newborn infant: Sonographic and clinical features. *Radiology* 1984;151:383–390.
49. Weindling AM, Rochefort MJ, Calvert SA, et al: Development of cerebral palsy after ultrasonographic detection of periventricular cysts in the newborn. *Dev Med Child Neurol* 1985;27:800–806.
50. Sinha SK, D'Souza SW, Rivlin E, et al: Ischemic brain lesions diagnosed at birth in preterm infants: Clinical events and developmental outcome. *Arch Dis Child* 1990;65:1017–1020.
51. Gilles FH: Neuropathologic indicators of abnormal development, in Freeman JM (ed): *Prenatal and Perinatal Factors Associated with Brain Disorders.* Washington, DC, U.S. Department of Health and Human Services (NIH Publication No. 85-1149), 1985, pp 53–108.
52. Blasco PA: Cerebral palsy: Clinical diagnosis and natural history, in Park TS, Phillips LH, Peacock WJ (eds): *Management of Spasticity in Cerebral Palsy and Spinal Cord Injury, Neurosurgery: State of the Art Reviews.* Philadelphia, Hanley & Belfus, 1989, vol 4, pp 371–378.
53. Shuman RM, Selednik LJ: Periventricular leukomalacia: A one-year autopsy study. *Arch Neurol* 1980;37:231–235.
54. Volpe JJ: Intraventricular hemorrhage in the premature infant: Current concepts: Part II. *Ann Neurol* 1989;25:109–116.
55. Keeney SE, Adcock EW, McArdle CB: Prospective observation of 100 high-risk neonates by high-field (1.5 tesla) magnetic resonance imaging of the central nervous system: II. Lesions associated with hypoxic ischemic encephalopathy. *Pediatrics* 1991;87:431–438.
56. Hope PL, Gould SJ, Howard S, et al: Precision of ultrasound diagnosis of pathologically verified lesions in the brains of very preterm infants. *Dev Med Child Neurol* 1988;30:457–471.
57. Towbin A: *The Pathology of Cerebral Palsy.* Springfield, IL, Charles C. Thomas, 1960.

58. Borit A, Herndon RM: The fine structure of plaques fibromyeliniques in ulegyria and in status marmoratus. *Acta Neuropath* 1970;14:304–311.

59. Roland EH, Hill A, Norman MG, et al: Selective brainstem injury in an asphyxiated newborn. *Ann Neurol* 1988;23:89–92.

60. Hayashi M, Sato J, Sakamoto K, et al: Clinical and neuropathological findings in severe athetoid cerebral palsy: A comparative study of globo-luysian and thalamo-putaminal groups. *Brain Dev* 1991;13:47–51.

61. Myers RE: Two patterns of perinatal brain damage and their conditions of occurrence. *Am J Obstet Gynecol* 1972;112:246–276.

62. Christensen E, Melchior J: *Cerebral Palsy: A Clinical and Neuropathological Study*, Clinics in Developmental Medicine. London, Heinemann Medical, 1967, no 25.

63. Brann AW Jr, Myers RE: Central nervous system findings in the newborn monkey following severe in utero partial asphyxia. *Neurology* 1975;25:327–338.

64. Scott H: Outcome of very severe birth asphyxia. *Arch Dis Child* 1976;51:712–716.

65. Jain L, Fenne C, Vidyasagan D, et al: Cardiopulmonary resuscitation of apparently stillborn infants: Survival and long-term outcome. *J Pediatr* 1991;118:778–782.

66. Younkin D, Medoff-Cooper B, Guillet R, et al: In vivo 31 P nuclear magnetic resonance measurement of chronic changes in cerebral metabolites following neonatal intraventricular hemorrhage. *Pediatrics* 1988;82:331–336.

67. Volpe JJ, Herscovitch P, Perlman JM, et al: Positron emission tomography in the asphyxiated term newborn: Parasagittal impairment of cerebral blood flow. *Ann Neurol* 1985;17:287–296.

68. Brown JK: Editorial: Is honesty the best policy? *Dev Med Child Neurol* 1990;32:565–566.

69. Papiernick E, Bouyer J, Dreyfus J, et al: Prevention of preterm births: A perinatal study in Hagenau, France. *Pediatrics* 1985;76:154–158.

70. Oakley A: Can social support influence pregnancy outcome? *Br J Obstet Gynaecol* 1989;96:260–262.

71. Iams JD: Current status of prematurity prevention. *JAMA* 1989;262:265–266.

72. Creasy RK: Preventing preterm birth. *N Engl J Med* 1991;325:727–729.

73. Manning FA, Harman CR, Morrison I, et al: Fetal assessment based on biophysical profile scoring IV: An analysis of perinatal morbidity and mortality. *Am J Obstet Gynecol* 1990;162:703–709.

74. Anthony MY, Levene MI: An assessment of the benefits of intrapartum fetal monitoring. *Dev Med Child Neurol* 1990;32:547–553.

75. Johnston MV: Neurotransmitter alterations in a model of perinatal hypoxic-ischemic brain injury. *Ann Neurol* 1983;13:511–518.

76. Vannucci RC: Current and potentially new management strategies for perinatal hypoxic-ischemic encephalopathy. *Pediatrics* 1990;85:961–968.

Chapter 2

The Neurophysiologic Basis of Spastic Muscle Hypertonia

William Z. Rymer, MD, PhD

Introduction

The most widely used definition of spastic hypertonia is that provided by Lance,[1] who defines spasticity (in part) as "a motor disorder characterized by a velocity dependent increase in tonic stretch reflexes, with exaggerated tendon jerks, resulting from hyperexcitability of the stretch reflex. . . ."

The central unresolved issue motivating ongoing research about spastic hypertonia concerns the pathophysiology of this increased tonic stretch reflex response. In this chapter I will examine the potential sources of disturbed motoneuronal excitability in spasticity and present evidence strongly supporting one of the proposed classes of disturbance. A more extensive discussion of many of the issues is provided in a recent review.[2]

Hypothetical Mechanisms for Spastic Hypertonia

The increase in the magnitude of the reflex response to muscle stretch may arise from two fundamentally different sources: (1) an increase in the motoneuronal excitability caused by a sustained or tonic descending depolarizing input to spinal motoneurons, or (2) an increase in the synaptic responses elicited by muscle stretch.

In the first case, the neural elements of the spinal cord, such as motoneurons and interneurons, are inherently normal in their function. The augmentation in muscle reflex force arises primarily because the descending stimulus from higher brain centers places the motoneurons in a more excitable state, from which they can reach their recruitment threshold with less potent sensory stimuli than would normally be required.

In the second case, the tonic descending stimulus to motoneurons is not directly enhanced, but the excitatory synaptic response of motoneurons to muscle afferent inflow is much greater than normal, for a variety of possible reasons. Restating these two hypotheses in quantitative terms, the first case is essentially a change in threshold behavior of the stretch reflex; the second is a change in stretch reflex ''gain'' or amplification.

These differences in mechanical outcome between the two hypothetical mechanisms are summarized in Figure 1, which is a diagram of torque-angle plots that might be recorded for the different causal mechanisms. Torque-angle plots are established by applying a constant velocity extension to the relevant joint, and recording the resulting torque. Although the torque-angle relations are roughly linear over much of the range, they have a curvilinear region near the intercept with the angle axis (Fig. 1). The abscissa intercept angle defines the threshold angle of the tonic stretch reflex, and the slope of the torque-angle relation defines the net joint stiffness. The component of angular stiffness attributable to stretch reflex responses is a measure of stretch reflex gain.

The plot on the right of Figure 1 portrays the normal torque-angle relation, in which the threshold angle is reached only toward the end of the extension movement. This figure further shows that one mechanism of spastic hypertonia could be associated with a horizontal shift to the left of the torque-angle plot, without change in slope. This graph, labelled (θ_τ), indicates a reduction in stretch reflex threshold. The alternative mechanism, shown between the other plots, is an increase in reflex stiffness (κ), which is associated with an increase in slope of the torque-angle relation.

For the most part, investigators have relied on the hypothesis of augmentations in stretch reflex gain, or increased stiffness, without considering fully the potentially separate contributions of reductions in motoneuron or interneuronal thresholds, which may be of fundamentally different origin. For example, prior studies have concentrated on such mechanisms as augmented spindle afferent responses to stretch (induced potentially by increased fusimotor activity),[3-5] increased sprouting of muscle afferent terminals,[6,7] reduced presynaptic inhibition of muscle afferent synaptic input,[8] changes in the intrinsic electrical properties of motoneuron membrane,[9] or enhanced responses of motoneuron postsynaptic receptor sites to transmitter release. In theory, each of these mechanisms would be capable of inducing enhanced motoneuronal synaptic responses to muscle stretch and, therefore, could induce spasticity.

There are several difficulties associated with the increased reflex gain hypothesis. The examples described above presuppose a significant intrinsic segmental contribution to spastic hypertonia, which is somewhat counterintuitive because, in most instances, the proposed spinal disturbances would develop many spinal segments below the primary site of damage to the nervous system in the cerebral cortex or subcortical white matter. The mechanisms responsible for such remote alterations are unclear, with the possible exception of afferent sprouting, which may contribute to altered patterns of synaptic response, especially after extensive afferent denervation.

I believe the uncertainty regarding the type of physiologic disturbance arising in spasticity has arisen, at least partly, because of a lack

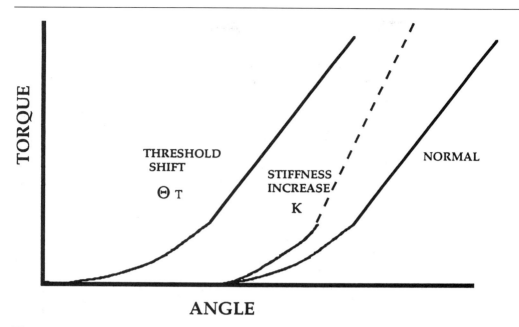

Fig. 1 *Diagrammatic representation of hypothetical torque-angle relations in normal and spastic elbow joints. Spastic muscles could be associated with leftward shifts in reflex threshold (θ_T), increases in reflex stiffness (κ), or changes in both variables simultaneously (not shown).*

of quantitative biomechanical and electromyographic (EMG) studies of spastic muscle. Although such studies are unlikely to yield specific information about the cellular basis of the neurophysiologic disturbance in spastic muscular hypertonia, they provide very powerful constraints that must be satisfied by any theories purporting to explain the mechanisms of spastic hypertonia.

Experimental Observations of Spastic Human Subjects

In my laboratory, studies on spasticity have focused largely on spastic hemiparesis resulting from stroke, because spastic hypertonia following stroke is often relatively consistent both in its spatial pattern of distribution and in its associated clinical features. In addition, the contralateral side of the hemiparetic-spastic subject provides an excellent control for characterizing the passive mechanical properties of a limb. No similar controls are available for spinal cord injured subjects or brain trauma subjects in whom the injury is almost always bilateral and often quite variable in its clinical presentation.

This choice does not indicate that the contralateral side of the spastic hemiparetic subject is functionally unimpaired; there is ample evidence to indicate that there are substantial functional motor and sensory deficits in this limb. Nonetheless, in the absence of overt spasticity, the contralateral limb is still a far better control than would be obtained by using some independent sample of limbs. Studies in stroke-induced spasticity were conducted in my laboratory over the last 5 years in an attempt to determine the relative impact of changes in stretch reflex gain versus stretch reflex threshold mechanisms.[10–12]

Load Application to Active Muscle

To evaluate stretch reflex gain, measurements of the stiffness of the joint are used to determine reflex gain[10] on the assumptions that augmented gain would be expressed as an enhanced torque response to a standard angular perturbation and that passive or nonreflexive sources of torque are comparable in spastic and contralateral limbs. The latter assumption must be applied with discretion, because it is sometimes incorrect, especially in chronically spastic-paretic muscle, in which passive joint and muscle stiffness may increase.

To eliminate the contributions arising from stretch reflex threshold reductions, the initial studies concentrated on applying loads to voluntarily preactivated muscle, in which the recruitment threshold of many motoneurons had already been reached.[10]

When spastic and contralateral arms of a stroke patient are subjected successively to identical elbow extension loads, initiated at the same background torque and elbow joint angle, the resulting torque increases are essentially indistinguishable on spastic and contralateral sides.[10] This observation indicates that there is no increase in joint stiffness in spastic muscle, and presumably no systematic increase in reflex gain, if the stated assumptions are correct. In effect, this approach chooses an ''operating point'' in the torque-angle space, and then evaluates stiffness about this point.

The use of preactivated muscle is necessary not only to eliminate the complex contribution of the motoneuronal threshold, a significant source of nonlinearity, but also to allow for the known dependence of reflex stiffness on muscle length and background torque.

In a small subset of the study population (approximately 15%), there were apparent increases in joint stiffness, but these were not accompanied by augmentations in EMG responses, suggesting that the effects were mediated largely by changes in the passive mechanical properties of muscle.

Load Application to Initially Passive Muscle

Studies of voluntarily preactivated muscle indicated that there was no evidence for augmented stretch reflex gain in this class of stroke patients, but did not directly implicate changes in reflex threshold.[11,12] This threshold issue was addressed by examining stretch reflex responses of initially passive spastic muscle to a range of angular velocities. These angular joint extensions were applied at velocities ranging from 0.25 to 2.0 radians/sec, over an amplitude of 1 radian.

A typical record of the responses of elbow muscles to constant velocity extension is shown in Figure 2, which displays the net elbow torque elicited during the extension, together with the EMG activity in two major elbow flexors: the biceps brachii and the brachioradialis. Each muscle shows a distinct angle of EMG onset, demarcated by the arrows, which can be used to estimate the threshold angle of the reflex in each muscle.

Study results indicated that there was a systematic reduction in stretch reflex threshold in spastic muscle in all subjects, and that this reduction was the primary mechanism by which joint torque varied with fluctuations in the severity of the spastic state (Fig. 2). For example, in one spastic subject who showed demonstrable fluctuations in the clinical severity of the spasticity, the changes in the torque angle plots as the degree of spasticity varied were consistent with horizontal shifts in the locus of the plot (indicative of threshold changes), rather than with changes in the torque angle slope or angular stiffness (which would indicate changes in reflex gain).

Although the responses of spastic elbow muscles to joint extensions of differing amplitudes were consistent with a straightforward stretch reflex threshold reduction, the responses to differing stretch velocities were less readily predicted. Specifically, an eightfold increase in angular velocity produced a very modest increase in peak joint torque (30% to 40%),[11] which appeared to be inconsistent with the velocity sensitivity of the reflex described by Lance.[1] This lack of reflex velocity sensitivity is entirely in keeping with earlier observations on stretch reflex dynamics, recorded in both normal human subjects and in animal models. The apparent discrepancy between this observation and Lance's definition arises because claims about velocity sensitivity of the reflex in Lance's studies were based on EMG recordings[13] rather than on measurements of the mechanical behavior, which give quite different results.

Electromyographic Responses of Spastic Muscle to Joint Extension

Two significant observations were made using EMG recordings in spastic muscle.[10-12] The first observation, described in part earlier, was that the augmented joint torque was not necessarily accompanied by an increased EMG response to muscle stretch.[10] In many instances EMG activity was actually reduced substantially, which indicates that there was probably a significant change in the number and/or size of active muscle fibers in these spastic muscles. Although I have no histologic confirmation, I believe that this EMG reduction results from a partial replacement of muscle fibers by some type of connective tissue, giving rise to a subclinical contracture. It should be acknowledged, however, that other investigators, such as Dietz and colleagues,[14,15] have suggested alternative explanations for this type of finding, which has been widely reported in leg muscles of cerebral palsy subjects as well.

The second observation concerns the dependence of EMG responses

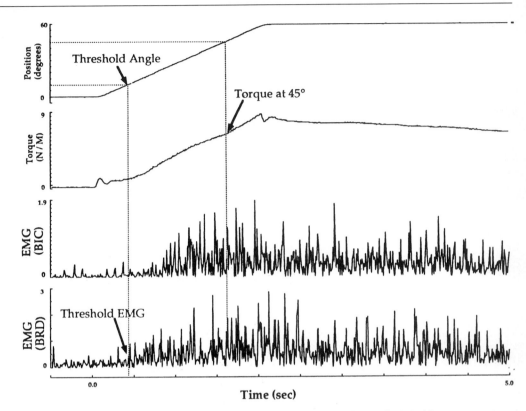

Fig. 2 *Response of elbow muscles in spastic arm of hemiplegic subject to constant velocity joint extension. The subject elbow is extended by a large DC motor, configured as a position servo. The traces show joint torque, which increases steeply after an initial modest rise, and EMG traces of biceps and brachioradialis. EMG traces are rectified. The joint angle of 45 degrees is demarcated to illustrate the torque and EMG values recorded at this angle. Estimates of this type may be useful for quantifying the severity of spasticity. EMG thresholds are also depicted with arrows.*

on the angular velocity of joint extension. Although the torque responses to joint extension increased relatively little with increasing angular velocity, the EMG responses increased by a larger amount.[11] This effect turned out to be largely a result of a change in the EMG threshold of the stretch reflex with increasing extension velocity. In other words, the stretch reflex threshold was acquired at a smaller joint angular extension with increasing angular velocity, thereby giving rise to an augmented EMG response. This EMG increase was not automatically reflected in a commensurate change in joint torque.

The origins of this reflex threshold dependence on angular velocity are not entirely clear; however, the changes are presumably attributable to the dynamic sensitivity of the recruitment threshold in motoneurons. In other words, the recruitment threshold of a motoneuron is not simply a function of the absolute level of motoneuronal depolarization; it is also influenced by the rate of change of membrane potential, which is likely to be more rapid during rapid muscle extensions, presumably because of higher discharge rates of muscle spindle afferents during rapid muscle stretch. In any event, once motoneurons are activated, there is no evidence that the EMG response shows any greater dependence on amplitude or velocity than is present in normal subjects, so the arguments for normal tonic stretch reflex gain remain unshaken.

Mechanisms of Spastic Hypertonia

As a result of these observations in hemiparetic spastic human subjects, it is reasonable to argue that the primary disturbance in the physiology of spastic muscle hypertonia in this neurologic disorder is a reduction in effective motoneuronal threshold that results, in all likelihood, from sustained depolarization of spinal motoneurons. This depolarization is attributable to enhanced net descending excitatory drive from higher centers, especially via vestibulospinal and reticulospinal pathways. It remains unresolved whether this augmented drive is caused solely by increased excitatory descending input from pathways, such as the vestibulospinal and reticulospinal pathways, or whether it reflects a reduced inflow from descending or regional inhibitory systems. Whatever the origin, the disturbances lie primarily in supraspinal centers, such as brain stem or cerebral white matter, and there is no requirement to superimpose additional alterations in intrinsic spinal segmental properties. I believe that this analysis represents a very potent simplifying conceptual scheme, which also will help guide diagnosis and therapeutic interventions in various types of spasticity.

Qualifications and Reservations

The experimental observations supporting this analysis are based exclusively on spastic hypertonia in patients following hemiparetic stroke and may have limited relevance to spasticity of spinal cord injury or of cerebral palsy. In each of the latter cases, the degree of structural disruption that takes place may be so extensive that anatomic and neurophysiologic reorganization of afferent, interneuronal, or motoneuronal systems is conceivably more likely. This means that hypotheses relying on intrinsic spinal disturbances are perhaps more realistic for this type of neural damage. However, if hypotheses of altered segmental responsiveness are to be substantiated, there should be demonstrable mechanical or EMG evidence for enhanced reflex gain.

Implications for Quantification of Spasticity

If stretch reflex gain is not enhanced in spasticity, there is no advantage to measuring stiffness of joints in response to angular perturbation.

Instead, the primary variable that needs to be quantified is the stretch reflex threshold. This threshold function may be quantified by direct or indirect means. Because threshold detection may be a statistically complex and uncertain procedure, as may be visualized from Figure 2, direct estimates of EMG onset or of torque departures from baseline may be impractical for routine clinical use. Furthermore, the EMG threshold may well differ for the different muscles, as is shown for the biceps and brachioradialis muscles (Fig. 2). It follows that spasticity estimates that derive measures of threshold less directly may ultimately be more practical for everyday clinical use.

Specifically, I would argue that joint torque-angle plots using the locus or horizontal position of the plot with respect to its intercept with the angular axis are probably the most straightforward measure. The angle axis intercept is a simple though potentially less accurate measure than is the threshold estimate alone. Alternatively, related mechanical variables such as joint torque at a specified angle (for example, 45 degrees as in Figure 2), the work performed, or the integral of joint torque with respect to time, are quite similar and comparably effective variables. This is because the work performed or the torque integral will increase in inverse proportion to the threshold angle.

None of these measures, however, is likely to be readily applicable across different subjects, because the absolute joint torque is closely dependent on the particular anatomy of the limb. Threshold estimates will likely be more useful for relative measures in which the clinician wishes to track the severity of the spastic state within a given subject over time. This is potentially the most important use of such a quantitative scale.

References

1. Lance JW: Symposium synopsis, in Feldman RG, Young RR, Koella WP (eds): *Spasticity: Disordererd Motor Control*. Chicago, Year Book Medical Publishers, 1980, pp 485–494.
2. Katz RT, Rymer WZ: Spastic hypertonia: Mechanisms and measurement. *Arch Phys Med Rehabil* 1989;70:144–155.
3. Rushworth G: Spasticity and rigidity: An experimental study and review. *J Neurol Neurosurg Psychiatry* 1960;23:99–118.
4. Dietrichson P: Phasic ankle reflex in spasticity and Parkinsonian rigidity. The role of the fusimotor system. *Acta Neurol Scand* 1971;47:22–51.
5. Dietrichson P: Tonic ankle reflex in Parkinsonian rigidity and spasticity. The role of the fusimotor system. *Acta Neurol Scand* 1971;47:163–182.
6. Chambers WW, Liu CN, McCouch GP: Anatomical and physiological correlates of plasticity in the central nervous system. *Brain Behav Evol* 1973;8:5–26.
7. McCouch GP, Austin GM, Liu CN, et al: Sprouting as a cause of spasticity. *J Neurophysiol* 1958;21:205–216.
8. Iles JF, Roberts RC: Presynaptic inhibition of monosynaptic references in the lower limbs of subjects with upper motoneuron disease. *J Neurol Neurosurg Psychiatry* 1986;49:937–944.
9. Hochman S, McCrea DA: The effect of chronic spinal transection on homonymous Ia EPSP rise times in triceps surae motoneurons in the cat. *Abstracts Soc Neuroscience* 1987;186:12.

10. Lee WA, Boughton A, Rymer WZ: Absence of stretch reflex gain enhancement in voluntarily activated spastic muscle. *Exp Neurol* 1987;98:317–335.

11. Powers RK, Campbell DL, Rymer WZ: Stretch reflex dynamics in spastic elbow flexor muscles. *Ann Neurol* 1989;25:32–42.

12. Powers RK, Marder-Meyer J, Rymer WZ: Quantitative relations between hypertonia and stretch reflex threshold in spastic hemiparesis. *Ann Neurol* 1988;23:115–124.

13. Burke D, Gillies JD, Lance JW: The quadriceps stretch reflex in human spasticity. *J Neurol Neurosurg Psychiatry* 1970;33:216–223.

14. Dietz V, Quintern J, Berger W: Electrophysiological studies of gait in spasticity and rigidity: Evidence that altered mechanical properties of muscle contribute to hypertonia. *Brain* 1981;104:431–449.

15. Dietz V, Berger W: Normal and impaired regulation of muscle stiffness in gait: A new hypothesis about muscle hypertonia. *Exp Neurol* 1983;79:680–687.

Chapter 3
Direct Measurement of Spasticity

Stephen R. Skinner, MD

Introduction

Children with cerebral palsy have abnormal central nervous system control over skeletal muscle. Spasticity is the major manifestation of this problem for many of these children. Simply explained, spasticity is an abnormal increase in the sensitivity of skeletal muscle to active or passive stretching. In the clinical setting, spasticity is assessed by examining the resistance to passive range of motion of the limbs, observing the response to tendon taps, or quickly stretching muscles to elicit clonus.

Many of the treatments applied to children with cerebral palsy are intended to decrease spasticity. Such treatments include physical therapy techniques, orthotic devices, pharmacologic agents, and surgical procedures. To evaluate therapeutic efficacy, some quantitative measurement of spasticity is desirable. In a clinical setting, one may apply the Ashworth scale,[1] which estimates resistance of muscles to passive motion, or attempt to grade the deep tendon reflex response, or count the beats of clonus in response to a quick stretch. While clinically useful, these assessments are somewhat subjective and are not easily assigned numeric values for statistical analysis.

The search for a quantitative measurement of spasticity has been the subject of many laboratory investigations. Measurements should be reproducible, accurate, practical, and expressed in numeric values. In this chapter I will attempt to review several approaches to the quantitative assessment of spasticity.

Physiology of Spasticity

The stimulus for clinically detectable muscle contraction is discharge of the alpha motoneuron, which innervates most of the fibers of a muscle. Within muscles there are stretch receptors known as muscle spindles, which are important for detection of the change in length of the muscle as well as the rate of that change in length. Information from the muscle spindles is conveyed to the central nervous system to play a major role in the regulation of muscle tone. Two types of fibers are found in muscle spindles. Named for the appearance of their central nuclei, they are nuclear chain fibers, which are responsible for detection of change in length, and nuclear bag fibers, which are responsible for detecting the velocity of muscle motion. The motoneurons to the fibers inside the muscle spindles are gamma efferent neurons. Gamma efferent neurons adjust the resting tension within the muscle spindle. Changes in the length of the spindle are transmitted to the spinal cord by type Ia and type II afferent neurons, which innervate the nuclear chain fibers. Changes in the rate of length change are transmitted by type Ia afferent neurons, which innervate nuclear bag fibers. These afferent neurons send excitation signals to the alpha motoneuron in the spinal cord, activating contraction of the muscle. The muscle's synergists are excited and the antagonists are inhibited. Within the spinal cord, many neurons interface with the alpha motoneuron, acting to excite or inhibit the activity of the final common pathway of muscle contraction.[2]

In patients with spasticity, there is inappropriate firing of the alpha motoneuron, causing muscle contraction at abnormal times and of abnormal strength. The alpha motoneuron is abnormally sensitive to input from the type Ia and type II afferent neurons, probably because inhibitory input from other pathways is lost.

Clonus is the rhythmic repetitive contraction of a muscle in response to quick sustained stretching. The frequency of clonus is usually between 5 and 8 Hz, and is specific to a particular muscle in a particular patient. Bursts of alpha motoneuron activity alternate with relaxation of the muscle and volleys of afferent neuron discharges. Both peripheral and central factors determine whether a muscle will respond to stretching with clonus.[3]

Approaches to Quantifying Spasticity

Not surprisingly, most efforts to quantify spasticity in patients are based on the characteristics that are examined clinically. Various techniques and devices have been developed to measure the resistance of muscles to passive stretching. Similarly, many investigators have attempted to quantify the deep tendon reflex. Electromyography (EMG) has proved to be a useful tool in studies of muscle physiology and abnormal function in spastic patients. Some investigators have used electromyographic techniques to quantify spasticity. Each approach to the quantification of spasticity has advantages and limitations when applied to children with cerebral palsy.

Electromyographic Techniques

After a volley of alpha motoneuron discharges, the activated motor units contract, and action potentials can be detected by EMG. The relationship between the EMG signal and the force of muscle contraction is complicated and probably differs from muscle to muscle, depending on the mechanism of increasing tension within the muscle.[4] EMG activity in spastic muscle has been monitored in a variety of laboratory testing protocols, but because characteristics of the EMG signal are dependent on the techniques used to record them, those characteristics have rarely been used to quantify spasticity. Stam and Tan[5] used the amplitude of the EMG response to tendon taps from spring-loaded and hand-held reflex hammers, reporting that the response was proportional to the stimulus. Similarly, Miglietta and Lowenthal[6] mounted an electromechanical hammer a fixed distance from the patellar tendons of their spastic subjects so that contact between the hammer and the tendon triggered an oscilloscope. They measured the amplitude of the EMG response to the hammer impulse in a study in which they examined the effects of certain medications on spasticity in adult patients. In experiments designed to examine the effects of vestibular influence and proximal joint position on ankle spasticity, Perry and associates[2] used action potential peak counts and counted beats of ankle clonus in response to quick passive stretch. While the objective of this study was to investigate effects of abnormal neurophysiology on the clinical examination of spastic patients, EMGs were used to quantify the stretch response.

The major problem with all of these techniques is that there is not a generally accepted technique for relating EMG signal to muscle force in spastic patients. Unless physiologists are able to demonstrate a clear correlation between muscle force and some characteristic of the EMG, studies in which investigators attempt to use EMG to quantify spasticity will continue to be criticized.

In 1918, Hoffmann[7] described an electrical potential, which could be evoked by an electrical stimulus over a sensory nerve, that was too low to evoke a normal muscle action potential (an M wave on EMG). This potential has become known as the H wave. It is thought that the H response reflects the level of excitability of the alpha motoneuron at the spinal cord level.[8,9] As such, the H response should be a good indicator of spasticity. Several characteristics of the H wave have been used to study spasticity in patients. These include the amplitude of the H wave, the refractory period between stimuli required to elicit successive H waves, the ratio of H to M waves in response to stimulus, comparison of H and M wave amplitudes, and the threshold of stimulus required to elicit the H wave. The afferent stimulus in H wave testing is delivered to the nerve proximal to the muscle spindle. Bernardelli and associates[10] concluded that the H reflex and the deep tendon reflex both utilize type Ia afferent neurons.

In normal individuals, the H reflex can be detected only from plantarflexor muscles in response to stimulation of the posterior tibial nerve. In spastic patients, the reflex can be identified after stimulation of other nerves. In normal individuals, H reflex measurements have been used for basic physiologic studies.[8,10,11] The H response has also been measured in studies of cerebellar stimulators in children with cerebral palsy[12] and in the evaluation of pharmacologic agents.[9]

There are several limitations to the use of the H response in quantitative assessment of spasticity. While most authors agree that the response reflects excitability of the alpha motoneuron, there is controversy about which characteristics of the H wave are most useful. Some authors have been disappointed because H reflex characteristics did not change despite apparent clinical improvement.[9,12] The H response bypasses the muscle spindle, which surely plays an important role in spasticity.[13] Values of some characteristics of the H wave in spastic individuals overlap normal values, and the H response can be altered by a variety of local environmental factors.[9] Still, many investigators continue to use H response testing to quantify spasticity.

Measurements of Resistance to Motion

Resistance to motion is a major characteristic of spastic muscle, which contributes to functional disability. It is not surprising that many investigators have attempted to quantify this resistance.

One obvious parameter to study is motion itself, in response to a known stimulus. The "pendulum drop test" is a method for studying knee motion that uses gravity as a constant stimulus. The patient lies on an examining table while the investigator holds the knee in full extension. The leg is dropped and the oscillations of knee motion are measured. Through a mathematical formula, the amplitude and frequency of the motion are combined to yield a number, which can be compared with results from the same subject at another time. Robinson and associates[14,15] used this technique to study the effects of surface electrical stimulation in patients with spinal cord injury. They were impressed with the sensitivity of the pendulum drop test, but observed that clinical spasticity varies at different times of the day in patients with spinal cord injuries. The test is easy to perform, but can be applied only to the knee.

In other studies examiners looked directly at passive range of motion, measuring not only the displacement of the limb segment, but also some value of the force required to achieve that displacement. Leavitt and Beasley[16] reported a technique in which an electrogoniometer was used to measure knee motions. The subjects were prone on an examining table. The examiner used a tensiometer strapped to the shank to flex and extend the knee. Both tensions and resulting motions could be recorded. Burke and associates[17,18] used a similar apparatus, substituting a load cell for the tensiometer, to study quadriceps and hamstring spasticity. Halpern and associates[19] described a technique that they called myotonometry, which, they claimed, could be used over a variety of joints. Goniometers were used to measure joint motions while the examiner moved the limb with a load cell to record the forces required. Time, force, joint position, and EMG were all recorded in their study. Simons and Bingel[20] developed an ingenious and somewhat elaborate apparatus to study spasticity in the upper extremity. The subject was seated with the arm horizontal on a table. A bicycle wheel was mounted on the table, aligning the wheel axle with the elbow axis. A goniometer was applied to the elbow, and a force meter was fixed to the goniometer.

EMGs of the biceps and triceps were recorded. The examiner could manually turn the wheel, which flexed or extended the elbow. Joint angles and forces were recorded. Because all of the above techniques require manual application of the range of motion, they closely mimic the clinical situation. Because the examiner determines the forces, tests can be performed without discomfort to the subject. However, these techniques also leave room for criticism. The arcs of motion can be fairly large, and the resistance to passive motion is very dependent on the muscle length.[21] Particularly at the extremes of joint ranges, factors other than spasticity contribute to the resistance to motion. The mechanical properties of connective tissues themselves are important variables that cannot be isolated by this type of testing. Spasticity is velocity dependent, and it is difficult to control velocity when an examiner manually performs the range of motion tests.

Mechanical devices have been used to impart controlled passive motion to limb segments. With a motorized apparatus, the investigator can vary the displacement, force, and velocity of movement during studies of spasticity. It is fairly easy to strap the human foot to a plate attached to a motor, so many of these devices are used to study spasticity about the ankle. Studies of plantarflexors allow comparisons between resistance to motion data and the H reflex, even in normal individuals.

Otis and associates[22] used a dynamometer to put the ankle through a range of motion from 35 degrees of plantarflexion to 10 degrees of dorsiflexion, measuring the torque in resistance to this displacement. The apparatus was under manual control, and the velocity of motion could be varied. They tested both normal individuals and spastic patients. In both groups, they found that torques varied with joint position and that there appeared to be a correlation between the slope of the velocity/torque curve and body height. Spastic patients displayed a greater torque in response to increasing stretch velocity than normal subjects. These investigators repeat-tested most of the normal subjects and patients, finding the results to be quite repeatable.

Motorized footplates have been used to move the ankle in a sinusoidal oscillation.[23] In the Spasticity Measurement System developed by Lehmann and associates[13] to quantify spasticity, the ankle is moved through a 5-degree arc of motion near the subject's maximum clinical position of dorsiflexion, and torque is measured in response to the motion. The torque response is divided into an elastic component, which is dependent on displacement but not velocity, and a viscous component, which is relatively unaffected by displacement but dependent on velocity. The inertia related to the mass of the foot is mathematically discounted. The frequencies of oscillation used range from 3 to 12 Hz. In a study of hemiplegics, patients were tested before and after nerve blocks to the posterior tibial nerve, demonstrating reduction in spasticity after the blocks. In a later study using the same devices, children with cerebral palsy were tested and compared with normal children and adults.[24] The spastic children displayed a frequency-dependent viscoelastic response similar to that seen in spastic adults.

In addition, an increase in stiffness of the ankle in normal subjects was observed with increasing age. Rack and associates[25] used a motor and crank handle device to put the ankle through sinusoidal arcs of motion at variable amplitudes and frequency, measuring joint position, force, and EMG. They actually found more variability in the results from normal subjects than in results from spastic patients.

Laboratory measurements of the resistance to passive motion seem to be repeatable and reliable. If performed carefully, the tests seem to be safe for the subject. Children have been successfully tested. Investigators may be able to separate resistance due to muscle spasticity from mechanical resistance of tissues if tests are performed using short arcs of motion and sinusoidal oscillations, but such testing does not examine resistance to motion over a functional arc for most joints.

Measurements of Deep Tendon Reflexes

The knee jerk reflex was discovered in 1875 independently by Erb and Westphal.[26,27] However, they disagreed about the meaning of the response of the knee to tapping on the tendon. Westphal thought that knee extension was a purely mechanical response to stretching the patellar tendon, while Erb believed that the knee jerk was a true reflex. Jendrassik's[28] discovery that the knee jerk response could be potentiated by clasping the hands together just before the hammer blow helped establish the physiologic nature of the reflex. The patellar tendon reflex became diagnostically useful because of its absence in tabes dorsalis. Hyperactivity of the deep tendon reflex is often observed in the clinical evaluation of spastic patients. Quantitative measurements of the reflex have been used in many laboratories.

To measure the reflex, investigators have addressed the measurement of the stimulus. The simplest approaches attempt to standardize the hammer blow, without actually measuring the impact on the tendon. Manual tapping has been performed, but it is hard to estimate the intensity of the stimulus.[11] The hammer can be dropped from a fixed distance, relying on gravity to standardize the blow,[26,29] or a spring-loaded hammer can be constructed to deliver a standardized blow to a tendon.[27,30–32] Mechanical hammers have been built, which are placed a known distance from the tendon to be struck, but without measuring the impact of the hammer blow.[6] Investigators using such devices generally must assume that the hammer impact is standardized. In other laboratories, hammers have been constructed and outfitted with strain gauges or force transducers mounted on them to record the force of hammer impact. These may be hand-held reflex hammers[5] or electromechanical devices.[8,9,33–38] Figure 1 illustrates the electromechanical hammer apparatus developed by Yoshida and associates.[38] Stam and Tan[5] found that the variability of impact forces was less with mounted hammers than with hand-held devices, but that the reflex response was similar for a comparable force. Burke and associates[11] took a different approach to measuring stimulus, attaching an accelerometer over the Achilles tendon of the subject to record the impact of the hammer.

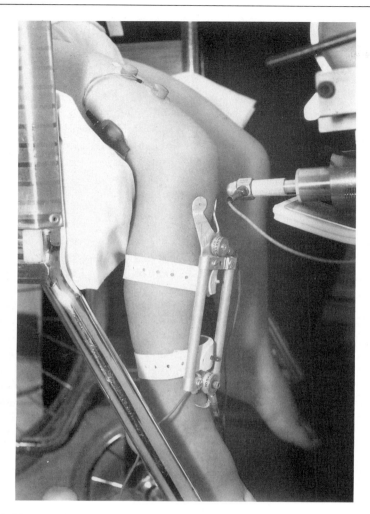

Fig. 1 *Photograph of patellar reflex apparatus used at San Francisco Shriners Hospital for Crippled Children. The child sits in a chair with the leg free to swing. An electromechanical hammer is aligned with the center of the patellar tendon. The force transducer mounted on the hammer records the force of the hammer blow. A small angular accelerometer strapped to the shank records angular acceleration of the limb in response to the tendon tap. A surface quadriceps electrode records EMG, which is used to identify valid data.*

In addition to the stimulus, quantifying the deep tendon reflex requires measurement of the response. Responses to tendon taps may be investigated by examining EMG latency or the myoelectric signal itself.[5,6,8,26] The motion of the free-swinging limb can be measured, as described by Erdman and Heather[30] in a portable testing system that uses oscillations of a light beam onto a mirror or photographic film to quantify the ankle jerk. The force of the reflex response to a tendon tap can be measured by fixing the distal limb segment in an apparatus that includes a strain gauge or load cell. Investigators have fixed the shank or the foot to study the Achilles or patellar reflex.[9,11,20,30,33,34,36,37] Fixing the distal limb and measuring the force of response eliminates error from the effect of spastic antagonists, which will affect data if the limb is allowed to swing freely. However, any slack in the fixed system must be taken up before force measurements are recorded.

In my colleagues' and my laboratory, the angular acceleration of the shank is measured in response to a patellar tendon tap.[37] A small angular accelerometer is attached to the shank, which is permitted to swing freely after the hammer blow. This device is illustrated in Figure 1. Only the area under the initial positive acceleration curve is measured in an attempt to reduce error imposed from hamstring spasticity. Figure 2 illustrates the recordings of the electromechanical hammer force, quadriceps EMG, and accelerometer recordings for a child with spastic cerebral palsy.

There are inherent problems when using the deep tendon reflex to quantify spasticity. While the muscle spindle is included in the reflex loop, only part of the type Ia afferent neuron input to the alpha motoneuron is represented in the deep tendon reflex. The contribution of the type II afferent neurons is probably not reflected. The deep tendon reflex can be changed by an enormous number of variables. These include time of day, drugs, alcohol, smoking, conversation, loud noises, cutaneous stimulation, anxiety, exercise, physical fitness, pain, weather, age, and sex.[6,27,29] There is substantial variation from tendon tap to tendon tap so that ten to 20 taps are recommended in order to obtain a representative sampling.[27] Tap-to-tap variations have even been reported in subjects under ether anesthesia, suggesting that the variability is related to spinal or subcortical factors, rather than voluntary activity.[37] Not all clinically spastic patients demonstrate hyperreflexia in laboratory testing. Simons and Sweetser[37] found that 30% of the hemiplegic patients in their study had normal reflex responses. One patient with a spinal cord injury reported by Yoshida and associates,[38] did not demonstrate hyperreflexia in the laboratory despite clinical spasticity.

Pediatric Considerations

Some features of laboratory testing present particular challenges when applied to children. Many children with cerebral palsy resist physical restriction and may not cooperate with testing protocols that restrain motion. Children often have difficulty holding still for testing. If the child moves, tendon taps may miss the target or proper resting tension in strain gauges may be lost. Elaborate testing apparatus may not be tolerated by children, and long protocols exceed the patience of little children. Because subject anxiety affects laboratory results, efforts must be made to keep children calm during testing.

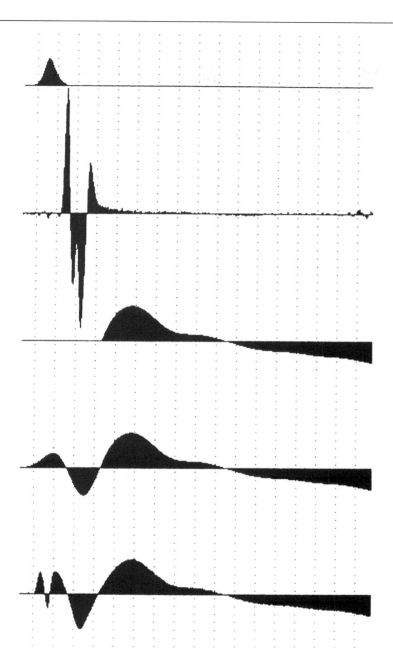

Fig. 2 *Output from patellar tendon test at San Francisco Shriners Hospital for Crippled Children. The top line represents the force of the tendon tap; the second line is the quadriceps EMG; and the third line is the angular acceleration, filtered and without artifacts. The area under the initial positive acceleration is used to quantify the reflex response. The fourth line is filtered acceleration with movement artifacts from the hammer blow, and the fifth line is raw accelerometer output.*

Studies of Therapeutic Efficacy

Laboratory measurements of spasticity have been used to evaluate the effects of therapy techniques, pharmacologic agents, nerve blocks, and surgical procedures. Test results have not always supported clinical impressions.

Robinson and associates[14,15] used the pendulum drop test to evaluate quadriceps spasticity in patients with spinal cord injuries who were treated by surface electrical stimulation. Electrical stimulation caused fatigue of the muscle, which reduced spasticity measurement values. Over a long term, the treatment had little effect.

Pedersen[9] used a variety of laboratory tests to evaluate medications in the treatment of spasticity. These included ankle jerk reflex tests with an electromechanical hammer and strain gauges on the foot, H response tests, and EMGs. Most tests demonstrated beneficial effects of medications, but the H response failed to change with administration of diazepam, which the author believed had a beneficial clinical effect. Erdman and Heather[31] used their portable reflex apparatus to demonstrate a beneficial effect of diazepam in patients with spinal cord injury. Miglietta and Lowenthal,[6] in an earlier study of a variety of drugs, used a mechanical hammer on the patellar tendon and measured the amplitude of the resultant quadriceps EMG. They concluded that most of the drugs were useful in reducing spasticity. Leavitt and Beasley[16] used passive motion with tensiometers and goniometers in a study of a variety of medications, all of which were found to be helpful to spastic patients.

Lehmann and associates[13] used the Spasticity Measurement System of sinusoidal oscillation of the ankle in adult patients with spasticity before and after nerve blocks to the posterior tibial nerve. They demonstrated unequivocal reductions in the resistance to passive motion after the nerve blocks.

McLellan and associates[12] included studies of the H response in their evaluation of cerebellar surface stimulation. They were disappointed with the results of the testing because laboratory tests failed to substantiate apparent clinical benefits of the treatment.

In my colleagues' and my laboratory, patellar tendon reflex testing was combined with functional clinical evaluation and gait analysis to study children with cerebral palsy in a prospective study of selective dorsal rhizotomy. The apparatus used was the electromechanical hammer and angular accelerometer device described by Yoshida and associates.[38] The investigators marked the center of the patellar tendon with ink and discarded ''misses'' by the hammer due to movement of the children. Quadriceps EMGs were recorded, but were used to discard tendon taps when pretap signal was recorded or sustained ''cheating''was suspected. As illustrated in Figure 3, selective dorsal rhizotomy significantly reduced the angular acceleration of the shank in response to a hammer force at six and 12 months after surgery. This study is ongoing, to follow children two and three years after the operation, but has shown significant changes in all but one child, who was areflexic prior to rhizotomy.

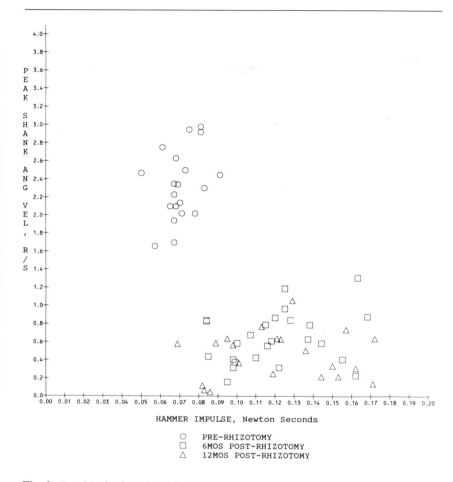

Fig. 3 *Graphic display of patellar reflex response for a child with cerebral palsy treated by selective dorsal rhizotomy. Preoperative reflex response was greater with lower hammer force than it was six or 12 months after rhizotomy.*

Discussion

Laboratory testing to quantify spasticity is challenging. Studies have focused on the stretch response, but a vast array of neural inputs from a variety of pathways impact the alpha motoneuron. There are large individual variations in responses observed in both normal subjects and spastic patients. Moreover, relatively wide ranges of normal standards seem to mandate that each subject serve as his/her own control, and environmental and emotional factors can dramatically change test results. Wide intersubject and intrasubject variations mandate multiple repetitions and large series to achieve statistical significance.

Each technique has limitations. Studies of the H reflex bypass the muscle spindle, looking at excitability of the alpha motoneuron after artificial type Ia afferent neuron stimulation. Investigations of the resistance to passive motion probably overemphasize type II afferent neuron input. Over large ranges of motion, it is difficult to separate the mechanical properties of the tissues from the physiologic changes of spasticity; when confined to small sinusoidal oscillations of joints, the tests do not cover a functional range of motion. The responses to tendon taps probably only measure the input of the nuclear bag fibers to the alpha motoneuron via Ia afferent neurons. The relationship between hyperreflexia and functional spasticity is unclear. Some evidence suggests that the results of passive motion studies and reflex testing do not correlate.[20] There is no clear "best test" or comprehensive quantitative measure of spasticity. We still have much to learn.

Almost any sort of laboratory testing of spastic children is difficult. Short attention spans, fears and anxieties, and poor cooperation challenge investigators. Clinicians disagree about the importance of function and form of motions and activity. It is not easy to discern which types of laboratory tests are most meaningful.

Still, laboratory measurements of spasticity can be used to evaluate the results of therapeutic intervention. The fact that laboratory tests do not always corroborate clinical impressions makes the laboratory tests all the more valuable. Clinicians cannot always agree about the effectiveness of therapeutic intervention. In the long run, only quantitative data and statistical analysis can be expected to settle controversies and measure the effects of what we do for children with cerebral palsy.

References

1. Ashworth B: Preliminary trials of carisoprodal in multiple sclerosis. *Practitioner* 1964;192:540–542.
2. Perry J, Giovan P, Harris LJ, et al: The determinants of muscle action in the hemiparetic lower extremity. *Clin Orthop* 1978;131:71–98.
3. Dimitrijevic MR, Nathan PW, Sherwood AM: Clonus: The role of central mechanisms. *J Neurol Neurosurg Psychiatry* 1980;43:321–332.
4. Solomonow M, Baratta R, Zhou BH, et al: Historical update and new developments on the EMG-force relationships of skeletal muscles. *Orthopedics* 1986;9:1541–1543.
5. Stam J, Tan KM: Tendon reflex variability and method of stimulation. *Electroenceph Clin Neurophysiol* 1987;67:463–467.
6. Miglietta OE, Lowenthal M: Measurement of the stretch reflex response as an approach to the objective evaluation of a spasticity. *Arch Phys Med Rehabil* 1962;43:62–68.
7. Hoffman P: Uber die Beziehungen der Sehnenreflexe zur willkurlichen Bewegung und zum Tonus. *Z Biol* 1918;68:351–370.
8. Bishop B, Machover S, Johnston R, et al: A quantitative assessment of gamma-motoneuron contribution to the Achilles tendon reflex in normal subjects. *Arch Phys Med Rehabil* 1968;49:145–154.
9. Pedersen E: Clinical assessment and pharmacologic therapy of spasticity. *Arch Phys Med Rehabil* 1974;55:344–354.
10. Bernardelli A, Hallet M, Kaufman C, et al: Stretch reflexes of triceps surae in normal man. *J Neurol Neurosurg Psychiatry* 1982;45:513–525.
11. Burke D, McKeon B, Skuse NF: Dependence of the Achilles tendon reflex on the excitability of spinal reflex pathways. *Ann Neurol* 1981;10:551–556.

12. McLellan DL, Selwyn M, Cooper IS: Time course of clinical and physiological effects of stimulation of the cerebellar surface in patients with spasticity. *J Neurol Neurosurg Psychiatry* 1978;41:150–160.

13. Lehmann JF, Price R, DeLateur BJ, et al: Spasticity: Quantitative measurements as a basis for assessing the effectiveness of therapeutic intervention. *Arch Phys Med Rehabil* 1989;70:6–15.

14. Robinson CJ, Kett NA, Bolam JM: Spasticity in spinal cord injured patients: 1. Short-term effects of surface electrical stimulation. *Arch Phys Med Rehabil* 1988;69:598–604.

15. Robinson CJ, Kett NA, Bolam JM: Spasticity in spinal cord injured patients: 2. Initial measures and long-term effects of surface electrical stimulation. *Arch Phys Med Rehabil* 1988;69:862–868.

16. Leavitt LA, Beasley WC: Clinical application of quantitative methods in the study of spasticity. *Clin Pharmacol Ther* 1964;5:918–941.

17. Burke D, Gillies JD, Lance JW: The quadriceps stretch reflex in human spasticity. *J Neurol Neurosurg Psychiatry* 1970;33:216–223.

18. Burke D, Gillies JD, Lance JW: Hamstrings stretch reflex in human spasticity. *J Neurol Neurosurg Psychiatry* 1971;34:231–235.

19. Halpern D, Patterson R, Mackie R, et al: Muscular hypertonia: Quantitative analysis. *Arch Phys Med Rehabil* 1979;60:208–218.

20. Simons DG, Bingel AGA: Quantitative comparison of passive motion and tendon reflex responses in biceps and triceps brachii muscles in hemiplegic or hemiparetic man. *Stroke* 1971;2:58–66.

21. Rebersek S, Stefanofska A, Vodovnik L, et al: Some properties of spastic ankle joint muscles in hemiplegia. *Med Biol Eng Comput* 1986;24:19–26.

22. Otis JC, Root L, Pamilla JR, et al: Biomechanical measurement of spastic plantarflexors. *Dev Med Child Neurol* 1983;25:60–66.

23. Gottlieb GL, Agarwal GC, Penn R: Sinusoidal oscillation of the ankle as a means of evaluating the spastic patient. *J Neurol Neurosurg Psychiatry* 1978;41:32–39.

24. Price R, Bjornson KF, Lehmann JF, et al: Quantitative measurement of spasticity in children with cerebral palsy. *Dev Med Child Neurol* 1991;33:585–595.

25. Rack PMH, Ross HF, Thilmann AF: The ankle stretch reflexes in normal and spastic subjects. *Brain* 1984;107:637–654.

26. Kroll W: Patellar reflex time and reflex latency under Jendrassik and crossed extensor facilitation. *Am J Phys Med* 1968;47:292–301.

27. Simons DG, Dimitrijevic MR: Quantitative variations in the force of quadriceps responses to serial patellar tendon taps in normal man. *Am J Phys Med* 1972;51:240–263.

28. Jendrassik E: Beitrage zur Lehr vonden Sehnenreflexen. *Deutches Arch Klin Med* 1883;33:177–199.

29. Tipton CM, Karpovich PV: Exercise and the patellar reflex. *J Appl Physiol* 1966;21:15–18.

30. Erdman WJ, Heather AJ: A method for the quantitative measurement of spasticity and its response to therapy. *Arch Phys Med Rehabil* 1958;39:630–633.

31. Erdman WJ, Heather AJ: Objective measurement of spasticity by light reflection. *Clin Pharmacol Ther* 1964;5:883–886.

32. Heather AJ, Smith TA, Graebe RA: New device for the quantitative measure of spasticity. *Arch Phys Med Rehabil* 1965;46:332–336.

33. Clarke AM: The effect of stimulation of certain skin areas on the extensor motoneurons in the phasic reaction of a stretch reflex in normal human subjects. *Electroenceph Clin Neurophysiol* 1966;21:185–193.

34. Clarke AM: Effect of the Jendrassik manoeuvre on a phasic stretch reflex in normal human subjects during experimental control over supraspinal influences. *J Neurol Neurosurg Psychiatry* 1967;30:34–42.

35. Fryer G, Lamonte RJ, Simons DG: Technical Note: An electronically controlled automatic reflex hammer. *Med Biol Eng* 1972;10:125–129.

36. Simons DG, Lamonte RJ: Automated system for the measurement of reflex responses to patellar tendon tap in man. *Am J Phys Med* 1971;50:72–78.

37. Simons DG, Sweetser TH: Effects of hemiparesis and handgrip on the mean response and variability of the knee-jerk. *Am J Phys Med* 1973;52:221–242.

38. Yoshida MK, Lamoreux LW, Johanson ME, et al: Quantitative assessment of patellar tendon reflex using an angular accelerometer, in Wallinga W, Boom HBK, de Vries J (eds): *Electrophysiological Kinesiology*. New York, Exerpta Medica, 1988.

Chapter 4

Spasticity and Gait: Knee Torques and Muscle Cocontraction

Christopher L. Vaughan, PhD
Kristen A. Bowsher, MS
Michael D. Sussman, MD

Introduction

Children who have cerebral palsy with spastic diplegia tend to have increased stretch reflexes of the muscles, a loss of selective muscle control, a dependence on primitive reflexes, and an imbalance between agonist and antagonist muscles crossing their joints.[1] These clinical features of spasticity obviously contribute to various pathologic gait patterns. Spasticity has been defined by Rymer and Powers[2] as "a motor disorder characterized by a velocity-dependent increase in tonic stretch reflexes, with exaggerated tendon jerks resulting from hyperexcitability of the stretch reflex."

Several approaches have been taken to develop a feasible and reliable method of quantifying the degree of spasticity, both in children with cerebral palsy and in adults with other disorders that result in spasticity. These approaches have been both subjective (eg, resistance to passive movement as in the work of Bohannon and Smith[3]) and objective.[2,4-6] While the objective approaches have been reasonably successful in quantifying the severity of spastic hypertonia, they all suffer from the same problem: The patient must be constrained in a specific posture or custom-designed device. In some individuals with cerebral palsy, however, spasticity only becomes apparent (and therefore problematic) when they attempt to perform some functional activity such as walking.[7] Research to quantify spasticity during functional tasks has been extremely limited.[8]

The overall goal of this research is to develop a quantitative measure of spastic diplegia in children with cerebral palsy using the tools of a gait analysis laboratory. Based on a review of the literature, we have determined that the parameters having the greatest potential are joint torque[2,5] and the degree of cocontraction in muscles crossing that joint.[7] Our aim is to measure knee joint angle, knee joint torque, and electromyographic (EMG) activity of the muscles crossing the knee joint for both normal children and those with spastic diplegia. Our interest is, therefore, to understand how a child having cerebral palsy differs from normal children at a freely-selected pace, and also to examine whether an increase in pace exaggerates any differences.

Table 1 Patient characteristics

Subject*	Age	Sex	Mass (kg)	Right Leg Length (m)
N1	5	F	18.2	0.570
N2	11	F	40.9	0.768
N3	11	M	38.6	0.743
N4	14	M	34.1	0.780
N5	11	M	41.4	0.816
N6	10	F	35.5	0.760
N7	8	M	24.5	0.675
N8	12	F	49.5	0.853
N9	11	F	43.6	0.835
N10	12	F	35.0	0.832
CP1	11	F	28.4	0.762
CP2	7	F	20.5	0.579
CP3	4	F	17.7	0.540
CP4	8	F	26.4	0.725
CP5	11	F	60.9	0.820
CP6	14	M	47.7	0.841

*N indicates normal child and CP indicates child with cerebral palsy.

Subjects and Methodology

Two populations were studied: a group of ten normal healthy children and a group of six children, each with a confirmed diagnosis of cerebral palsy. Clinical findings for the cerebral palsy group were consistent with mild to moderate spastic diplegia in all cases. All of these subjects were independent ambulators, and none of them used orthoses. None of the normal children had a history of, or showed any signs of, physical abnormalities. The normal group consisted of six girls and four boys between the ages of 5 and 14, while the cerebral palsy group consisted of five girls and one boy between the ages of 4 and 14 (Table 1).

Each subject performed six walking trials: three at a "normal" or self-selected pace, and three at a much faster pace. The instructions given were: "walk at your normal speed" and "walk as fast as possible, but do not run." Our intent with the trials at the higher speed was to try and elicit a spastic response from the children with cerebral palsy. All subjects walked barefoot on a level walkway 11 meters long with 4.5 meters of space between the ends of the walkway and the walls. During each trial, the positions of the joints in three-dimensional (3-D) space and bilateral surface EMG recordings of the quadriceps and hamstring muscle groups were collected simultaneously.

The displacement data were captured at 60 Hz for 3 seconds using a 3-D ExpertVision System (Motion Analysis Corporation, Santa Rosa, CA) and a body surface marker set developed at Helen Hayes Hospital in New York by Kadaba and associates.[9] The markers consisted of 15 small plastic balls (2 to 3 cm in diameter) covered with retroreflective material. They were attached, with double-sided tape, to the sacrum, anterior superior iliac spines, knee joint lines (posterior to the lateral femoral condyle), the lateral malleolus, the second metatarsal heads, and the heels. Four of the markers were attached to 7.5-cm wands: two to the thighs, midway between the hip and knee joints; and two to the shanks, midway between the knee and ankle joints. The design of the cuffs and length of the wands were such that unwanted oscillations (eg, at heel-strike) were minimized.

The EMG signals were captured using surface electrodes and an eight-channel telemetry unit (MIE Medical Research, England) so that the subject was not encumbered with an umbilical cord of trailing wires. There were six main components: pregelled silver/silver chloride surface electrodes (Lewis Medical Instruments, Rockville, MD); light weight preamplifiers (45 g including cable and connector); a transmitter unit (less than 0.6 kg) carried on the subject's back with a halter vest; a receiver unit; a high-pass filter (greater than 30 Hz) to remove any motion artifact; a 12 bit analog-to-digital convertor; and an IBM-compatible personal computer. The EMG electrodes were placed over both the right and left quadriceps and hamstring muscle groups. In addition to the rectus femoris, the quadriceps EMG electrodes probably also picked up signals from the vasti muscles, and possibly the sartorius. Likewise the hamstring EMG electrodes, being positioned slightly laterally, picked up signals primarily from the biceps femoris, but may also have recorded activity from the semitendinosus and semimembranosus muscles.

Anthropometric measurements were taken on each subject for the purpose of calculating body segment parameters (eg, segment masses and moments of inertia) and estimating joint centers.[10] These measurements included: total body mass, anterior superior iliac spine breadth, thigh length, thigh circumference, calf length, calf circumference, knee diameter, foot length, malleolus height, malleolus diameter, and foot breadth. The instruments used were a standard doctor's scale, calipers, and a flexible tape measure.

The 3-D coordinates of the external markers were read into a program called GAITMATH, developed by Vaughan and associates[10] and published with their book *Dynamics of Human Gait*. This program calculated internal joint centers and 3-D anatomical joint angles according to Grood and Suntay.[11] The raw data were smoothed and differentiated to provide linear and angular accelerations,[12] and these, in turn, were combined with the body segment parameters in a Newtonian formulation to calculate joint torques.[10] In this study, ground-reaction forces were not measured because a force plate system was not available at that time. We, therefore, concentrated on the swing phase of the gait cycle where the knee joint undergoes its greatest range of angular motion.

The raw EMG data were processed through a program that performed full wave rectification, low pass filtering with a cut-off frequency of 3 Hz, and then converted the magnitude to microvolts (based on the various gains and the characteristics of the analog-to-digital convertor). Finally, because the kinematic data were collected at 60 Hz while the EMG data were collected at 1,000 Hz, the EMG data were interpolated to synchronize the two data sets. Figure 1 shows an example of a raw data file and a filtered data file for the quadriceps.

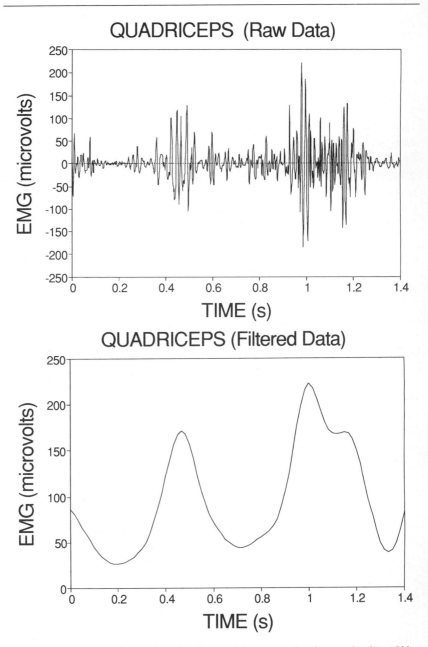

Fig. 1 *Electromyographic activity for the quadriceps muscle of normal subject N4, walking at a freely selected speed of 1.18 m/sec, showing how the data were processed:* **Top**, *Raw signal;* **Bottom**, *Low pass filtered signal. Note that this window of data includes more than one complete gait cycle.*

Table 2 Mean walking speed (standard deviation)

Subjects	Walking Speed (m/sec)		Percent Increase
	Free	Fast	
Normal (N = 10)	1.16 (0.26)	2.07 (0.32)	81% (22)
Cerebral Palsy (N = 6)	0.76 (0.21)	1.25 (0.28)	71% (52)

A cocontraction index (CCI) was created to contrast the level of muscle activity of the quadriceps with that of the hamstrings at each instant in time, and it represented the degree to which the two muscle groups were acting together (or cocontracting). In calculating the CCI it is not possible to compare the actual EMG values (in microvolts) of the quadriceps and hamstrings because of many factors, including electrode placement, skin resistance, subcutaneous fat, fiber type, and skin temperature. Therefore, we normalized the EMG values between 0 and 1, with 1 representing maximal activity. The formulae used to calculate the CCI were:

$$\text{activation level of } H_t = \frac{H_t - H_{min}}{H_{max} - H_{min}} \tag{1}$$

$$\text{activation level of } Q_t = \frac{Q_t - Q_{min}}{Q_{max} - Q_{min}} \tag{2}$$

$$CCI_t = 1 - |(\text{activation level of } H_t) - (\text{activation level of } Q_t) \tag{3}$$

where:

CCI_t	= cocontraction index for data point t,
H_t	= value of hamstrings EMG for data point t,
Q_t	= value of quadriceps EMG for data point t,
H_{max}, Q_{max}	= maximum EMG recording for all trials within a subject for the hamstrings and quadriceps, and
H_{min}, Q_{min}	= minimum EMG recording for all trials within a subject for the hamstrings and quadriceps.

A CCI of 1 meant that both muscle groups were firing at the same relative levels and a CCI of 0 meant that one muscle group was firing at a maximum level while the other muscle group was firing at its minimum value. Our definition for CCI is similar to that developed by Falconer and Winter,[13] except that these authors looked at a time interval (for example, stance phase). Our definition in equation (3) provides a value for CCI at each time instant.

Results and Discussion

Table 2 is a summary of the mean walking speeds of the normal children and those with cerebral palsy. There are a number of points to note from this table. First, the ten normal children, on average, walked at a higher speed than their counterparts with cerebral palsy, for both

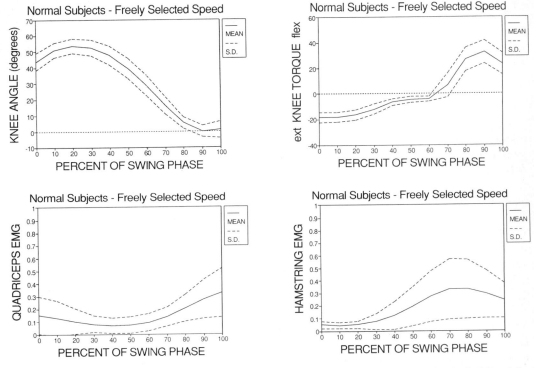

Fig. 2 *Mean data (with ± one standard deviation indicated by the dashed lines) for ten normal subjects walking at their freely selected speed: **Top left**, Knee joint angle; **Top right**, Resultant knee joint torque in the sagittal plane; **Bottom left**, Quadriceps EMG; and **Bottom right**, Hamstrings EMG. Note that these data are for the swing phase only; the torque data have been normalized by body weight and leg length; and the EMG data were normalized according to equations (1) and (2) in the text.*

the freely-selected and the faster pace, and showed a larger percent increase from the freely-selected to the faster pace (81% versus 71%). Second, the speed data for both sets of children tended to be quite variable, although this was skewed somewhat for the children with cerebral palsy by child CP1, who went from 0.52 m/sec to 1.48 m/sec, an increase of 185%. The fact that five of the six children with cerebral palsy had a far smaller increase in walking speed may have had an impact on the angle, torque, and EMG data that we acquired. Note that all of the data are for the subject's right knee joints during the swing phase of gait.

Figure 2 summarizes the mean data for the normal subjects walking at their freely-selected speed. The knee joint angle in Figure 2, *top left*, varies from 45 degrees at toe-off, flexes to over 50 degrees in mid-swing, and then returns to 0 degrees (ie, full extension) just prior to heel-strike. As indicated by the two standard deviation lines, there is good consistency from subject to subject. These data are in excellent agreement with other studies of normal children.[14,15]

The joint torques were normalized according to each subject's weight in Newtons and right leg length in meters (Table 1). The right leg length was calculated by adding the thigh length, calf length, and malleolus height.[10] The following formula was used for torque normalization:

$$\text{Normalized Torque} = \frac{\text{Torque (Nm)} \times 1000}{\text{weight [N]} \times \text{right leg length [m]}}$$

From Figure 2, *top right*, we note that at toe-off a knee extensor torque of about 20 units is needed to accelerate the calf forward. At 60% of the swing phase, the torque changes sign, becoming a flexor torque with a maximum value of over 30 units and decelerating the calf in anticipation of heel-strike. These torque data are also in good agreement with the data of Ounpuu and associates.[15] The quadriceps EMG data for the normal subjects at a freely-selected speed (Fig. 2, *bottom left*) has two high points: at toe-off, where it provides the knee extensor torque (Fig. 2, *top right*); and in late swing, where it is stabilizing the knee joint in anticipation of heel-strike. In contrast, the hamstrings EMG, as seen in Figure 2, *bottom right*, is relatively quiescent in early swing, but builds up to its maximum value at 75% of the swing phase, contributing to the knee flexor torque that decelerates the calf prior to heel-strike. It is interesting to note from Figure 2 that while the knee joint angle and torque data are relatively consistent (indicated by the "tight" standard deviation lines), the EMG data for quadriceps and hamstrings are quite variable. The trends, however, are quite clear.

Figure 3 contrasts the mean data for ten normal subjects walking at the freely-selected and fast speeds. For the sake of clarity, standard deviation curves have not been included. We observe that the knee joint angles are almost identical at the two speeds, the only slight difference being a 5 degree flexion angle at heel-strike for the fast pace versus full extension at the free walking speed. The torque data are similar in shape but differ only in magnitude: A larger extensor torque after toe-off and a larger flexor torque prior to heel-strike were associated with the fast pace. These torques are generated by musculature crossing the knee joint: The quadriceps are increased throughout for the fast pace but particularly at the beginning and end of the swing phase, as they vigorously accelerate and stabilize the calf respectively; the hamstrings increase substantially during the latter part of swing, providing the knee flexor torque to arrest the forward motion of the calf.

Figure 4 illustrates the mean cocontraction index (CCI) data for the ten normal subjects walking at both speeds. On average, the CCI decreased in the normal subjects with increased walking speed. However, because Figure 4 is a composite of ten subjects, and CCI varies as a function of time, as seen in Equation (3), it is probably more instructive to examine the data for a single subject. Figure 5, *left*, shows the EMG and CCI data for normal subject N1 at the freely-selected speed. We notice that the CCI is very high for the first 50% of swing,

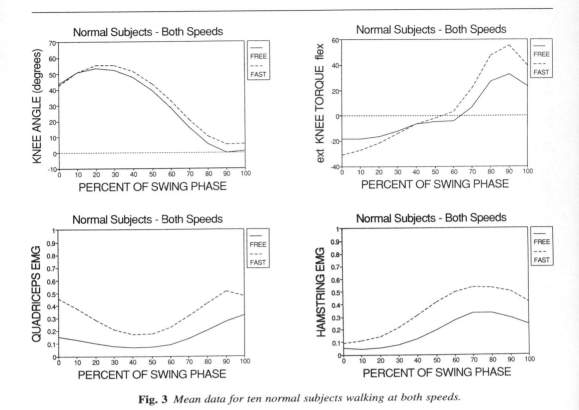

Fig. 3 *Mean data for ten normal subjects walking at both speeds.*

and then decreases somewhat during the latter half of the phase, as the quadriceps EMG builds up to stabilize the knee joint. At the fast speed (Fig. 5, *right*), the CCI drops off dramatically in two loops, reflecting the reciprocating action of the quadriceps and hamstrings muscle groups. Figure 5, *right*, is representative of all ten subjects, the only difference being the position (in time) of the high point, where the quadriceps and hamstrings EMG curves crossed over. In summary, at faster speeds normal subjects recruit only those muscles that they need, leading to a decrease in the CCI.

Figure 6 shows the mean data for the six subjects with cerebral palsy walking at their fast pace. The mean knee joint angle, which is quite variable (indicated by the standard deviation lines), varies from 40 degrees at toe-off to 20 degrees at heel-strike. This relatively ''flat'' curve is characteristic of the crouch gait of spastic diplegia.[1] The knee torque has a very similar shape to normal, starting off at 20 units of extensor torque at toe-off, changing sign, and reaching 20 units of flexor torque prior to heel-strike. The EMG data (Fig. 6, *bottom left* and *bottom right*) are relatively flat, increasing slightly before heel-strike, but extremely variable. This variability should be interpreted with caution, however, because we have gathered data for only six subjects, and

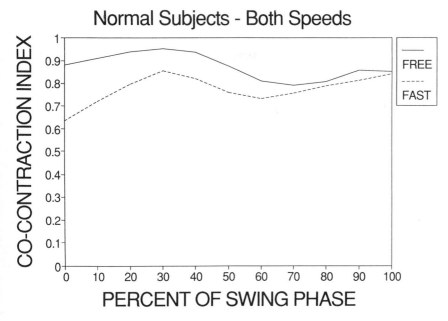

Fig. 4 *Mean cocontraction index data for ten normal subjects walking at both speeds. Note that this index is defined according to equation (3) in the text.*

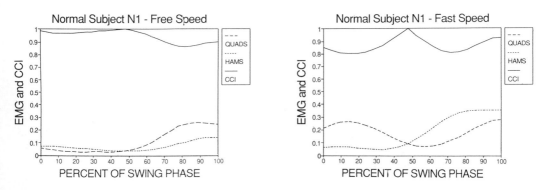

Fig. 5 *Quadriceps EMG, hamstrings EMG, and cocontraction index (CCI) data for normal subject N1 during swing phase:* **Left,** *Freely-selected speed (0.75 m/sec; and* **Right,** *Fast speed (1.48 m/sec). EMG normalization and CCI are defined in equations (1), (2), and (3).*

cerebral palsy——even of the spastic diplegic type—tends to lack homogeneity.

The effects of increased walking speed, intended to elicit a spastic response, are shown in Figure 7. We notice a very slight increase of

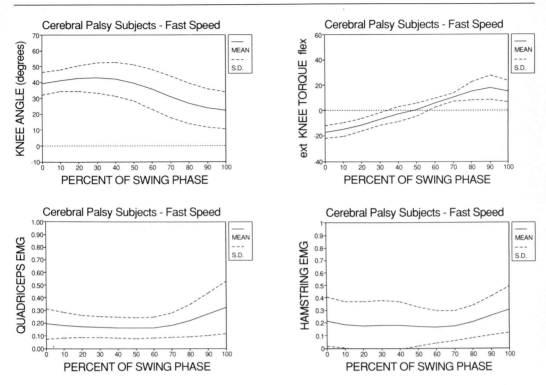

Fig. 6 *Mean data (with ± one standard deviation indicated by dashed lines) for six subjects with cerebral palsy walking at their fast speed:* **Top left**, *Knee joint angle;* **Top right**, *Resultant knee joint torque in the sagittal plane;* **Bottom left**, *Quadriceps EMG; and* **Bottom right**, *Hamstrings EMG. Note that the data are for the swing phase only; the torque data have been normalized by dividing by body weight and leg length; and the EMG data were normalized according to equations (1) and (2) in the text.*

knee joint angle at mid-swing, and a knee joint torque that is almost identical until late swing when the flexor torque for the fast speed exceeds the free speed by ten units. The EMG data appear to decrease slightly at the faster speed, but the large variability (Fig. 6) probably means that the difference is of no real significance. The cocontraction of quadriceps and hamstrings has been well-documented in the clinical literature.[16] Figure 8 illustrates the effect of walking speed on the CCI, where the increased speed leads to an increase in CCI. As before with the normal child (Fig. 5), it is instructive to examine the CCI data for an individual subject with cerebral palsy. Figure 9 shows the quadriceps and hamstrings EMGs and CCIs for subject CP4 at freely-selected and fast speeds. Both EMG patterns increase slightly from toe-off to heel-strike at both speeds, leading to consistently high CCI values, which vary between 0.85 and 1.0.

There have been other attempts to quantify spasticity using an index of muscular contraction. McClellan[17] studied the effects of the drug

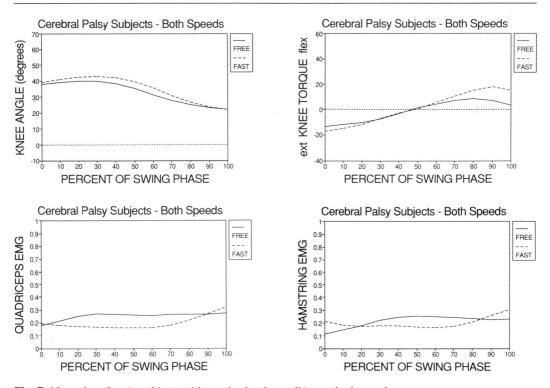

Fig. 7 *Mean data for six subjects with cerebral palsy walking at both speeds.*

baclofen on spasticity and determined his index by measuring the EMG within an individual muscle group rather than between two groups. His subjects performed cyclical flexion and extension while seated in a chair, and he showed that while the spastic subjects had a higher index than normal subjects, baclofen did not produce any significant changes in the index. Fung and Barbeau[8] developed a spastic locomotor disorder index that was defined, for a particular muscle, as the ratio of the EMG in the predetermined ''off'' window of the normalized gait cycle to that in the ''on'' window. This index tended to be elevated for spastic subjects. Whereas both the above methods were used to look at the effect of spasticity on an individual muscle, our approach has been to concentrate on cocontraction: the degree to which two muscle groups (agonist and antagonist) are acting together.

Conclusions

Based on the data presented in Table 2 and Figures 2 to 5, the following conclusions may be drawn for the normal children: (1) At both speeds of walking, the knee joint angle pattern was consistent with a range of 55 degrees. (2) At both speeds, the extensor knee joint torque

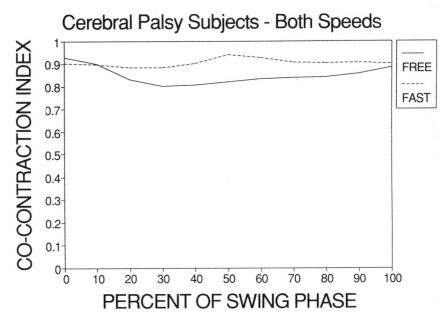

Fig. 8 *Mean cocontraction index data for six subjects with cerebral palsy walking at both speeds. Note that this index is defined according to equation (3) in the text.*

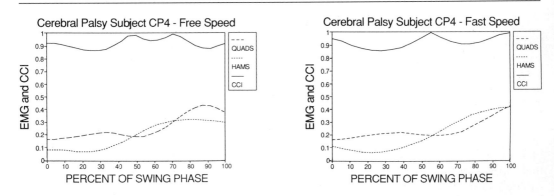

Fig. 9 *Quadriceps EMG, hamstrings EMG, and cocontraction index (CCI) data for cerebral palsy subject CP4 during swing phase: **Left**, Freely-selected speed (1.06 m/ sec), and **Right**, Fast speed (1.45 m/sec). EMG normalization and CCI are defined in equations (1), (2), and (3).*

dominated in early swing while the flexor torque dominated during terminal swing. (3) At an increased gait speed there was a larger flexor torque in late swing. (4) At both speeds, the quadriceps EMG decreased during early swing until mid-swing and then increased during late swing, while the hamstrings EMG was diminished for the first half of the swing phase and then increased from mid-swing to terminal swing. (5) At an increased gait speed, the quadriceps EMG increased early in the swing while the hamstrings EMG increased late in the swing. (6) At an increased gait speed, the cocontraction index decreased.

Based on the data presented in Table 2 and Figures 6 to 9, the following conclusions may be drawn for the children with cerebral palsy: (1) At both speeds of walking, the knee joint angle pattern was flat (but quite variable) with a range of about 20 degrees. (2) While the extensor torques were similar to normal, flexor torques tended to be much smaller, and increased speed of walking had little impact on the knee torques. (3) At both walking speeds, the EMG activity of both quadriceps and hamstrings was relatively low. (4) At both speeds of walking, the cocontraction index was very close to 1.0 (ie, quadriceps and hamstrings were active at the same time) throughout the entire swing phase.

While the data for the subjects with cerebral palsy were quite variable, the above conclusions do offer some insight into the strategies used by normal children and those with spastic diplegia to increase their speed of walking. Because we concentrated only on the swing phase of the gait cycle, it may be that the stance phase could provide further insights.

Acknowledgments

This work was done with the financial support of the Biomedical Research Support Grant 5-S07-RR05431–29, the Kluge Research Fund, and the Orthopaedic Research and Education Foundation.

References

1. Gage JR: Surgical treatment of knee dysfunction in cerebral palsy. *Clin Orthop* 1990;253:45–54.
2. Rymer WZ, Powers RK: Pathophysiology of muscular hypertonia in spasticity. *Neurosurgery: State of the Art Reviews* 1989;4:291–301.
3. Bohannon RW, Smith MB: Interrater reliability of a modified Ashworth scale of muscle spasticity. *Phys Ther* 1987;67:206–207.
4. Lamoreux LW, Yoshida MK: Accelerometer assessment of hyper-reflexia in patellar tendon reflex. *IEEE Ninth Ann Conf Eng Med Biol Soc* 1987;465:1–2.
5. Lehmann JF, Price R, deLateur BJ, et al: Spasticity: Quantitative measurements as a basis for assessing effectiveness of therapeutic intervention. *Arch Phys Med Rehabil* 1989;70:6–15.
6. Otis JC, Root L, Pamilla JR, et al: Biomechanical measurement of spastic plantar flexors. *Dev Med Child Neurol* 1983;25:60–66.
7. Myklebust BM: A review of myotatic reflexes and the development of motor control and gait in infants and children: A special communication. *Phys Ther* 1990;70:188–203.
8. Fung J, Barbeau H: A dynamic EMG profile index to quantify muscular activation disorder in spastic paretic gait. *Electroencephalogr Clin Neurophysiol* 1989;73:233–244.
9. Kadaba MP, Ramakrishnan HK, Wootten ME, et al: Repeatability of kinematic, kinetic and electromyographic data in normal adult gait. *J Orthop Res* 1990;7:849–860.

10. Vaughan CL, Davis BL, O'Connor JC: *Dynamics of Human Gait*. Champaign, IL, Human Kinetics, 1992.
11. Grood ES, Suntay WJ: A joint coordinate system for the clinical description of three-dimensional motions: Application to the knee. *J Biomech Eng* 1983;105: 136–144.
12. Vaughan CL: Smoothing and differentiation of displacement-time data: An application of splines and digital filtering. *Int J Biomed Comput* 1982;13:375–386.
13. Falconer K, Winter DA: Quantitative assessment of co-contraction at the ankle joint in walking. *Electromyogr Clin Neuorphysiol* 1985;25:135–149.
14. Sutherland DH, Olshen RA, Biden EN, et al: *The Development of Mature Walking*. Philadelphia, JB Lippincott, 1988.
15. Õunpuu S, Gage JR, Davis RB: Three-dimensional lower extremity joint kinetics in normal pediatric gait. *J Pediatr Orthop* 1991;11:341–349.
16. Gage JR, Perry J, Hicks RR, et al: Rectus femoris transfer to improve knee function of children with cerebral palsy. *Dev Med Child Neurol* 1987;29:159–166.
17. McClellan DL: Co-contraction and stretch reflex in spasticity during treatment with baclofen. *J Neurol Neurosurg Psychiatry* 1973;36:555–560.

Chapter 5

Biologic Basis of Cerebral Palsy

Cirill V. Mashilov, PhD
Boris M. Kogan, PhD

Cerebral palsy is a complex condition with a variety of etiologic factors. One of these may be abnormalities in the neuroendocrine system. We, therefore, determined the level of cortisol and its main regulator adrenocorticotropic hormone (ACTH) in plasma of patients. We also assessed the levels of prolactin as an indirect indicator of dopaminergic system activity, because dopamine is one of the most powerful regulators of prolactin secretion. In addition, somatotropic hormone is also of interest because it is controlled by the dopaminergic system. We have, therefore, also determined dopamine-β-hydroxylase activity.

Materials and Methods

We defined cerebral palsy as a disorder in which there is aberrant control of movement or posture with no recognized underlying neurologic pathology. Patients were subclassified into the following categories: (1) Spastic diplegia, impairment involving the legs to a greater degree than the arms; (2) Spastic hemiplegia, impairment involving the arm and leg on one side; (3) Double hemiplegia, involvement of both arms and legs equally, with emphasis greater in the arms than the legs; (4) Atonic/astatic syndrome, characterized by generalized hypotonia; (5) Hyperkinetic form, marked by presence of involuntary movement; and (6) Cerebellar form, impairment characterized by ataxia, usually associated with either spasticity or hypotonia.

We investigated 102 children. Of these, 66 had spastic diplegia (with 15 of these having hyperkinetic involvement), 12 patients had predominantly hyperkinetic form, and 19 patients had spastic hemiplegia.

For controls, we used 15 children with either posttraumatic infectious or allergic encephalopathy. A second control group included 15 patients with congenital spinal cord disease, including brain stem herniation, and 15 patients with spinal cord injuries. Risk factors, including prematurity, defined as a child born prior to 36 weeks gestation, and prenatal or perinatal problems were studied. We attempted therapy with carbidopa-levodopa in a group of 11 patients with spastic diplegia, two with spastic hemiplegia, and one patient with the hyperkinetic form. When blood samples were drawn, they were taken in the fasting state at 9:00 to 10:00 a.m. Most hormone levels were determined using commercially available RIA kits; dopamine-β-hydroxylase activity was determined using a spectrophotometric method.[1]

Student's t test was used for statistical analysis of results; paired student's t was used for analysis of dynamic observations.

Results and Discussion

For the purposes of this study, all children with hyperkinetic involvement, even if they also were classified as having spastic diplegia, are classified as hyperkinetic.

We found no age-specific deviations in detected hormone levels. A possible reason for this is that pathologic changes are greater than age-dependent ones, and our highly homogeneous groups are too small.

We found the plasma cortisol level (mean ± standard deviation) of patients with spastic diplegia (1059.86 ± 39.28 nM) to be statistically significantly ($p < 0.001$) higher than that of patients with electroencephalopathies (601.39 ± 48.71 nM), spastic hemiplegia (716.31 ± 101.44 nM), and hyperkinetic form (537.04 ± 48.71 nM). Because the prevalence of premature birth among patients with cerebral palsy is much higher than in the general population, we analyzed the relationship between plasma cortisol level and premature birth in our patients. We found cortisol levels in patients born prematurely (962.68 ± 51.64 nM) to be statistically significantly ($p < 0.001$) higher than in those born at term (662.95 ± 65.86 nM). Although most of the children born prematurely have spastic diplegia, the significant difference in two independently formed groups leads us to believe that high cortisol level, prematurity, and spastic diplegia are different consequences of one disorder. The hypothetical character of this disorder might be explained by the complicated functions, effects, and interactions of cortisol with other systems.

Liggins[2,3] theorized that fetal cortisol release initiates parturition. He showed in sheep that hypophysectomy, adrenalectomy, or blocked pituitary portal vessels lead to protraction of pregnancy, while in a fetus that has an intact adrenal cortex, injection of cortisol or ACTH leads to premature labor.[2,3] This theory leads to the supposition that prematurity and increased plasma cortisol levels in patients with spastic diplegia are of the same etiology and are caused by hypothalamic-pituitary-adrenal access (HPAA) injury. This supposition is indirectly confirmed by our finding that patients with spastic diplegia were the only group that had very high cortisol plasma content dissociated with ACTH (Fig. 1). Experimental results have shown that the offspring of adrenalectomized rats have increased production of corticosteroids, and we can suppose the same mechanisms are present in humans. Maternal hypercorticoidism, for example, might be initial, or caused by liver dysfunction, HPAA disorder, or high doses of estrogens reducing transcortin

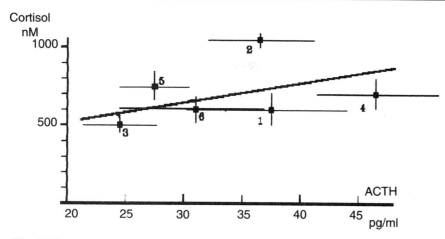

Fig. 1 *The cortisol response on ACTH stimulus in different groups of patients. Each point reflects one group: 1, group with encephalopathies; 2, with spastic diplegia; 3, with hyperkinetic form; 4, with spastic hemiplegia; 5, with congenital disorders of the spinal cord; 6, with spinal cord injuries.*

synthesis, a known risk factor for cerebral palsy.[4] The maternal cortisol level may be supported, and even increased, by the fetus. Adrenal cortex hyperfunction leads to its hyperplasia, which is often accompanied by preterm labor.[5] Of course, most children born prematurely are healthy and do not have spastic diplegia, and maternal hypercorticoidism and premature labor undoubtedly are not the cause of spastic diplegia. However, preterm labor is a spastic diplegia ''result'' caused by abnormal HPAA function. Thus, the premature birth of these children has a specific mechanism, and this mechanism may be intensified by maternal hypercorticoidism.

Also, among these patients with rather high plasma cortisol levels there are no clinical signs of hypercorticoidism. This state may be caused by transportation system defects or decrease of receptor sensitivity, or it may be a result of compensation changes related to dysfunction of another regulatory system.

Thus, the only evidence we have is an increased cortisol level in patients with spastic diplegia. This has not been observed in any other described group of patients we have investigated. For instance, there were no statistically significant differences between cortisol levels in the spinal cord disorder group (762.07 ± 95.5 nM), the spinal cord injury group (594.41 ± 73 nM), and the encephalopathy group.

Determination of somatotropic hormone (STH) levels presented a different picture. The plasma STH level in the encephalopathy group (8.19 ± 1.51 ng/ml) was very similar to that in the spastic hemiplegia group (5.79 ± 1.24 ng/ml). Plasma STH levels in patients with spastic diplegia (21.27 ± 1.74 ng/ml, $p < 0.001$) and those with hyperkinetic form (20.21 ± 4.51 ng/ml, $p < 0.002$) were statistically significantly higher than in both groups mentioned above. The dramatic increase in the plasma STH level of the spastic diplegia group may have at least two explanations. First, glucocorticoids stimulate STH-prohormone mRNA accumulation in pituitary cells,[6] which may be considered an activation of STH synthesis. Second, glucocorticoids inhibit somatomedin synthesis in the liver, which, in turn, leads to somatostatin deficit in the brain and a decrease in somatostatin inhibition of STH release. A deficit in somatomedin response to STH explains the absence of gigantism in these children. The STH level (19.68 ± 1.81 ng/ml) in the group of premature children was statistically significantly ($p < 0.002$) higher than in the group born at term (9.94 ± 1.89 ng/ml); this also indirectly indicates cortisol-STH intercommunication.

We believe the increase in the plasma STH level of patients with hyperkinetic form has another origin. Hyperkinetic form often is a result of hemolytic disease of the newborn, caused by materno-fetal blood group incompatibility. Usually, hemolytic disease of the newborn is accompanied by liver injuries. Because the liver influences somatomedin synthesis, altered liver function leads to the same consequences as in the group with spastic diplegia. However, hemolytic disease of the newborn is accompanied by injury to the basal ganglia, a brain region with a developed dopaminergic net. Undoubtedly, dopamine may influence STH secretion; however, opinions as to its influence vary.[7-9] This makes us believe that observed changes may be caused by the central dopaminergic system.

The plasma STH level in patients with spinal cord injuries (18.31 ± 3.33 ng/ml) is also significantly ($p < 0.001$) higher than in those with spinal cord disorders (5.69 ± 0.55 ng/ml), encephalopathies, and spastic hemiplegia. We consider this increase a compensation reaction of normally developed organisms, which counteracts atrophy processes caused by paralysis.

Data from girls 10 years of age and older were excluded from analysis of prolactin levels in all groups. Plasma prolactin levels in patients with spastic diplegia (193.71 ± 20.03 mIU/ml, $p < 0.001$), hyperkinetic syndrome (152.43 ± 40.42 mIU/ml, $p < 0.005$), and spastic hemiplegia (174.57 ± 26.10 mIU/ml, $p < 0.005$) were statistically significantly higher than in those with encephalopathies (74.13 ± 16.96 mIU/ml). Prolactin secretion is regulated by a number of factors other than dopamine; these are serotonin, thyrotropin-releasing hormone, growth hormone-releasing hormone, and endorphins. We believe these results indicate hypofunction of the hypothalamus dopaminergic net, because there is no clinical evidence of dysfunction in any of the above-mentioned prolactin-regulating factors.

We give the same interpretation to the significant increase in prolactin levels in the groups with spinal cord disorders (170.06 ± 23.13 mIU/ml) and spinal cord injuries (230.63 ± 35.74 mIU/ml) when compared to those with encephalopathies.

We also investigated another indirect indicator of catecholamine system function: the activity of dopamine-β-hydroxylase in patient's plasma. We found that dopamine-β-hydroxylase activity was statistically significantly lower in the groups with spastic diplegia (6.25 ± 0.3 nm/ml/min, p < 0.001), hyperkinetic form (8.19 ± 1.1 nm/ml/min, p < 0.01), and spastic hemiplegia (9.53 ± 0.76 nm/ml/min, p < 0.05) than in those with encephalopathies (18.00 ± 1.25 nm/ml/min). This indicator was also significantly lower in patients with spinal cord disorders (4.95 ± 0.5 nm/ml/min, p < 0.001) than in those with spinal cord injuries (13.63 ± 0.5 nm/ml/min). These results led us to assume that, among the groups investigated, congenital disorders are characterized by decreased noradrenalin secretion.

We investigated the same neuroendocrinological parameters in patients with clinical signs of dopamine deficit, who were being treated with carbidopa-levodopa. We divided this group into two subgroups for analysis of the results. The first subgroup included children never treated with carbidopa-levodopa and children who needed permanent pharmacologic support to prevent reversal of pronounced clinical improvement. The second subgroup included children who had been treated with carbidopa-levodopa. Clinical improvement was observed in both subgroups, but was more marked in the first one.

We observed more pronounced biochemical changes in the first subgroup, and, unexpectedly, the most sensitive indicator proved to be hypothalamic-pituitary-adrenal access. There were statistically significant (p < 0.05) decreases in cortisol (1149.18 ± 115.43 nM to 761.93 ± 166.55 nM) and ACTH (72.31 ± 18.40 pg/ml to 45.91 ± 11.63 pg/ml) levels. In addition, there was a strong tendency toward increasing STH levels and decreasing prolactin levels. These tendencies are not statistically significant because of the rather low number of observations and the great individual fluctuations in parameter levels. There is no doubt that these changes are connected with dopaminergic system function because the activity of carbidopa-levodopa is well known. In this subgroup there also was a statistically significant (p < 0.02) increase in plasma dopamine-β-hydroxylase activity from 10.77 ± 2.62 ng/ml/min to 14.25 ± 2.60 ng/ml/min, that provided evidence of increased noradrenaline secretion. This increase may be caused by noradrenaline accumulation resulting from a decrease in phenylethanolamine N-methyl transferase content, which in turn is caused by a decrease in glucocorticoid level.[10] It is possible that increased catecholamine secretion is accompanied by increased proenkephalin release.[11]

In the second subgroup, the initial plasma cortisol level (707.26 ± 158.46 ng/ml/min) was statistically significantly (p < 0.05) different from that of the first subgroup. The renewal of carbidopa-levodopa treatment led to a significant (p < 0.02) increase in cortisol level (1122.58 ± 98.46 ng/ml/min), and we must point out that this change is opposite to that in the first subgroup. There were no clear tendencies in other parameter shifts.

These results allow us to assume that the main common feature characterizing the patients in the first subgroup is the presence of an initial dopamine deficit. These patients have an adequate response to treatment and better clinical improvement. The second subgroup consists of children with a compensated dopamine deficit. Their compensation abilities were insufficient to normalize dopaminergic system functions, but proved to be enough to support them after carbidopa-levodopa treatment. That explains why their response to renewal of carbidopa-levodopa treatment was not as good as that of the first subgroup. Thus, there are two types of dopamine deficiency in these children: ''correctable'' and ''uncorrectable.''

Conclusions

We believe the data presented in this paper allow us to arrive at some conclusions. The first is that we have obtained biochemical evidence of the heterogenicity of cerebral palsy. Our results show that in mixed forms of cerebral palsy, hyperkinetic form is most prevalent biochemically, and that, apparently, at least one clinical form of cerebral palsy (spastic diplegia) has a specific pathogenesis and differs from others by more than localization of impairment. Second, we have obtained biochemical evidence that there is a group of patients wherein dopamine deficit plays the leading role in pathogenesis. Of course, even in this group the dopamine deficit is not the only pathogenic mechanism, but may play a significant role.

References

1. Nagatsu T, Udenfriend S: Photometric assay of dopamine-β-hydroxylase activity in human blood. *Clin Chem* 1972;18:980–982.
2. Liggins GC: Initiation of parturition. *Br Med Bull* 1979;35:145–150.
3. Liggins GC: Initiation of spontaneous labor. *Clin Obstet Gynecol* 1983;26:47–55.
4. Nelson KB, Ellenberg JH: Antecedents of cerebral palsy (Univariate analysis of risk). *Am J Dis Child* 1985;139:1031–1038.
5. Anderson AB, Laurence KM, Davies K, et al: Fetal adrenal weight and the cause of premature delivery in human pregnancy. *J Obstet Gynecol Br Commonw* 1971;78:481–488.
6. Teppermen J, Teppermen HM: *Metabolic and Endocrine Physiology*, ed 5. Chicago, Year Book Medical Publishers, 1987, part VI, chap 11.
7. Serri O, Deslauriers N, Brazeau P: Dual action of dopamine on growth hormone release in vitro. *Neuroendocrinology* 1987;45:363–367.
8. Hanew K. Sasaki A, Sato S, et al: Growth hormone inhibitory and stimulatory actions of L-Dopa in patients with acromegaly. *J Clin Endocrinol Metab* 1987;64:255–260.
9. Chihara K, Kashio Y, Kita T, et al: L-Dopa stimulates release of hypothalamic growth hormone-releasing hormone in humans. *J Clin Endocrinol Metab* 1986;62:466–473.
10. Ciaranello RD: Regulation of phenylethanolamine N-methyl transferase synthesis and degradation: I. Regulation by rat adrenal glucocorticoids. *Mol Pharmacol* 1978;14:478–483.
11. Costa E: The modulation of postsynaptic receptors by neuropeptide cotransmitters: A possible site of action for a new generation of psychotrophic drugs, in Usdin E, Bunney WE, Davis JM (eds): *Neuroreceptors: Basic and Clinical Aspects*. Chichester, NY, John Wiley & Sons, 1979, pp 15–27.

Consensus

Spasticity

Spasticity is defined as an increased resistance of muscle to stretch. The degree of spasticity increases with the amplitude and velocity of the stretch.

Neurophysiologic Basis of Spasticity

Supraspinal mechanisms are the cause of the net increased excitatory drive to the alpha motoneurons in brain-injured adults. In cerebral palsy, it is possible, but not conclusively proven, that spinal cord reorganization as well as supraspinal mechanisms contribute to increased alpha motoneuron excitability.

Research is needed to define molecular changes in the biochemistry and electrophysiology of the alpha motoneuron in conditions that have increased spasticity. This cellular-level research would enhance understanding of the secondary effects of spasticity as well as providing more effective therapies for spasticity. However, considerable technical obstacles must be overcome to enable this research. Another area of research involves comparing the physiology of spasticity in children with cerebral palsy to that seen in brain-injured adults.

Measurement of Spasticity

Clinical measurements of spasticity can be safely applied to many joints, but they do not provide objective, reproducible data. However, there are sensitive, objective laboratory tests that can be used to measure aspects of spasticity. Effective techniques of measuring spasticity in children include examination of torque/angle relationships and measurements of deep tendon reflexes elicited by mechanical hammers. These techniques are compromised by intrasubject variability, but may be useful in studying the natural history of neurologic disease or the efficacy of treatments designed to reduce spasticity. Present techniques are limited to tracking the severity of spasticity within a given subject over time. Furthermore, because present techniques grade spasticity under passive conditions, their correlation with the effect of spasticity on walking and other movements cannot be assessed, and, therefore, changes in spasticity may or may not reflect changes in function. Finally, it should be remembered that spasticity is not the entire problem in cerebral palsy and that spasticity may be beneficial to motor function in certain people with cerebral palsy.

Research is needed in several areas. Special problems in reproducing measurements in children must be addressed. This is especially true for younger and retarded individuals. New techniques or means of normalizing data obtained using existing methods are needed so that spasticity in different individuals can be compared. The relationship between spasticity as measured in the laboratory and the functional disabilities of the patient must be defined as well as the role of altered muscle mechanical properties in mediating spasticity.

Section Two
Deficits Other Than Spasticity

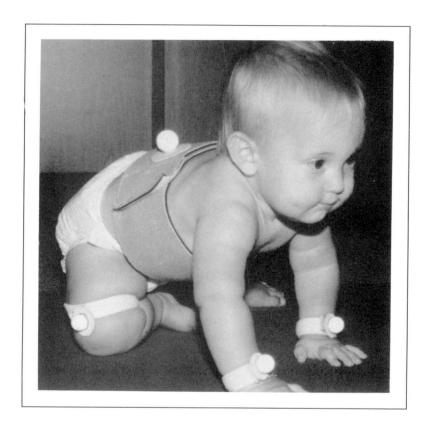

Chapter 6

Motor Dysfunction and Spatial-Cognitive Development

Robert L. Freedland, PhD
Bennett I. Bertenthal, PhD

Introduction

A revolution is underway in movement research as cognitive and perceptual processes are recognized as being related to motor skill acquisition. The emergence and refinement of motor skills can no longer be considered as an isolated process; cognitive and perceptual factors must be included within a functionally relevant environmental setting. The recent "Movement Science" series in *Physical Therapy* embodies this emerging perspective.[1-5] Kamm and associates[1] emphasize that infants demonstrate adaptive responses to changing environments, Goodgold-Edwards[2] argues that motor skill assessments should include such nonmotor components as cognitive and perceptual processes, and Mulder[3] proposes a model of rehabilitation that directly implicates cognitive and perceptual mechanisms. More specific to spastic diplegia, Fetters[4] emphasizes the importance of the functional context of movements in a study of cerebral palsy, while Harris[5] suggests that the evaluation of eye-hand coordination and visual tracking will assist in its early diagnosis.

If perceptual and cognitive processes are indeed interwoven with the normal acquisition of motor skills, we must determine how such processes will be affected by delayed or dysfunctional movements. Moreover, if subsequent development is dependent on such skills, even more dysfunctional responses may be perpetuated.[6] To provide some perspective on this issue, we examined empirical evidence that links one aspect of motor development, onset of crawling, with specific changes in cognitive and perceptual development. The emergence and development of crawling has played a prominent role in many different theories of early psychological development.[7] Yet, until recently, experimental investigation of self-produced locomotion (outside the specification of developmental norms) was largely ignored.[8]

The goals of this chapter are threefold: First, we introduce systems theory as a framework for discussing the relation between locomotor experience and early development. Next, we briefly review the evidence by discussing the methods and results from two specific paradigms—fear of heights and object localization. Finally, we address the implications of this perspective for understanding the development of children with motor delays, for example, children with spastic diplegia.

Developmental Causality in the Context of a Systems Approach

The systems approach to development provides a unique framework for investigating self-produced locomotion within the context of other developmental changes.[9–11] In this approach, no one factor is considered predictive of, or prescriptive for, development; instead, multiple factors influence the course of development. The systems approach recasts a variety of seemingly independent developmental processes into a stable and unified behavior. A singular rate-limiting factor, called a control variable, is typically responsible for the reorganization of this behavior from one stable mode of functioning to the next. Bertenthal and Campos[10] show how self-produced locomotion is such a control variable, responsible for the reorganization of a number of psychological skills including visual-vestibular relations, visual attention to the environment, social referencing, and differentiation of emotions.

Bertenthal and Campos[10] propose that self-produced locomotion makes available to the infant new experiences that necessitate the reorganization of some specific skills in novel and more flexible forms. For example, a prelocomotor infant is relatively successful in coding the location of objects in terms of a body-centered frame of reference because objects, such as the mother or a favored toy, remain in the same relation to the immobile infant for an extended period of time. However, when infants begin crawling, they are continuously changing their orientation relative to previously seen objects. They now need a location-coding strategy that does not depend on their immobility, and soon after the development of self-produced locomotion infants do acquire a new strategy based on stable landmarks in the environment. From a logical perspective, this is a necessary developmental transition fueled by the infants' changing experience with locomotion. (Later we will discuss some of the empirical evidence for this interpretation.)

If self-produced locomotion is assumed to be the control variable that underlies the development of a skill, the nature of this influence over time might be characterized as facilitation, attunement, or induction.[12] Self-produced locomotion would be considered facilitative if its onset changed only the acquisition rate of another skill. In this case, the new skill would develop eventually, even in the absence of locomotion. The emergence of self-propelled locomotion would be defined as attunement if, in its absence, only a rudimentary expression of the skill emerged because complete differentiation and refinement of the skill requires locomotor experience. Finally, induction specifies that no expression of the skill would exist in the absence of self-produced locomotion.

These three processes—facilitation, attunement, and induction—

imply more than correlation between the emergence of self-produced locomotion and the development of other skills; they implicate self-produced locomotion as causal in that development. Establishing a causal connection between the emergence of self-produced locomotion and the expression of a developing skill is important because of its theoretical and clinical implications, but it is extremely difficult and elusive to establish that one of two coinciding phenomena leads to the other.

The principal difficulty in establishing locomotor experience as a causal variable is that it covaries with age and other developmental variables. As such, it is difficult to know whether differences between prelocomotor and locomotor infants are a function of locomotor experience or of some other age-related variable. One strategy for effectively resolving this age-experience confound rests upon the finding that crawling emerges within a fairly broad developmental window.[13] Because same-age infants show considerable variation in crawling experience, the researcher can design an experiment in which the variability of locomotor experience is pitted against the variability attributed to age. For example, Bertenthal and Campos[10] used a lag design in which infants between 6.5 and 9.5 months of age were grouped as a function of 11 or 44 days of locomotor experience to disentangle the effects of these two variables. By comparing differences as a function of age and also as a function of locomotor experience, these two researchers were able to evaluate the relative contributions of the two variables to the development of a specific skill.

Establishment of a causal relation for locomotor experience is assisted by two natural manipulations. One of these manipulations involves testing prelocomotor infants who have had experience with baby walkers. In essence, this investigation corresponds to an enrichment study in which infants are provided early experience with the critical variable. The other manipulation involves testing orthopaedically handicapped infants who are delayed in the acquisition of self-produced locomotion. This corresponds to a deprivation study in which the orthopaedically handicapped infants are limited in their experience with the critical variable.

In general, converging evidence through different paradigms, such as those described above, is necessary for inferring a causal relationship between self-produced locomotion and the development of other skills.

Locomotor Experience and the Development of Spatial-Perceptual Skills

Fear of Heights on the Visual Cliff

There is considerable evidence showing that fear of heights follows the acquisition of self-produced locomotion. Campos and associates[7,8,10] explored the emergence of this fear through the use of a testing apparatus dubbed the visual cliff.[14] In essence, this apparatus corresponds

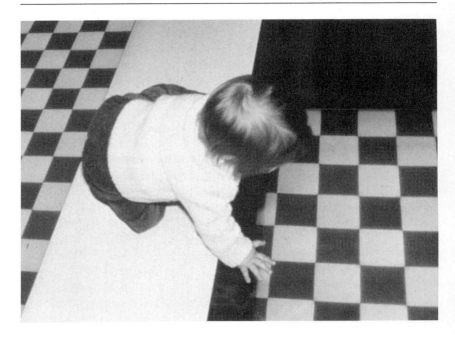

Fig. 1 *Child on visual cliff apparatus.*

to a large glass table-top (4 × 8 ft) suspended 4 feet above the floor. A center-board divides the glass into two 4 × 4-ft surfaces. On one side of the center-board (henceforth referred to as the shallow side), a checkerboard pattern is placed directly below the glass to give the impression of a solid surface of support. On the other side of the center-board (henceforth referred to as the deep side), the checkerboard pattern is placed 4 feet below the glass surface to give the impression of a vertical descent.

The visual cliff was originally intended to assess depth perception in young infants. It has since been established that infants acquire depth perception long before the onset of self-produced locomotion. Campos and associates[7,8,10] adapted this apparatus (Fig. 1) to measure infants' interpretation of the visual cliff. This interpretive response depends upon a host of skills, including visual-vestibular relations, visual attention to environmental changes, social referencing, and emotional differentiation. Because these are some of the same skills hypothesized to change as a function of self-produced locomotion, these researchers predicted that infants would appreciate the functional significance of an apparent drop-off or vertical descent only after the onset of locomotion, and that this appreciation would be expressed as a fear of heights.

This research used three measures of fear. The first of these, which can be used for both locomotor and prelocomotor infants, was inferred

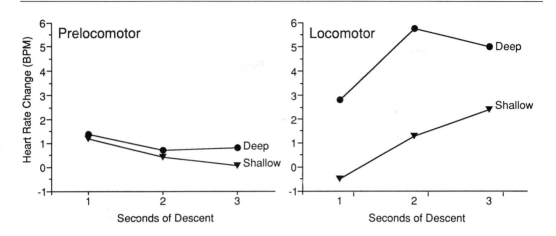

Fig. 2 *Average heart rate change (beats per minute) for 7.3-month-old infants during descent onto the deep and shallow sides of the visual cliff as a function of locomotor experience. (Adapted with permission from Bertenthal et al.[10].)*

by heart rate acceleration during a slow vertical descent onto each side of the apparatus. When age was held constant (average of 7.3 months), prelocomotor infants showed no sign of heart rate change when lowered onto the shallow or deep sides of the visual cliff. Conversely, locomotor infants showed a fear response, evidenced by a heart rate acceleration when placed over the deep side (Fig. 2).

A second method of testing locomotor infants' responses to the visual cliff, involved placing them on the center-board while their mothers stood at the edge of either the deep or shallow side and encouraged their infants to crawl across the cliff. In this experiment, infants were brought to the lab at either 11 or 44 days of parent-reported locomotor experience. Infants in this study were assigned to one of three age groups based on the age of onset of crawling (6.5, 7.5, and 8.5 months (± 2 weeks)). The crossing of these two design parameters created an experimental lag design of 6 groups (3 ages by 2 levels of locomotor experience).

Regardless of age, 60% to 80% of the infants with greater locomotor experience (41 days) refused to cross the deep side to their parents, whereas only 30% to 45% of the infants with less locomotor experience refused. When latency to begin moving from the center-board toward their parents was assessed, regardless of age, infants with greater locomotor experience took longer to move across the deep side (Fig. 3).

Although these results are quite compelling, they are by no means definitive. To establish a causal role for locomotor experience, it is necessary to manipulate the criterion experience experimentally. This manipulation was accomplished by testing prelocomotor infants who had locomotor experience in baby walkers versus age-matched control

73

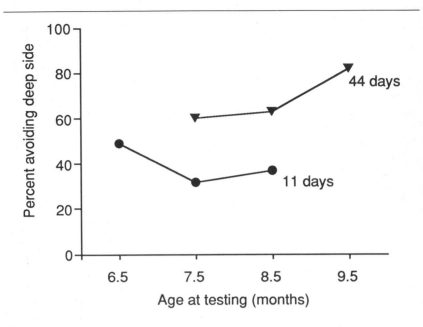

Fig. 3 *Percentage of infants who avoided the deep side of the visual cliff as a function of locomotor experience and age. (Adapted with permission from Bertenthal et al.[10].)*

subjects who did not receive any walker experience. The original goal was to test infants after their parents reported 40 hours of walker experience. Because some of the infants began crawling before they were tested, it was necessary to subdivide the groups further as a function of crawling experience. (Note that the range of crawling was quite small and no infant had been crawling for more than a week.)

As can be seen in Figure 4, infants with a double dose of locomotor experience (crawling and walker experience) displayed the greatest evidence of fear as indexed by heart rate acceleration. Conversely, prelocomotor infants who had no walker experience showed a significant deceleratory response when lowered onto the deep side of the cliff. Typically, heart rate deceleration is associated with interest and attention, but not fear. These experiments indicate that wariness of heights, as measured by the visual cliff, is functionally linked to the acquisition of locomotion.

Localization of Objects

One obvious consequence of locomotion during infancy is a greater level of visual attention to self and objects within the three-dimensional spatial layout of the environment. Otherwise, infants would continuously bump and stumble into objects.[8] In contrast, prelocomotor infants passively moving through the environment do not require the same

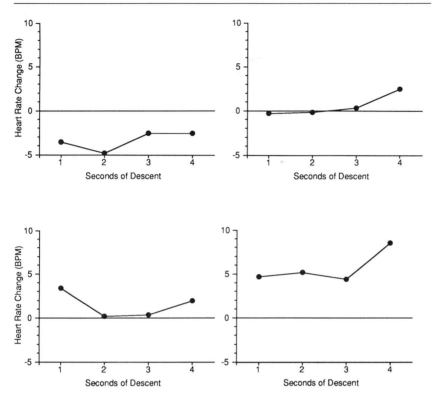

Fig. 4 *Average heart rate change (beats per minute) during descent onto the deep side of the visual cliff as a function of locomotor experience.* **Top left,** *Precrawling infants without walker experience;* **Top right,** *Precrawling infants with walker experience;* **Bottom left,** *Crawling infants without walker experience; and* **Bottom right,** *Crawling infants with walker experience. Note deceleratory response for precrawling infants without walker experience and acceleratory response for crawling infants with walker experience. (Adapted with permission from Bertenthal et al.[10])*

level of attention to the spatial layout. Bai and Bertenthal[15] predicted that self-propelled locomotion would improve infants' performance in tasks that require attention to the spatial displacement of self and objects. The paradigm took advantage of two spatial-cognitive skills. The first is called "object permanence," whereby an object continues to exist, even when it is out of view.[16] By 8 months, infants demonstrate early evidence of object permanence by searching for objects that are completely hidden from view. The second skill is a shift from egocentric coding (referencing objects relative to the self) at 6 months to allocentric coding (referencing objects to environmental landmarks) at 9 months.

Bai and Bertenthal[15] postulated that, before self-produced locomotion, infants would tend to reference objects relative to themselves. Once they begin to locomote, however, objects do not remain in a fixed position relative to their body-centered frame of reference. Accordingly, infants would seek out more stable environmental cues.[17]

To test this prediction, Bai and Bertenthal[15] used a spatial rotation task, consisting of a rotatable circular table and a chair that could be rotated around the table. Two containers were placed on the table; one to the right and one to the left of the infant. A toy was hidden under one of the containers. Before the infant could search for the toy, either the table or the chair was rotated by 180 degrees, which moved the container with the toy to the opposite side of the infant. Infants who consistently searched in the correct container were apparently sensitive to their change in spatial orientation.

From our perspective, the most important finding from this study is that 8-month-old infants who were crawling on hands and knees performed significantly better at this task than belly crawlers or precrawling infants. Search performance was over 70% correct for hands and knees crawlers, but only 30% and 25% correct for belly crawlers and precrawling infants, respectively.

The results of this study are important for two reasons. First and foremost, they provide converging evidence with the visual cliff studies that independent mobility is systematically related to not one but rather a number of discrete spatial-cognitive tasks. Second, the findings provide converging evidence with other recent studies[18] suggesting that it is the specific form or topography of the crawling behavior, rather than merely the quantity of the crawling behavior, that is relevant to understanding the developmental changes that have been reported in the literature.

Developmental Changes in the Control and Coordination of Crawling

As a first step in learning why the form of crawling should be systematically related to performance on our criterion variables, we conducted a short-term longitudinal study of six infants who were beginning to crawl. The crawling patterns of these infants were assessed with a motion analysis system so that detailed changes in limb movements could be determined reliably.

Six healthy, full-term infants were tested weekly in the Gait Laboratory at the University of Virginia's Kluge Children's Rehabilitation Center. Independent sitting and minimal evidence of forward progress were used as criteria for entering the study. Average age at the initial visit was 7.7 months. Testing continued until infants reached a predefined crawling plateau, followed by three additional visits every other week.

Infants were assessed using a motion analysis system that tracked limb movements over the course of a 10-second trial. Five reflective markers were strategically secured to the infant using elastic-velcro bands (Fig. 5). One marker was secured on each wrist and one marker was positioned on the outer side of each knee. An additional spherical

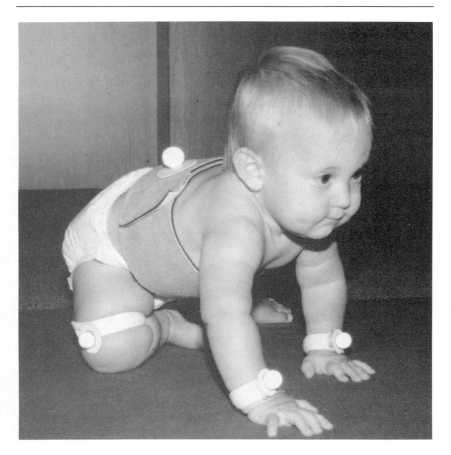

Fig. 5 *Infant with reflective markers.*

marker was centered on the infant's back. The motion analysis equipment is capable of integrating the XYZ positions of the reflective markers over a runway of 2.75 meters, resulting in the capture of from 3 to 10 complete gait cycles. The vector displacement of each limb includes both a rotational and a translatory component. By using the back marker as a translatory referent, we can separate out the translatory component from each limb, resulting in a cyclic limb movement pattern relative to the back marker. For example, the wrists are closest to the back marker at the beginning of the swing phase and move to their furthest point away from the back at the beginning of the stance phase. Conversely, the knees are farthest from the back at the beginning of the swing phase and move closest to the back at the beginning of the stance phase. In order to preserve the true phase relations between the limbs, no smoothing algorithms were performed on the resultant vector displacements.

The vector displacements of each limb allow us to calculate and compare swing and stance phase offsets between the four limbs. Sum-

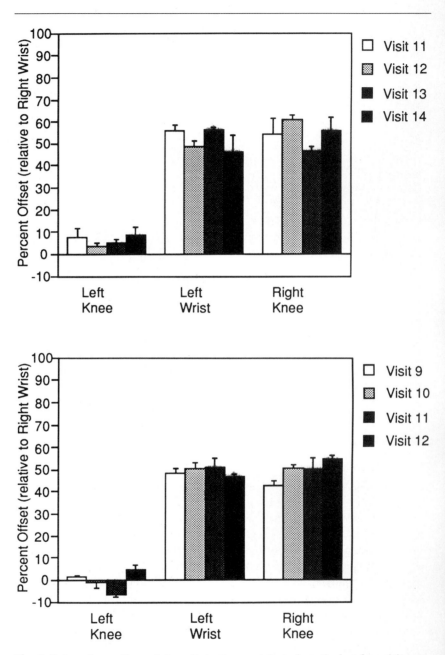

Fig. 6 *Swing phase offsets of three limbs for two infants from the last four visits. Top, Infant 1; Bottom, Infant 2. Successive visits are patterned from white to black. Values of 50% indicate limbs that are 180 degrees out of phase with the right wrist.*

maries of the swing phase from the last four visits (approximately 2 months) of two subjects are presented in Figure 6. Particularly striking is the tremendous stability shown in the phase relations of the limbs. Note that the swing and stance phase of the two wrists are 180 degrees out of phase, while the contralateral knee remains closely entrained with each wrist. This movement sequence compares favorably with Hildebrand's[19] description of infant crawling as a symmetrical "lateral sequence, diagonal couplet" gait. Figure 7 outlines the percent stance and swing maintained through each gait cycle. The wrist swing components within each cycle average about 30%, while the average swing component of the knees is closer to 40%. Hildebrand[19] also observed this wrist/knee difference, adding that this was ". . . the greatest discrepancy I have noted for any animal."

The phasing of the limbs by infants is but one of at least seven different quadrupedal gait patterns reported in the literature. One of the alternative gait patterns, corresponding to a horse's slow walk, involves moving only one limb at a time. This particular pattern is optimally designed for minimizing loss of balance by maintaining a tripod-like base of support during all phases of the gait cycle. For this reason, a number of developmental researchers suggest that this particular gait pattern should precede one in which diagonally opposite limbs, for example, right wrist and left knee, move simultaneously and 180 degrees out of phase with the other two limbs. Nevertheless, preliminary findings reveal no evidence of this more conservative gait pattern preceding a gait pattern in which diagonally opposite limbs move together. Interestingly, the latter gait pattern is dynamically more efficient, because gravity is used to thrust the infant forward during times when balance is lost. It thus appears that infants choose the dynamically more efficient gait pattern over the one that ensures greater balance.

In contrast to the sequencing of the limbs, which appears to be independent of experience, preliminary evidence reveals that the speed of limb movement increases with experience. Limb velocity was calculated by multiplying amplitude (displacement/cycle) by temporal frequency (cycles/sec). Data from the last four visits for two infants are summarized in Figure 8. As illustrated by this figure, infants increased their limb velocity across visits. Despite this increased velocity, the pattern of coordination between the four limbs (ie, phase relations) remained constant.

From a dynamic systems perspective, we interpret velocity as corresponding to a control variable, whereas the gait pattern corresponds to an order or coordinative variable. A tentative conclusion suggested by the current data is that the order variable in crawling does not show developmental changes, whereas control variables, such as speed of crawling, do show systematic changes with development. This conclusion is beginning to undergo additional testing in which we are examining how infants modulate their crawling as a function of different perturbations (eg, adding weight to individual limbs).

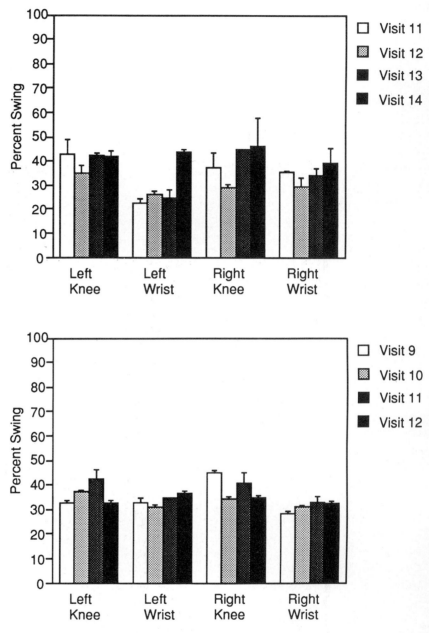

Fig. 7 *Percent swing phase per gait cycle for two infants from the last four visits.*
***Top**, Infant 1; **Bottom**, Infant 2. Successive visits are patterned from white to black.
Swing durations of 40% imply stance durations of 60%.*

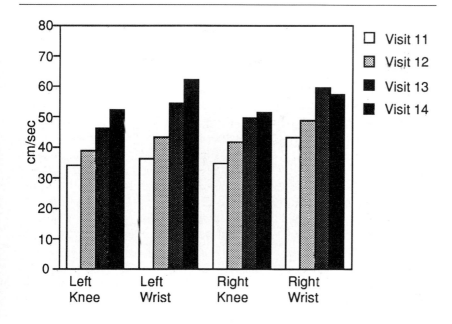

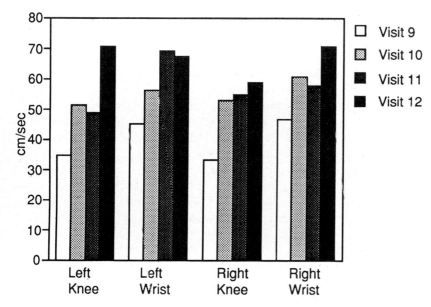

Fig. 8 *Limb velocity for two infants from the last four visits.* **Top,** *Infant 1;* **Bottom,** *Infant 2. Successive visits are patterned from white to black for each of the four limbs. Note increasing limb velocity with later visits for both infants.*

Implications for Infants and Children with Spastic Diplegia

The clear and unequivocal conclusion emerging from the research reviewed above is that locomotor experience exercises a rate-limiting effect on the early development of spatial-cognitive skills. However, the evidence suggesting a causal relation between locomotor experience and the development of specific spatial-cognitive skills is restricted to a relatively narrow age range during infancy. This qualification is important when considering the implications of our research on the development of spatial-cognitive skills in children with severe motor delays, such as those with spastic diplegia. Clearly, this population of children will begin independent mobility at much later ages than children without motor handicaps. Indeed, Robson[13] reports that children with mild forms of diplegia do not begin crawling until 20 months of age, and do not typically walk without assistance until 3 to 7 years of age.

Motor handicapped infants could use other experiences and skills that emerge during infancy to develop the spatial-cognitive skills assessed in the reviewed studies. Indeed, this possibility is entirely consistent with our earlier discussion of experience exercising different roles in development. Currently, it is not clear whether locomotor experience represents a facilitative, attuning, or inductive role in the development of spatial-cognitive skills.

Although the specific process by which locomotor experience contributes to the development of other skills remains unclear, the literature provides preliminary evidence that delayed locomotor experience exercises a rate-limiting effect on spatial-cognitive development for at least 3 to 6 months. Two separate investigations are relevant to this issue.[10,20]

In the first study, reported by Bertenthal and Campos,[10] an otherwise normal infant born with two dislocated hips was placed in a full-body cast to correct the defect. In spite of this orthopaedic problem, the infant's development quotient (DQ) was well above average (128 according to the Bayley Scales of Infant Development). This infant was tested monthly on the visual cliff, beginning at 6 months of age and continuing until 10 months of age. During the first two months of testing, all movement was prohibited by the cast. Before the third visit, the cast was removed and replaced by a Pavlik harness (this orthopaedic device is much lighter than a cast and allowed for movement of the upper body). Still, this infant did not have any opportunity to crawl until the parents were instructed to remove the harness for 4 hours a day. The mother reported that her infant began moving on the floor during the time that he was unencumbered by the harness. By his final visit, the harness had been removed and the infant was crawling proficiently.

The results of the visual cliff testing are summarized in Figure 9. There was no evidence of fear, as indexed by heart rate acceleration, until the final visit. By comparison, most infants without orthopaedic handicaps show fear of heights on the visual cliff by 7 to 8 months of

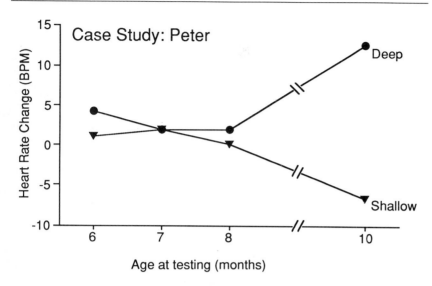

Fig. 9 *Average heart rate change (beats per minute) during descent over the deep and shallow sides of the visual cliff for an orthopaedically handicapped infant. (Adapted with permission from Bertenthal et al.[10].)*

age. Although it is difficult to generalize from a single-subject case study, the results are consistent with evidence that spatial-cognitive skills emerge from experiences fueled by independent locomotion. When these experiences are delayed by two to three months, so is the development of fear of heights on the cliff.

The findings from the second study are equally dramatic. Telzrow and associates[20] tested seven infants with myelodysplasia on an object search task similar to the one used by Bai and Bertenthal.[15] All seven of these infants were delayed in the acquisition of crawling (mean age: 10.4 months; range: 8.5 to 13.5 months). Admittedly, the presence of other central nervous system complications in these infants makes inferences about the cause of some deficit difficult to assess. Nevertheless, we find the results from this study quite provocative, because a consistent relation between locomotor experience and performance on the spatial search task was reported. In the two months prior to locomotion, infants showed correct search on only 15% of the trials. Conversely, following the onset of locomotion, infants showed correct search on 72% of the trials. This difference is quite dramatic, and it is even more impressive when one considers that locomotor onset is but one of many changes that might have affected performance.

We believe that, taken together, these findings provide converging evidence that infants who show delays in locomotion are likely to show delays in the development of specific spatial-cognitive tasks. A number of social and affective skills have also been linked to the onset of self-produced locomotion,[10] and it is thus conceivable that locomotor-delayed infants will show delays in the development of these skills as well.

Our discussion was confined specifically to the effects of self-produced locomotion on spatial-cognitive development, because the literature does not yet extend to other motor skills. Nevertheless, the logic of our argument for proposing a relation between locomotor experience and other skills certainly transcends any specific skill. In essence, we assert that new motor skills provide children with new and more flexible opportunities to learn about the physical and social world. New levels of cognitive and social understanding emerge in response to the new challenges and experiences associated with the use of these new skills. Although some experiences that are missed because of a specific motor handicap are compensated for by other experiences, it is sometimes difficult to arrive at the same developmental outcome when lacking a specific motor skill, because many developmental processes are context specific.[19] The context specificity of development is greatest in the early years because cognitive skills allowing generalizability from one situation to another have not yet emerged.[21] Accordingly, we suggest that, at the very least, early delays in motor development place infants and toddlers at risk for later developmental delays.

References

1. Kamm K, Thelen E, Jensen JL: A dynamical systems approach to motor development. *Phys Ther* 1990;70:763–775.
2. Goodgold-Edwards SA: Cognitive strategies during coincident timing tasks. *Phys Ther* 1991;71:236–243.
3. Mulder T: A process-oriented model of human motor behavior: Toward a theory-based rehabilitation approach. *Phys Ther* 1991;71:157–164.
4. Fetters L: Measurement and treatment in cerebral palsy: An argument for a new approach. *Phys Ther* 1991;71:244–247.
5. Harris SR: Movement analysis: An aid to early diagnosis of cerebral palsy. *Phys Ther* 1991;71:215–221.
6. Scherzer AL, Tscharnuter I: *Early Diagnosis and Therapy in Cerebral Palsy: A Primer on Development Problems*, ed 2. New York, Marcel Dekker, 1990.
7. Bertenthal BI, Campos JJ, Barrett KC: Self-produced locomotion: An organizer of emotional, cognitive, and social development in infancy, in Emde R, Harmon R (eds): *Continuities and Discontinuities in Development*. New York, Plenum Press, 1984.
8. Campos JJ, Bertenthal BI: Locomotion and psychological development in infancy, in Morrison F, Lord C, Keating D (eds): *Applied Developmental Psychology*. New York, Academic Press, 1989, vol 2, pp 230–258.
9. Thelen E: Self-organization in developmental processes: Can systems approaches work?, in Gunnar M, Thelen E (eds): *Systems and Development: The Minnesota Symposium on Child Psychology*. Hillsdale, NJ, Erlbaum, 1989, vol 22, pp 77–117.
10. Bertenthal BI, Campos JJ: A systems approach to the organizing effects of self-produced locomotion during infancy, in Rovee-Collier C, Lipsitt LP (eds): *Advances in Infancy Research*. Norwood, NJ, Ablex, 1990, vol 6, pp 1–60.
11. Thelen E, Ulrich BD: Hidden skills. *Monogr Soc Res Child Dev* 1991;56:(1, Whole No. 223).
12. Gottlieb G: The psychobiological approach to developmental issues, in Haith M, Campos JJ (eds): *Handbook of Child Psychology: Infancy and Developmental Psychobiology*. New York, John Wiley & Sons, 1983, pp 1–26.

13. Robson P: Prewalking locomotor movements and their use in predicting standing and walking. *Child Care Health Dev* 1984;10:317–330.

14. Walk R, Gibson E: A comparative analytical study of visual depth perception. *Psychol Monogr* 1961;75:(15, Whole No. 519).

15. Bai DL, Bertenthal BI: Locomotor status and the development of spatial search skills. *Child Dev*, 1992;63:215–226.

16. Piaget J: *The Construction of Reality in the Child*. New York, Basic Books, 1954.

17. Bremner JG: Egocentric versus allocentric spatial coding in nine-month-old infants: Factors influencing the choice of code. *Dev Psychol* 1978;14:346–355.

18. Kermoian R, Campos JJ: Locomotor experience: A facilitator of spatial cognitive development. *Child Dev* 1988;59:908–917.

19. Hildebrand M: Symmetrical gaits of primates. *J Phys Anthropol* 1967;26:119–130.

20. Telzrow R, Campos JJ, Shepherd A, et al: Spatial understanding in infants with motor handicaps, in Jaffe KM (ed): *Childhood Powered Mobility: Developmental, Technical and Clinical Perspectives*. Washington, DC, RESNA, 1987.

21. Siegler RS: *Children's Thinking*, ed 2. Englewood Cliffs, NJ, Prentice-Hall, 1990.

Chapter 7

Sensorimotor Deficits Associated With Posture Control in Children With Cerebral Palsy

Marjorie H. Woollacott, PhD
Patricia A. Burtner, MOT, OTR

Introduction

In normal development and mastery of motor coordination abilities, such as balance control and locomotion, children pass through specific behavioral stages. For example, in normal infants postural control of the head develops within the first few months of life, followed by the emergence of control of the trunk with independent sitting at about 6 months, the onset of independent stance at about 12 months of age, and the development of walking soon after. At about 4 to 6 years of age, the ability to balance under sensory conflict conditions emerges. A number of neural systems contribute to the development of normal posture control, including the somatosensory system, the visual and vestibular systems, the motor system, and the higher level adaptive neural systems.

Developmental studies of children with cerebral palsy have consistently demonstrated that these neurologically impaired children achieve motor milestones at a much later chronological age than their normal peers. The factors contributing to this delay could include delayed maturation or dysfunction in any of the above neural systems. The aim of this chapter is to review the research on the contribution of each of these systems to the development of balance in the normal child and to compare this with research on postural development in children with cerebral palsy.

Development of Independent Stance and Walking in Normal Children

It has been hypothesized that there are specific phases in the development of any behavior.[1,2] These include: (1) movements initially showing excessive degrees of freedom, (2) movements being simplified as the new skill level is mastered, and (3) movements being re-elaborated as the child learns to reach the same endpoint through variable means. To determine if this hypothesis was true for the developmental stages seen in balance control, Woollacott and Sveistrup[3] explored

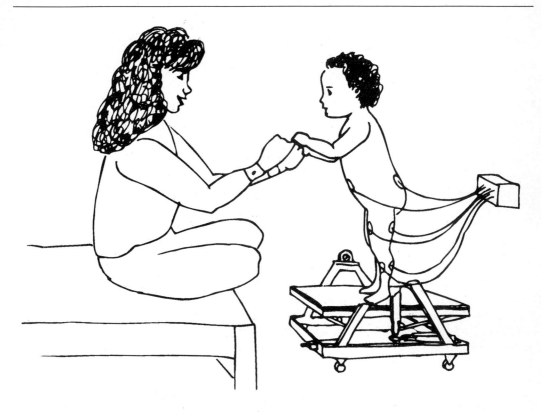

Fig. 1 *Diagram of child standing on the moveable platform. If a child was unable to stand independently, the parent gave partial support. As seen in the diagram, EMGs were recorded from the muscles of the leg and trunk.*

changes in balance abilities in infants from 7 to 14 months of age as they made the transition to independent stance and locomotion.

During the experiments the infants stood on a platform that could be moved unexpectedly in the anterior or posterior direction, and thus disturb balance (Fig. 1). The platform moved 3 cm forward or backward with a velocity of 10 to 30 cm/sec. Postural muscle response characteristics were determined by analyzing onset latencies, variability, and activation frequency of muscle responses (measured by surface electromyograms) from the gastrocnemius, hamstrings, trunk extensors, tibialis anterior, quadriceps, and abdominal muscles of the left leg. Movement patterns were determined by analyzing changes in hip, knee, and ankle angles through video recordings. Before the infant was able to stand independently, she/he was supported either by holding on to a rod placed in front of her/him or to a toy castle, which was placed at chest height.

With the initial emergence of pull-to-stand behavior at about 7 to 9 months, the infants showed excessive movement at the ankle, knee, and

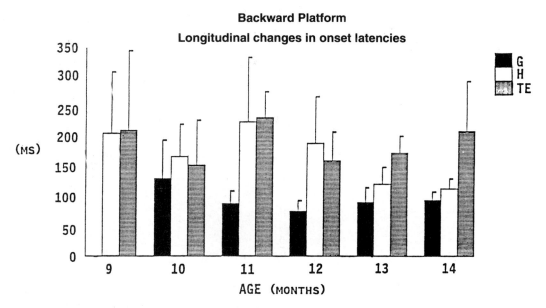

Fig. 2 *Bar plots of the means and standard deviations of onset latencies for the gastrocnemius (G), hamstrings (H), and trunk extensor (TE) muscles activated during backward platform movements and used to compensate for forward sway. Data collected from one normal infant from 9 to 14 months of age. (Reproduced with permission from Woollacott et al.[3])*

hip joints in response to platform perturbations, and postural responses were disorganized, with delayed and highly variable onset latencies in all muscles recorded. For example, for platform perturbations in the posterior direction, causing anterior sway, the gastrocnemius, hamstrings, and trunk extensor muscles were infrequently activated, were very slow in onset latency, and were highly variable. Figure 2 shows muscle response latencies of a child from 9 to 14 months of age. Note the absence of gastrocnemius activity at 9 months when the child was at the pull-to-stand stage. This behavior changes with experience in dependent stance (Fig. 2, 10 months). However, at the onset of independent stance, the muscle response patterns show a regression, toward longer onset latencies and higher variability (Fig. 2, 11 months).

With improved ability at independent stance and the onset of independent walking, the postural response organization became consistent and latencies were shortened to more mature levels. Also, the mature distal to proximal sequencing of muscles, which is seen in older children and adults, became consistent. Variability of response onsets was reduced, and responses were activated whenever the child's balance was disturbed.

For platform perturbations in the anterior direction, causing posterior sway, a similar developmental progression was noted; the mature mus-

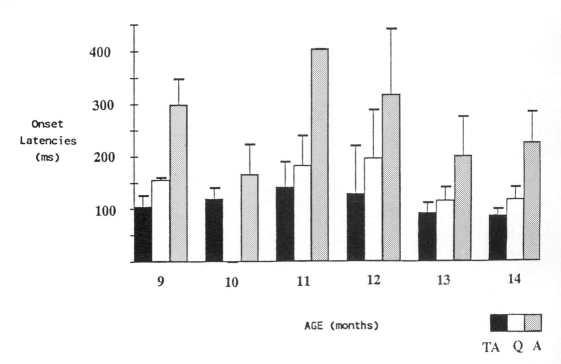

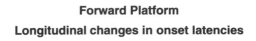

Fig. 3 *Bar plots of the means and standard deviations of onset latencies for the tibialis anterior (TA), quadriceps (Q), and abdominal (A) muscles activated during forward platform movements and used to compensate for backward sway. Data collected for one normal infant from 9 to 14 months of age.*

cle response organization (tibialis anterior to quadriceps to abdominal), gradually developed with experience in stance and walking (Fig. 3).

Though infants with little experience walking show some characteristics of adult postural response organization, they still have many immature characteristics. Forssberg and Nashner[4] reported that responses of children in this age range show more antagonistic coactivation and also are more variable and slower than those of adults. The slower electromyographic responses and faster rates of sway acceleration seen in young children (due to their smaller size) also cause sway amplitudes that tend to be larger, with more oscillations than are seen in older children. In addition, the responses of 15- to 31-month-olds are consistently large in amplitude and longer in duration than those of adults.[5]

Early Development of Stance in Children With Spastic Diplegia

To determine the extent to which development of postural muscle responses in the child with spastic diplegia differed from that of the normal child, we performed studies on two young children with spastic diplegic cerebral palsy. Children were asked to stand on the platform during forward and backward platform perturbations, both with and without ankle-foot orthoses. These children were each 3.7 years old and were both able to walk while using a walker, but they were still in the pull-to-stand stage of balance development, because neither could stand independently. Both subjects were in good health with height and weight at the 5th percentile. Their motor development level was within the 8 to 10 month range, with normal joint range of motion, normal hearing and vision, and normal cognitive development.

Child 1 showed spasticity primarily in the hamstrings and gastrocnemius-soleus muscles. She showed equinus in stance, but with time would relax into a more plantigrade posture. She showed a definite asymmetry in gait with internal rotation/adduction on the left. She began to pull to stand independently at 19 months, and began ambulation training in a walker at 20 months. Child 2 showed significant spasticity in the lower extremities in the adductor, hamstrings, and gastrocnemius-soleus muscles. She was plantigrade in quiet stance, but developed mild equinus as well as internal rotation at the hips bilaterally during walking. She began to pull to stand at 18 months and began ambulation training in a walker at 22 months.

Figure 4, *top*, shows the response latencies of the gastrocnemius, hamstrings, and trunk extensors muscles of the two children for posterior platform perturbations, while standing without and with orthoses. Without orthoses both children show inappropriately organized muscle responses, with no clear distal to proximal order of response onset. Response latencies were also very late: gastrocnemius, 217 $\pm$ 15 msec; hamstrings, 170 msec; and trunk extensors, 230 $\pm$ 10 msec for child 1. When orthoses were worn, the response latencies were shortened slightly: gastrocnemius, 188 msec; hamstrings, 200 msec; and trunk extensors, 147 $\pm$ 18 msec. However, the response organization was not improved. The orthoses also reduced the excitability of the muscles: For both children there was a reduction in percentage of trials in which a response was elicited in the different muscles.

It is interesting that the gastrocnemius is normally considered the agonist muscle for responses to posterior platform perturbations, because the platform movement causes a forward sway, and the activation of the gastrocnemius serves to bring the center of mass back over the base of support. However, for these children the tibialis anterior muscle, which is the antagonist, was almost always activated before the gastrocnemius muscle. This is no doubt due to the fact that it is the gastrocnemius and hamstrings muscles that show abnormal function.

Figure 4, *bottom*, shows the response latencies of the tibialis anterior, quadriceps, and abdominal muscles of the two children for anterior

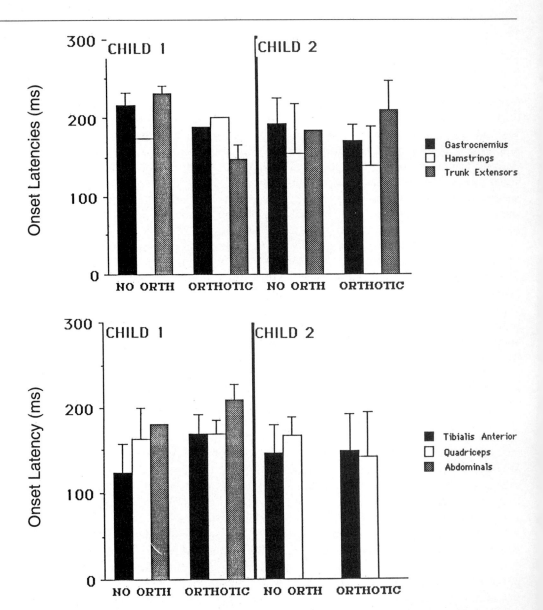

Fig. 4 *Data are for two 3.7-year-old children with spastic diplegia, under conditions of using orthoses and standing without orthoses.* **Top**, *Bar plots of means and standard deviations of onset latencies for the gastrocnemius, hamstrings, and trunk extensor muscles activated during posterior platform movements.* **Bottom**, *Bar plots of means and standard deviations of onset latencies for the tibialis anterior, quadriceps, and abdominal muscles activated during anterior platform movements.*

platform perturbations. (Note that there was no response in the abdominal muscle of child 2.) For this perturbation direction, the muscles are activated in an appropriate ascending order and at shorter, more normal latencies, for both children when they are standing without orthoses. This again may be due to the children showing more normal function in the tibialis anterior and quadriceps muscle groups. Tibialis anterior and quadriceps muscles were recruited before gastrocnemius and hamstrings for both directions of platform perturbations. The children thus did not show a directionally specific response to platform movements.

For anterior platform perturbations, the orthoses appeared to interrupt the ascending synergy (tibialis anterior to quadriceps pattern) for both children. They also increased the actual onset time of the responses for child 1, probably as a result of the locked position at the ankle.

In comparing the responses of the children with spastic diplegia with those of normal children, we note the following similarities and differences in response characteristics: (1) Responses of the children with spastic diplegia appear to have very late onset latencies, similar to those of a 7- to 9-month-old normal child in early pull-to-stand behavior. This is in spite of the fact that these children with spastic diplegia had been able to pull to stand for at least 1½ years. (2) Responses of these 3.7-year-olds with spastic diplegia are very different from those of normal children of 13 months or older, who have achieved independent stance and walking abilities. By 13 months of age and the onset of independent walking, normal children show greatly reduced response latencies in the muscles of the postural synergy; responses occur in 100% of the trials and in an ascending response sequence. The 3.7-year-olds with spastic diplegia continued to show very sporadic responses, of long latencies and often in an inappropriate response sequence.

However, a confounding variable in comparing the data for the normal children and children of the same age with spastic diplegia is the fact that the mechanics of the perturbation are different for a child that is supported than for a child that is standing independently, in that part of the perturbation can be absorbed by the arms when a child is holding on to a stable surface. It is unclear how much of the difference we see between the two groups of children is due to this biomechanical difference in the stance characteristics.

An additional study by Nashner and associates[6] on 7- to 9-year-old children with cerebral palsy (groups of children with spastic hemiplegia, ataxia, and spastic diplegia) has shown similar muscle response organization problems in response to platform perturbations. The children with spastic hemiplegia showed both slower onset latencies and a reversal of response organization in the involved leg, with the sequence being proximal to distal. This was observed for both directions of platform perturbation. The children with spastic diplegia showed more intersubject variability. One of these children resembled those with spastic hemiplegia, with response reversals for both directions of platform perturbation, but distributed bilaterally. A second child showed a highly variable response sequence, but only in muscles compensating for backward sway. The ataxic children showed a delayed, but correctly ordered, sequence of muscle responses for both directions of platform perturbation.

Visual Contributions to Postural Control in Normal Children and Spastic Diplegic Children With Cerebral Palsy

Research on the contribution of vision in the control of posture has shown that normal children first learning to stand are highly influenced by the visual environment, and will sway, stagger, or fall when subjected to visual cues indicating sway, even though vestibular and somatosensory cues do not signal movement.[7,8] In a study examining the changing contributions of visual inputs to postural sway during the development of pull-to-stand behavior, independent stance, and locomotion it was noted that visual contributions to postural control gradually increase from the onset of independent sitting through pull-to-stand behavior, and then peak at the onset of independent walking.[9] This dependence on visual input diminishes with continued experience in walking, so that 3-year-olds are almost unaffected by erroneous visual cues indicating sway.

To determine the extent to which the 3-year-old children with diplegia were affected by visual cues, they were asked to stand in a room with walls and ceiling that moved (60 cm at approximately 0.48 m/sec) in the anterior or posterior direction, but with a stable floor. Their sway was measured by a video camera and later calculated as a percentage of their maximum body sway within their limits of stability. Both children with spastic diplegia lost balance on all six trials for both directions of visual box movement, and thus behaviorally resembled the children at the newly walking stage of balance development.

These results are similar to those found by Bai and associates[10] in examining the responses of a 3-year-old child with ataxic cerebral palsy to repeated presentation of optical flow information from the moving room. This child continued to stagger or fall on almost every trial, within a series of 30 successive trials.

Development of Intersensory Integration

Experiments analyzing the onset latency and variability of leg muscle responses of normal 4- to 6-year-olds detected an unusual change in the response characteristics of this age group.[5] The 4- to 6-year-olds showed a regression in their postural response organization, in that postural response synergies were more variable and longer in latency than in the 15- to 31-month-old or 7- to 10-year-old age groups. In addition, the 4- to 6-year-olds showed a delay in the activation latency of proximal leg muscle synergists for both anterior and posterior platform perturbations. These timing delays between distal and proximal leg muscles produced increased motion at the knee joint during compensatory body sway. The activation of the proximal leg muscles of 4- to 6-year-olds was not rapid enough to compensate for the inertial lag associated with the mass of the thigh and trunk.[5] What caused this apparent regression in response onsets to slower latencies? It has been hypothesized that this is the time when normal children develop intersensory integration abilities and that their normal postural responses become more variable as they learn to shift from using one sensory input to another.

To test the ability of children of different age ranges to adapt to altered sensory conditions, one can ask the child to stand quietly for 5 seconds under conditions of progressively decreased redundancy of inputs relevant for balance control. These include: (1) normal somatosensory ankle joint, visual, and vestibular inputs; (2) normal somatosensory ankle joint inputs and vestibular inputs with eyes closed; (3) ankle joint inputs minimized by rotating the platform in direct relationship to body sway, but normal vision and vestibular inputs; and (4) ankle joint inputs minimized (as above), eyes closed, and vestibular system normal. Children's performances were measured by determining body sway as a percent of theoretical maximum sway, with 100% indicating loss of balance.

Shumway-Cook and Woollacott[5] demonstrated that even under normal stance conditions 4- to 6-year-olds swayed more than the older children or adults. (The youngest children would not tolerate the unusual sensory conditions without crying.) With eyes closed their balance decreased further, but they retained stability. However, when the platform was rotated with body sway to keep the ankle joint at about 90 degrees, the 4- to 6-year-olds swayed significantly, and one lost balance. In the final condition, in which ankle joint inputs were minimized and eyes were closed, leaving only vestibular cues to contribute to stability, four of the five children in this age group lost balance while none of the older children or adults needed assistance.

Thus, normal children under 7 years of age are unable to balance easily when both somatosensory and visual cues are removed, leaving only vestibular cues to control posture. They also appear to have difficulty in shifting from the use of ankle joint somatosensory cues to visual cues when ankle joint inputs were made incongruent with body sway. This may also indicate the inability of the 4- to 6-year-old to resolve intersensory conflict during postural control.

Intersensory Integration in Children With Cerebral Palsy

Intersensory integration abilities have also been studied in 7- to 9-year-old children with spastic hemiplegia, spastic diplegia, and ataxia.[6] Children with ataxia demonstrated an inability to accurately maintain upright balance under conditions in which there were conflicting sensory inputs from vision and somatosensation. Shumway-Cook[11] notes that because motor-coordination processes were largely normal in children with ataxic cerebral palsy, these equilibrium problems could not be caused by lack of coordination among muscle synergists responding to loss of balance. Instead, the problems seem to be the result of abnormalities in central processes responsible for the integration of sensory inputs. None of the children with spastic hemiplegia showed these problems, and only one of three with spastic diplegia showed these inter-sensory integration deficits. Thus, because these children are 7 to 9 years old, they show a normal progression in the maturation of inter-sensory integration abilities.

Summary

In summary, we have reviewed research on both the normal development of postural control and the development of posture control in children with cerebral palsy from a systems perspective in which we (1) examined the contributions of sensory, motor, and higher integrative functions to normal postural development, and (2) examined the extent to which dysfunction in these systems contributed to postural abnormalities in the child with cerebral palsy.

It was shown that normal infants develop the muscle response synergies underlying postural control gradually, with the responses first appearing at about 7 to 9 months of age with the onset of pull-to-stand behavior. With the emergence of pull-to-stand behavior, infants showed excessive movement at the ankle, knee, and hip joints, and postural responses were disorganized, with delayed and highly variable onset latencies. Response organization improved with experience in dependent stance. At the onset of independent stance, response patterns again showed increased variability. However, with increased experience and the onset of independent walking, the response organization became consistent, and latencies were shortened to more mature levels.

Children with spastic diplegia, who were at a similar level of behavioral development (pull to stand) but were 3.7 years of age, showed similar response organization, with delayed onset latencies and highly variable responses when not wearing orthoses. In addition, for posterior platform perturbations, response sequences tended to show reversals in order of activation, with proximal muscles being activated before distal muscles. Though orthoses shortened response latencies slightly, they did not improve response organization, and they actually decreased the number of trials in which responses were activated. Muscle responses to anterior platform perturbations were more consistently organized in an appropriate distal to proximal sequence.

Visual contributions to postural control in these children were very strong, with children falling whenever inappropriate visual sway cues were presented.

Studies on postural response organization in 7- to 9-year-old spastic hemiplegic children have shown that these children also have delayed response onsets and inappropriate response organization in their affected leg.[11] Ataxic children have delayed onset latencies, but have close to normal response organization.

Intersensory organization abilities have been examined for children with spastic hemiplegic, spastic diplegic, and ataxic cerebral palsy.[11] All children studied with spastic hemiplegia and most with spastic diplegia show close to normal intersensory integration abilities. However, children with ataxia have severe problems in this area, indicative of deficits in higher integrative functions.

References

1. Bernstein N: *Coordination and Regulation of Movements*. New York, Pergamon Press, 1967.
2. Fentress JC: Developmental roots of behavioral order: Systemic approaches to the examination of core developmental issues, in Thelen E, Gunnar MR (eds): *Systems and Development: The Minnesota Symposium in Child Psychology*. Hillsdale, NJ, Erlbaum, 1989, vol 22, pp 35–76.
3. Woollacott M, Sveistrup H: Changes in the sequencing and timing of muscle response coordination associated with developmental transitions in balance abilities. *Hum Movement Sci*, 1992;11:23–36.
4. Forssberg H, Nashner L: Ontogenetic development of postural control in man: Adaptation to altered support and visual conditions during stance. *J Neurosci* 1982;2:545–552.
5. Shumway-Cook A, Woollacott M: The growth of stability: Postural control from a developmental perspective. *J Motor Behav* 1985;17:131–147.
6. Nashner LM, Shumway-Cook A, Marin O: Stance posture control in select groups of children with cerebral palsy: Deficits in sensory organization and muscular coordination. *Ex Brain Res* 1983;49:393–409.
7. Lee DN, Aronson E: Visual proprioceptive control of standing in human infants. *Perception Psychophysic* 1974;15:529–532.
8. Bertenthal BI, Bai DL: Infants' sensitivity to optical flow for controlling posture, in Butler C, Jaffe K (eds): *Visual-vestibular Integration in Early Development: Technical and Clinical Perspectives*. Washington, DC, RESNA, 1988, pp 43–61.
9. Sveistrup H, Foster E, Woollacott M: Changes in the effect of visual flow on postural control across the lifespan, in Wollacott M, Horak F (eds): *Posture and Gait: Control Mechanisms*. Eugene, OR, University of Oregon Books, 1992, vol 2, pp 224–227.
10. Bai DL, Bertenthal BI, Sussman MD: Children's sensitivity to optical flow information for the control of stance, in *Abstracts of the Third Annual East Coast Clinical Gait Laboratory Conference*. Bethesda, MD, NIH, 1987.
11. Shumway-Cook A: Equilibrium deficits in children, in Woollacott M, Shumway-Cook A (eds): *Development of Posture and Gait Across the Life Span*. Columbia, SC, USC Press, 1989, pp 229–252.

Chapter 8

Diplegic Gait: Is There More Than Spasticity?

George T. Rab, MD

This chapter focuses on questions surrounding the neurologic causes of diplegic gait. Although spasticity is the hallmark of this form of cerebral palsy, ambulation abnormalities can rarely be explained on the basis of spasticity alone. Comparing it with the ambulation of the spinal cord spastic patient, who has a more ''pure'' form of spasticity, confirms the unique nature of diplegic gait.

Anatomic Factors

The relationships between diplegia and prematurity, low birthweight, hypoxemia, peri- and intraventricular hemorrhage, and other pre- and postnatal events have been outlined.[1,2] Correlation between pathologic, ultrasonographic, computed tomographic, and magnetic resonance imaging (MRI) findings suggests a likelihood of damage to the white matter in the vicinity of the internal capsule and basal ganglia of the brain, although there is much variability in the individual anatomic lesion. In the infant, periventricular leukomalacia is characterized on MRI by delayed myelinization;[3] MRI performed between 2 and 10 years continues to show unilateral and bilateral atrophy in the peritrigonal regions of many diplegic children with disorders of gait, with extension of white matter atrophy along the lateral ventricle in children with more extensive involvement (Fig. 1, *top*).[4] This region contains pyramidal tract axons to the lower extremity in the internal capsule (Fig. 1, *bottom*), but it is an oversimplification to assume that only fibers originating from the motor cortex are affected. Major nuclear components of the extrapyramidal system are almost certainly involved in the lesion. Thus, spasticity is a feature of diplegia associated with prematurity, but not the only one; Levitt[5] suggests that if spasticity were removed from the diplegic child, the handicap would remain.

Lower forms of mammalian and animal life apparently have locomotor generators at brainstem and spinal cord levels, which can function in some form to produce locomotion without cortical control. The ''chicken without a head'' is known to all farm children. Decerebrate

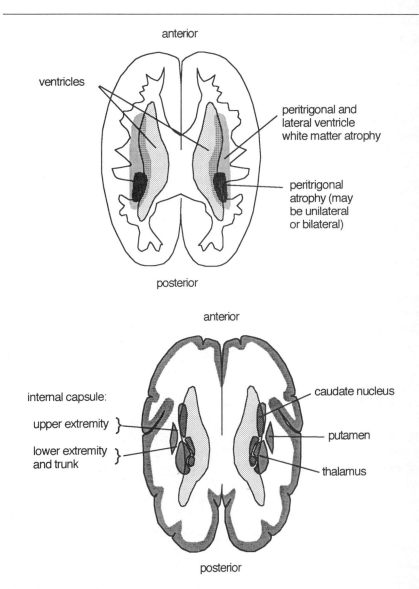

Fig. 1 *Top, Schematic representation of magnetic resonance imaging scan demonstrating white matter atrophy in diplegic children over age 2. The extent of lesions correlates with the severity of diplegia. (Modified from Yokochi et al.[4]) Bottom, Periventricular leukomalacia can damage pyramidal and extrapyramidal structures in the brain.*

cats can be made to walk, trot, or run with mid-brain stimulation.[6] The locomotor generator is thought not to be significant in the human, although electromyographic and kinematic studies of normal infants compared with infants with cerebral palsy suggests striking uniformity during the supported stages of early reflex locomotion; however, later plantigrade step patterns did not develop in the children with cerebral palsy.[7] Harrison,[8] citing the remarkably stereotypical walking pattern of most diplegic children, suggested that interneuronally mediated activity dominates in cerebral palsy. She felt that abnormalities of motor control conceivably could be caused by different agents at different ages; that is, brain damage, abnormal muscle growth, and joint contractures might each be the dominant factor in abnormal control at different developmental levels.[8]

The role of spinal cord reflexes, intersegmental connections, inhibitory and excitatory control is complex. However, changes following dorsal rhizotomy, described elsewhere in this volume, may provide further insight into the role of some of these factors.

Diplegia associated with full-term birth, although it sometimes mimics that seen in premature infants, usually differs in important clinical ways from the clinical situation in the premature child, and there is evidence that the neurologic lesion is different.[9] For those reasons, diplegia associated with full-term birth will not be considered here.

Neurologic Symptoms and Their Assessment

Tone

Tone refers to the continuous low-level electrical and mechanical activity of skeletal muscle. It appears during sleep. Tone is an extrapyramidal phenomenon, under control of the basal ganglia and lower brainstem and spinal centers. In a superficial way, tone acts as a neurologic volume control, increasing as a subject goes from supine to sitting to standing. This variation may be exaggerated in the child with diplegia, and frequently changes with development. Dystonic posturing, a distortion of tone, includes bizarre flailing of limbs (ballismus), writhing action (athetosis and chorea), or more subtle positional abnormalities of the extremities. Dystonia is extrapyramidal in origin and is generally associated with lesions of the basal ganglia, although the exact lesions that produce it have not been characterized.

Rigidity

Rigidity may be thought of as a generalized pathologic increase in tone. It is extrapyramidal, but its cause is unknown. Diplegic children who exhibit rigidity in the supine position are likely to have abnormally high tone in sitting or standing positions, with resultant difficulty walking. This characteristic, despite the obvious increase in motor tone, is not true spasticity.

Spasticity

While dysfunction of the pyramidal tract, known as spasticity, is straightforward conceptually, its detection and measurement are elusive. The clinical features of spasticity include increase in deep tendon reflexes and muscle stretch (clasp-knife) behavior, clonus, and presence of the Babinski sign. Attempts to actually quantify spasticity have been limited to easily accessible joints, such as the ankle, in controlled experimental environments.[9,10] As motor tone rises (as with standing or walking), spasticity may be exaggerated or it simply may be misdiagnosed. Many astute clinicians have mistaken the hyperreflexia of the tension athetoid patient for spasticity, while there is actually no involvement of the pyramidal tracts in these patients.

Weakness

Weakness may be muscular or neurologic in origin and is measured by subjective muscle testing, which is difficult in children. In diplegia, the assumption that damage to the pyramidal tract leads to a decrease in upper motor neuronal discharge and weakness is probably accurate, but it is difficult to prove. Experimental lesions of the basal ganglia can produce profound hypotonia. Infants who later develop spasticity may start out hypotonic. Muscles that lack the inhibitory influence of higher centers on their lower motor neuron pool, and thereby exhibit spasticity, may show profound weakness when the spinal reflex arc is interrupted by dorsal rhizotomy.

Muscle weakness can be localized (for example, a weak anterior tibialis muscle working against spastic ankle plantarflexors) or generalized, and can lead to penalties in energy cost. The role of weakness in the development of fixed contractures is undefined, but experience with patients with poliomyelitis suggests that weakness can cause skeletal deformities. How best to quantitate the neurologic contributions of combined weakness and spasticity in the same muscle group is an unanswered question.

Contracture

Muscle appears to grow in length mainly at the musculotendinous junction. Ziv and associates[11] use the presence of contracture in spastic mice during growth to explain how spasticity during growth can lead to fixed deformities. Explanation of the way passive stretching of spastic muscles counteracts this tendency to form contractures is still controversial.

Chronic spastic muscle imbalance and shortening can lead to fixed joint contractures. Contractures of joints or muscle do not occur as result of dystonia or athetosis; their presence is, in a way, a measure of the overall level of spasticity in a child. If such contractures interfere with ambulation, they may be treated surgically.

Ataxia

Ataxia is a disorder of balance that may be cerebral or cerebellar in origin. Children with ataxia are frequently seen in cerebral palsy clinics, and often are mildly retarded. Mild ataxia as a symptom is fairly common in the child with diplegic cerebral palsy, but it usually is not the primary motor disability.

Balance

Disorders of balance are extremely common in diplegic children. These disorders range from mild disturbances of posterior equilibrium to gross loss of equilibrium in both anteroposterior and mediolateral planes. Gross loss of balance requires assistance of a walker or crutches, depending on the severity of the symptom and the function of the upper extremities.

When a normal individual loses balance, as on the pitching deck of a boat, his/her natural tendency is to crouch and reduce the height of the body's center of gravity. Unfortunately, this tendency, which may be exaggerated in the diplegic child, has not been experimentally quantified. It is conceivable that some diplegic children crouch because of poor balance, rather than predominance of hip and knee flexors, and consequently such children would be inappropriate subjects for hip flexor and/or hamstring lengthening surgery.

Energy Cost

Walking consumes energy, and diplegic children expend more energy and walk more slowly than do normal children.[12] It is a common finding that diplegic children, operated on to improve their gait, may ambulate postoperatively with a different (cosmetically improved?) gait but increased energy consumption.

The relationship between weakness and energy cost in the older diplegic child is of great importance prognostically. Many of these children, who were marginal ambulators using walking aids during their younger years, cease to be able to walk in adolescence. Their contractures suddenly worsen, and wheelchair use becomes the preferred mode of mobility. Operations to correct the severe contractures are doomed to failure if the child's energy expenditure exceeds a reasonable level for functional walking or if the child lacks motivation to walk.

Examples of Diplegic Gait

Diplegic gait is easily recognizable by the experienced observer. However, describing and quantifying the typical diplegic gait is much more difficult. In the past decade, gait analysis laboratories have been developed in which it is possible to record three-dimensional joint motions, walking speed, step length, and muscle electrical activity during walking. In some laboratories it is possible to measure oxygen consumption or pulse rate or to calculate joint moments, power, or muscle length variation. The information generated from these laboratories has had a profound effect on the understanding of diplegic gait, and on criteria for selecting patients for treatment as well as measuring effects thereof.

By convention, measurement and description of the gait cycle begin and end at the instant of foot contact; a stride is the time between foot contact on two successive steps of the same limb. Excellent summaries of kinematic (motion) analysis of normal and cerebral palsy gait appear in the literature;[13,14] these will not be repeated here.

Following are gait analyses of two children with diplegia associated with premature birth. They represent different extremes of the disorder, but their study brings out the many questions surrounding diplegia.

Case 1

Case 1 is an 8-year-old girl who is intellectually normal and attends regular school. She had physical therapy as a younger child, and has worn ankle-foot orthoses to control ankle position.

When first seen at age 6 years and 3 months, she walked independently on tiptoe, with slight scissoring and internal rotation of the hips. She had a tendency to hyperextend both knees during stance phase. She had bilateral ankle clonus without loss of passive dorsiflexion, and her hamstrings were tight at a straight-leg raise of 45 degrees symmetrically. Her anteroposterior balance was fair, and she had a tendency to run into objects in order to stop forward progress.

By age 8 years, she had changed her walking pattern to one of crouch. Her balance was marginally better. Her passive range-of-motion had changed little, except that she had lost 15 degrees of dorsiflexion of the ankles and had developed 10-degree hip flexion contractures. Both femurs exhibited internal torsion, and hip abduction was limited to 20 degrees in extension.

Results of her three-dimensional gait study are summarized in Figure 2; for simplicity, only one side is shown although her abnormalities were fairly symmetric. She exhibits the classical findings of crouch-internal rotation gait: hip extension is lost in late stance; the hip is persistently adducted and internally rotated; knee extension is lost throughout stance, with additional swing-phase flexion insufficient to clear the foot easily; the ankle comes only to neutral dorsiflexion in stance, which leads to toe-walking because of the persistently flexed knee; the ankle plantarflexes markedly during swing (without orthoses), correlating with highly variable, low amplitude electromyograms of the anterior tibialis muscle.

There is certainly clinical evidence of spasticity, with ankle clonus and increased deep tendon reflexes in the lower extremities. She was treated with ''weakening'' procedures that are standard orthopaedic operations for spastic gait: iliopsoas aponeurotic lengthening, medial and lateral hamstrings aponeurotic lengthening, gracilis lengthenings, distal rectus femoris transfer to the sartorius, and rigid polypropylene ankle orthoses. When she underwent gait analysis one year postoperatively, all of the above motions were improved, and she looked more normal. Her parents were pleased with the result. However, her walking velocity was 10% lower, despite an 18-month interval of growth between studies.

Was her walking abnormality due to spasticity? Is she better off now from an energy standpoint? Why did she go from a hyperextended knee gait at age 6 to a flexed, crouch gait at age 8 (a quite common evolution for the diplegic child, in my experience)?

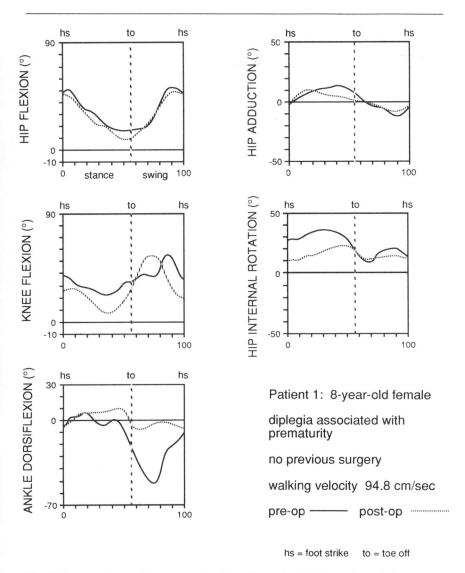

Patient 1: 8-year-old female

diplegia associated with prematurity

no previous surgery

walking velocity 94.8 cm/sec

pre-op ——— post-op ·················

hs = foot strike   to = toe off

Fig. 2 *Preoperative and postoperative three-dimensional joint motions during walking for diplegic patient, Case 1, described in text.*

When her ankle is fixed at neutral during weightbearing there is continuous activity in the triceps surae. However, during swing, this muscle group is silent. Although she could actively dorsiflex the ankle upon request, during walking the electrical activity was highly variable and frequently absent. The complex neurologic roles of extensor mass movement, balance reactions, and inhibition at central or spinal cord levels responsible for failure to dorsiflex the ankle during swing are open to speculation; spasticity alone cannot be indicted easily.

Hamstring spasticity is frequently blamed for crouch gait. Figure 3 shows the calculated length of several muscles during the gait cycle shown in Figure 2. These lengths are generated from a three-dimensional skeletal computerized model of muscle origins and insertions correlated with kinematic data. The semitendinosus shows slight prolongation of stance phase electrical activity, but certainly not the overflow associated with spasticity. Furthermore, the muscle is shortening rapidly throughout stance, which is a normal pattern, not a situation likely to stimulate an exaggerated stretch reflex. The rectus femoris elongates passively, then undergoes a swing phase active shortening; this indicates that the rectus femoris is performing work—hip flexion and leg acceleration during swing—but not that it is spastic. The adductor longus is electrically active only when short; it functions isometrically during stance and does not logically fit the pattern of a spastic muscle as I define it.

This child's change in energy consumption was not studied scientifically. She seems to walk more upright and more slowly after surgical correction of her spastic gait; it is difficult to quantitate the abnormalities responsible.

Case 2

Case 2 is a 14-year-old spastic diplegic girl with a history of intracerebral hemorrhage at birth, and who required shunting for hydrocephalus. She underwent bilateral achilles tendon lengthenings elsewhere at age 9. She walks with two Lofstrand crutches, and sometimes a walker. She would like to use a wheelchair more because it is fast, but her parents and therapist have discouraged it because they wish her to remain a walker.

Her supine physical exam reveals 5 degree hip and knee flexion contractures and evidence of tight hamstrings (popliteal angles 90 degrees bilaterally). There is mild resistance to movement of the limbs, but it is easily broken, indicating minimal rigidity, and there is no clonus. Deep tendon reflexes are brisk but not pathologic. Prone rectus test produces a mild reflex hip flexion.

Results of a three-dimensional walking study, carried out while she was using her crutches, are shown in Figure 4. Note that her walking velocity is extremely reduced—less than 20 cm/sec, and that stance phase is 87% of her total gait cycle (Normal = 62%). Her overlengthened heel cords contribute to excessive dorsiflexion of the ankle in mid and late stance, and there is poor coordination of all her joint motions, with very little variation at the hip and progressive loss of knee extension in stance.

Except for prolongation of hamstring activity in stance, surface electromyograms of vasti, rectus femoris, hamstrings, and adductor muscle groups were appropriately timed. Her pulse went to 130 beats/min after walking 125 feet.

It is obvious that spasticity per se is not the problem. There is actually little clinical evidence to indicate spasticity. Weakness and increased

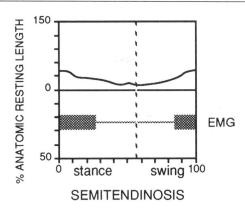

SEMITENDINOSIS

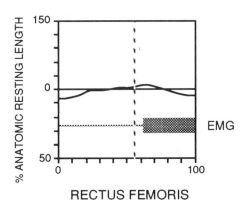

RECTUS FEMORIS

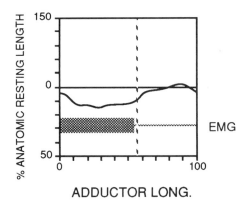

ADDUCTOR LONG.

Patient 1: muscle length - EMG relationship

Fig. 3 *Calculated muscle length variation and recorded electromyogram activity during walking cycle shown in Figure 2. Muscle lengths are normalized and expressed as a multiple of resting anatomic length.*

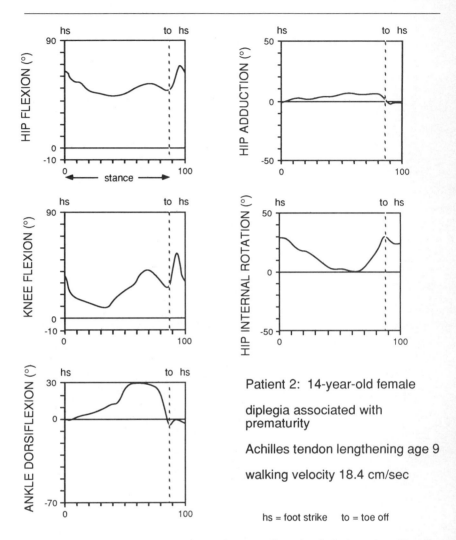

Patient 2: 14-year-old female

diplegia associated with prematurity

Achilles tendon lengthening age 9

walking velocity 18.4 cm/sec

hs = foot strike   to = toe off

Fig. 4 *Three-dimensional joint motions during walking for diplegic patient, Case 2, described in text.*

energy consumption are the major physical issues limiting her ability to walk. It was recommended that she concentrate on transfer skills and use a wheelchair.

Summary

Spasticity has long been considered the primary culprit in cerebral palsy. Early studies of the central nervous system of patients with cerebral palsy included a high percentage of specimens from patients with severe neonatal anoxia resulting in extensive cortical damage, leading to an erroneous concept of pathoanatomy, which has been clarified in the last quarter century. Until recently, there was much confusion about classification, with low-birthweight premature children classified as quadriplegics. Cerebral injury associated with prematurity usually results in diplegia with pyramidal tract involvement as a common, almost constant, feature. However, the unique features of the typical diplegic make it necessary to look beyond spasticity for an explanation of gait disorders.

Research to enlarge the knowledge base in these areas will have to come from many directions. Studies of prenatal high-risk infants in utero may shed light on pathologic processes. Ultrasound, MRI, and other new imaging modalities are improving rapidly in resolution, and documentation of anatomic defects and understanding of the dynamics of myelinization will improve. Three-dimensional gait analysis, energetics studies, and long-term natural history studies will certainly elucidate the need for intervention and the efficacies and failures of therapy.

We should strive to enlarge, rather than to simply refine, knowledge. Better assessment of balance and reflex mechanisms in diplegia will provide data as to which abnormalities are internally programmed and which are reactive to environment, position, and other stimuli. Better definition of neurologic abnormalities and better tools to quantitate them are needed, as well as new methods for exploring the central nervous system and its diseases.

References

1. Stanley F, Alberman E: *The Epidemiology of the Cerebral Palsies,* Clinics in Developmental Medicine. Philadelphia, JB Lippincott, 1984, vol 87.
2. Nelson KB, Ellenberg JH: Neonatal signs as predictors of cerebral palsy. *Pediatrics* 1979;64:225–232.
3. Dubowitz LM, Bydder GM, Mushin J: Developmental sequence of periventricular leukomalacia. Correlation of ultrasound, clinical, and nuclear magnetic resonance functions. *Arch Dis Child* 1985;60:349–355.
4. Yokochi K, Aiba K, Horie M, et al: Magnetic resonance imaging in children with spastic diplegia: Correlation with the severity of their motor and mental abnormality. *Med Child Neurol* 1991;33:18–25.
5. Levitt S: *Treatment of Cerebral Palsy and Motor Delay.* Oxford, Blackwell Scientific Publications, 1982, pp 1–47.
6. Shik ML, Severin FC, Orlovskii GN: Control of walking and running by means of stimulation of the mid-brain. *Biofizika* 1966;11:659–666.
7. Leonard CT, Hirschfeld H, Forssberg H: Independent development of walking in children with cerebral palsy. *Dev Med Child Neurol* 1991;33:567–577.
8. Harrison A: Spastic cerebral palsy: Possible spinal interneuronal contributions. *Dev Med Child Neurol* 1988;30:769–780.
9. Price R, Bjornson KF, Lehman JF, et al: Quantitative measurement of spasticity in children with cerebral palsy. *Dev Med Child Neurol* 1991;33:585–595.

10. Otis JC, Root L, Pamilla JR, et al: Biomechanical measurement of spastic plantarflexors. *Dev Med Child Neurol* 1983;25:60–66.

11. Ziv I, Blackburn N, Rang M, et al: Muscle growth in normal and spastic mice. *Dev Med Child Neurol* 1984;26:94–99.

12. Campbell J, Ball J: Energetics of walking in cerebral palsy. *Orthop Clin North Am* 1978;9:374–377.

13. Perry J: Cerebral palsy gait, in Samilson RL (ed): *Orthopaedic Aspects of Cerebral Palsy,* Clinics in Developmental Medicine. Philadelphia, JB Lippincott, 1975, vol 52/53, pp 71–88.

14. Sutherland DH: Gait disorders in childhood and adolescence. Baltimore, Williams & Wilkins, 1984.

Consensus

Orthopaedic surgery concentrates primarily on treatments that pertain to the complications of spasticity. However, eight deficits other than spasticity may affect the patient's overall treatment and, specifically, may affect surgical decision making. These include cognitive deficits, visual spatial deficits, poor balance, weakness, dyspraxia (motor planning problems), impaired selective motor control, social and emotional problems, and dystonia and dyskinesia. Each of these deficits was evaluated to determine if it could be objectively measured, if it was relevant to the outcome of orthopaedic or other surgical procedures, and if there is current research regarding the deficit.

Many of these deficits are particularly important to those interested in rhizotomy. Four deficits—lack of balance, weakness, dystonia, and lack of selective motor control—can have a major impact and should be considered relative contraindications to rhizotomy in a specific patient.

Cognitive and Visual Spatial Deficits

Cognitive deficits and visual impairments are not by themselves contraindications to orthopaedic surgery nor do they necessarily affect surgical outcome unless these deficits are extremely severe. For example, a visually impaired child with spastic diplegia may benefit by orthopaedic surgery but a completely blind child probably should not have surgery to correct a crouched gait. Moderate cognitive deficits are not a contraindication to orthopaedic surgery whereas extreme retardation is a contraindication unless the goal is improvement in nursing care or relief of pain.

Poor Balance

Balance and the lack thereof are extremely important determinants of function, which are affected by multiple sensory systems, including the somatosensory, visual, and vestibular systems. New methods are being investigated to measure patient balance and posture control. One research method involves measuring a child's ability to balance while standing on a moving platform under different sensory conditions while determining electromyographic activity in response to the platform perturbations. The clinician can assess balance through the Romberg test or by comparing sway on a firm support to that on a foam support, which reduces sway-related ankle-joint input. Balance is extremely important for the ultimate function of the child with spastic diplegia and may influence the outcome following surgery; however, balance, or the lack thereof, need not affect the surgeon's decision to perform appropriate orthopaedic surgical procedures for individual patients. Orthopaedic procedures may affect the patient's balance in a positive way because balance is a combination of central three-dimensional sensation and having a stable base of support. The more stable the lower extremities, the better the overall balance and the better the patient's ability to adapt to central balance errors.

Weakness

A contracted muscle can still be a weak muscle. Although weakness will affect outcome following surgery it is very difficult

111

to measure in the patient with spastic diplegia. Excessive weakness will be manifested when tone is reduced following rhizotomy and is a contraindication to rhizotomy.

If the patient has selective motor control, weakness can be measured using equipment designed to measure muscle strength and joint torques. It is very difficult for a child without selective motor control to perform the tasks necessary for objective measurement of muscle strength.

Evaluating the child's ability to squat will provide a gross evaluation of strength. Strength can also be assessed by observing the child's ability to kick a ball (requires good balance) or climb stairs. Pulse rate can be used to estimate the energy of walking and, if normal, might suggest the patient actually has adequate strength. Although there is a preliminary suggestion that baclofen may decrease spasticity to the point where the patient has sufficient selective motor control for determination of muscle strength, this is not yet proven.

Dyspraxia (Motor Planning Deficits)

Many children with spastic diplegia have deficits in motor planning, which is defined as the ability to plan out an act such as opening and walking through a door or turning around. Making plans to move body segments in an appropriate order and direction requires cognitive skills. In normal individuals this planning becomes automatic and cognitive skills are not required for most routine daily activities. Many diplegia patients continue to require cognitive skills for almost all routine motion planning activities. The patient's ability to plan ahead and perform specific acts can be evaluated objectively. Although motor planning research may be more applicable to evaluation of upper extremity function, it might also be applicable for transfer and walking.

Impaired Selective Motor Control

Impaired selective motor control is a major problem for a majority of patients with spastic diplegia. If a child is able to control individual joints, for example, to dorsiflex the

ankle without flexing the hip and knee, a better prognosis for most orthopaedic treatment might be expected. If, however, the patient does not demonstrate selective motor control, surgical results may not be as good.

Selective motor control is age-related. Normal children do not develop full maturation of selective motor control until 6 or 7 years of age. The fact that it is inappropriate to expect children with spastic diplegia to develop complete selective motor control before reaching this age may assist the orthopaedic surgeon in choosing the appropriate age for surgical intervention. For example, if a procedure requires the patient to selectively contract a muscle postoperatively, the orthopaedic surgeon might consider delaying surgery until the patient reaches age 6 or 7. Upper extremity surgery is commonly delayed until the child can cooperate with a postoperative physical therapy program.

Social and Emotional Problems

Social and emotional problems that may coexist with the physical problems in children who have spastic diplegia can adversely affect the patient's outcome. When considering and recommending various procedures to a family, an orthopaedic surgeon must take into account the fact that the family's expectations must be realistic and that their cooperation is essential for a good outcome. If a family's expectations are beyond what can be delivered by the orthopaedic surgeon, either the family must be counseled or the surgeon should proceed with caution. The effects that hospitalization, immobilization, and rehabilitation would have on the actual social and emotional health of the child and family must be considered along with the preoperative assessment. Orthopaedic surgeons must remember that there is a relationship between the psychological health of the child and the treatment they are planning.

Summary

Many deficits beyond spasticity are present in diplegic cerebral palsy. These other deficits are especially important in the assessment of the overall function of the patient if the objective of intervention is to help develop a happy patient who is able to interact in an intact family. To this end, the orthopaedic surgeon must work with other professionals, including pediatricians, neurologists, neurosurgeons, social workers, and therapists.

Section Three
Outcome Assessment

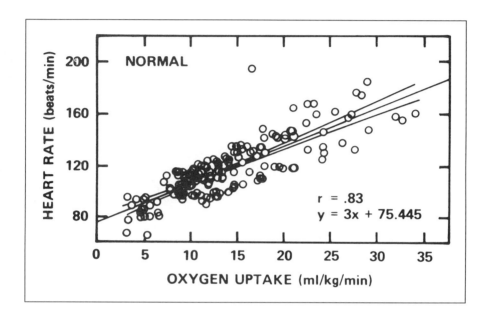

Chapter 9

Designing Outcome Studies in Cerebral Palsy

James C. Torner, PhD

Introduction

Determining that an intervention is efficacious involves proving that it has resulted in improvement in function and can be performed without significant risk. The evaluation is based on valid, unbiased measurement relative to a desired goal or in comparison with a current standard. A reasonable goal for children with spastic cerebral palsy is increased mobility and freedom from pain. Outcome studies must measure the improvement as well as the risk associated with the decision for and performance of a given therapy. These studies must be designed to determine which intervention is best, given the characteristics of the child and the goal of the intervention. Because several domains and disciplines are involved in the management of cerebral palsy, existing studies have not supplied an answer as to which is the best plan for children with spastic cerebral palsy.

Several study designs have been used for evaluating interventions. While most studies have been prospective in the areas of case selection, data collection, and outcome evaluation, they lack comparison populations. Simeonsson and associates,[1] Parette and Hourcade,[2] and Harris[3] have reviewed designs for studies of early interventions for treatment of cerebral palsy. Historical controls and nonrandomized studies have all too frequently been used. Over half the studies had no control groups; less than half had statistical support for evidence of therapeutic efficacy, while the majority concluded the intervention was effective. Randomized studies have been attempted but comparability of groups and sample sizes are inadequate, primarily because these studies are conducted within a single institution. The advantage is that the investigators can supervise and/or perform the intervention, but the disadvantages are the lack of sufficient numbers and generalizability of subjects.

Considerations

Natural History and Clinical Course

Data from surveys of patient populations suggest that approximately 75% of patients with cerebral palsy show a predominantly spastic component, and half of these have diplegia. Greater than half of patients with spastic diplegia have moderate or severe disability.[4] Overall about one quarter of patients with cerebral palsy are walkers who may benefit from a surgical intervention to correct spasticity.

The plan for intervention depends on recognition of cerebral palsy and knowledge of its natural history. The diagnosis of spasticity resulting from cerebral palsy coincides with neuronal development and learning to walk. Evans and associates,[5] in their study of cerebral palsy in 520 children in the South Thames Region of England, noted that nearly half of the patients with cerebral palsy were diagnosed by age 1, and 80% were diagnosed by age 2, but children still were being diagnosed as having cerebral palsy at age 4. Recognition of the disease is related to the severity of the spasticity.

Not all spasticity should be considered permanent. In the Collaborative Perinatal Project, classification of cerebral palsy was evaluated at 1 and 7 years of age.[6] Patients who outgrew cerebral palsy varied by severity and type of abnormality. Additional factors related to outgrowing cerebral palsy were race, sex, IQ, seizures, speech abnormality, visual abnormality, hyperactivity, and socioeconomic skills. This background and prognostic factors form the clinical course by which interventions are pursued and compared.

The time of intervention, therefore, depends on recognition of the presence and severity of spasticity. In addition, selection of treatment often has been based on the failure of prior therapies. A child may undergo physical therapy, pharmacologic treatment, and surgical procedures based on failure of an earlier therapeutic maneuver. This process of selection may influence the effectiveness of the intervention. Parental and clinical decisions are made based on this early success or failure, expected outcomes, and long-term cost of the intervention. Hence, the decision and selection for treatment is influenced by the desire for achievement of goals that were not fulfilled or by the desire to achieve a different goal. The timing, in relation to natural history and therapeutic history, must be considered in evaluation of the intervention.

Patient Selection

Criteria for patient selection can be a major facet of the success or failure of an intervention, particularly where treatments are not randomly assigned. Criteria based on prior therapy, clinical grade, and characteristics of the patients should be stated specifically to adequately describe the patient population in which the intervention is intended. Standard accepted criteria for classification of spasticity resulting from cerebral palsy and for grading of severity must be used. The Ashworth scale[7] has been used widely to classify severity. Because its evaluation is subjective, reliability between investigators may be a problem. Further precision in measurement may be achieved through technical evaluation by gait analysis.[8–10] However, lack of standardization between gait laboratories may preclude uniform classification based on this assessment. The efficacy of any intervention can be tested across classifications or with subgroups. Recently, Albright and associates[11] used intrathecal baclofen in children with cerebral palsy and suggested that assessment of response to this technique may be useful as a screening evaluation for patients who might be selected to undergo rhizotomy.

Predictors of Outcome

Further classification of characteristics based on functional components and predictors, such as type of spasticity, etiology, age, neurologic function, walking performance, and potential parental compliance, may be important in discriminating between patients likely to benefit from the treatment and those at risk of complications. Many of these children have mental, verbal, and other abnormalities.[5,6] The likelihood of success may be increased in children with a more normal clinical profile. The spectrum of spasticity and associated conditions needs to be evaluated, and careful documentation of the patients who benefit from treatment is necessary.

Treatment Description

Treatment protocols need to be standardized and performed in a variety of settings based on case mix and therapeutic expertise. Pharmacologic treatment is dose-dependent and varies in terms of efficacy, tolerance, and side effects. Studies have been done using diazepam, baclofen, dantrolene, tizanidine, and other related medications.[12,13] Phase II studies (those first conducted in clinical subjects) evaluate the safety and determine dose and frequency of administration. Phase III studies (those conducted based on a safe dose determined from Phase II studies) evaluate the efficacy in larger, often multicenter populations. Where possible, the dosage should be standardized. In spasticity, a dose-titration may be necessary to produce the desired effects. Adequate guidelines for administration based on response must be determined and described.

Physical therapy is somewhat individualized, but methods and intensity are programmatic. Crucial methods necessary for muscle training need to be specified so they can be replicated. While casting and splinting is somewhat device dependent, specifications for application and duration are needed. Surgical interventions such as dorsal rhizotomy are technique dependent and surgeon specific. Methods developed by surgical investigators are typically evaluated in nonrandomized studies with historical controls, and very few are assessed in randomized trials. The uncontrolled studies within institutions have shown an improvement in gait and function.[14] However, investigators should be trained to replicate the technique so that it can be evaluated with larger, more generalizable populations. Objective measures, such as electromyography, are needed to determine efficacy of surgical techniques. Standard preintervention care and postintervention care should be specified and evaluated. Decision trees need to be done to document the selection, based on prior therapy and patient characteristics.

Outcome Assessment

Outcome must focus on the goal. Improvement in performance, function, and quality of life are primary objectives.[15]

Technical outcomes need to be evaluated to determine if the treatment has brought about the desired mechanistic change, for example, muscle tone and strength. Similarly, safety studies should investigate short-term and long-term complications. Functional outcomes can be assessed through such measures as walking ability, range of motion, and performance of daily activities. Functional components, such as hip subluxation and pain relief, are also important. Measurement must be objective, and blinding is often impossible. Use of standard developmental indices facilitates assessment versus normal development as well as interstudy comparisons. An example of such a scale is the Bayley Index.[16] Independent evaluations using either technology-dependent methods, such as gait analysis, or blinded evaluators are needed before and after treatment.

Long-term function must also be assessed: Has the outcome for the intervention led to improved performance in motor skills 5 to 10 years later? Has the psychosocial environment been benefited by the intervention in the interaction with parents, with siblings, and with classmates, and has there been improvement in self-esteem and general measures of quality of life? Quality of life outcomes in children are important measures of spasticity interventions because they measure the social and functional adaptation resulting from the therapy. Three assessments are possible: (1) childhood developmental change, (2) parental concept of change, and (3) clinician's or professional's concept of change.[17]

Assessment of childhood development presents a problem because it involves measurement of a moving target. Psychosocial measures may be more suited for long-term assessment, for example, when the child reaches teenage years. Parental satisfaction may be a reflection of the child's performance and happiness, but it also may reflect the parents' desired goals for the therapy. The clinician or professional may assess the neurodevelopment, the cognitive development, and the social development of the child as well as his/her interaction with parents and peers. Standard measures for these observational evaluations should be developed and used. In general, the timing (age of the child) of the quality of life assessment and the person doing it need to be considered in the evaluation of long-term effects.

Another outcome measure is the cost-effectiveness of the therapy. The cost of the procedures and related therapy is evaluated in terms of the benefit obtained versus the cost of the disability left untreated. Direct short-term costs of surgical procedures must be compared to long-term cost of physical therapy or pharmacologic treatment. Indirect costs of family support, transportation, and lost income must be included in the evaluation. These measures may be used to determine the net worth of interventions.

Study Designs

Many treatment evaluation studies use a pre-post, prospective design. The pretreatment evaluation and posttreatment change are compared, and if a positive difference is found the treatment is considered suggestive of improved function or performance. These designs measure technical or mechanistic change in function, for example, tone, strength, or gait, because the design uses the subject as his/her own control and minimizes subject variation. An estimate of a certain magnitude of change is needed to estimate the sample size.

Unless there is a control group that underwent either no treatment, sham treatment, or standard treatment, comparisons of functional outcome may be affected by other factors influencing development. Control groups allow for the simultaneous evaluation of change. Few studies have used a standard treatment as control with random assignment. These studies are necessary to gauge how much improvement new interventions will achieve compared to standard therapies as well as to lessen the bias of subject selection. Sample sizes need to be determined based on the difference expected in the primary functional assessment.

Palmer and associates[18] performed a model randomized study of physical therapy. Background and functional characteristics were compared at baseline and demonstrated the adequacy of randomization. Functional assessments, including measures of motor skills and developmental status, were done at fixed intervals. These measures were compared in groups undergoing standard neurodevelopmental therapy or a play session, and the results favored the group involved in the play session.

Crossover studies for spasticity control are feasible and have been used for reversible interventions. In particular, physical therapy and pharmacologic therapies have been evaluated using these methods. These studies can be very powerful, precision versus sample size, in evaluating mechanistic and short-term control of spasticity. They do not provide, however, the long-term evaluation or final therapeutic dosage needed to evaluate long-term toxicity and benefit.

Conclusions

Designs of spasticity intervention studies need to be goal oriented. Similar to goals set for individual patients, trial of interventions need short-term and long-term goals as criteria for success. Preintervention-postintervention differences are suggestive but not necessarily reflective of improvement on goal accomplishment. Studies evaluating effectiveness need to use: (1) a standard definition of spasticity; (2)

uniform criteria for selection of subjects who are expected to benefit from therapy; (3) a standard measure of severity of spasticity for baseline assessment; (4) uniform data collection tools including pretherapy assessment of spasticity and prognostic factors; (5) a description of treatment and variation of application; (6) a description of necessary continued or supportive care; (7) assessment of complications and therapeutic failures; and (8) uniform or standardized outcome measures of mechanism, function, disability, quality of life, and cost.

Achieving a multidisciplinary consensus for standard classifications and assessments is difficult. Advances in technological assessment of spasticity through gait analysis have improved the measurement of therapeutic change. However, assessment of change varies from investigator to investigator. Randomized studies of various alternatives, for example, orthopaedic and neurosurgical procedures, must be undertaken to determine the appropriate decision based on the patient's needs. These studies need to include evaluation of long-term outcomes to determine if short-term gains in tone reduction and gait improvement are sustained and are better than improvements determined by the natural history and/or the clinical course with alternative managements. Quality of life measures need to be used to determine whether the procedures improve the social and mental well-being in children with spasticity. While the initial question open to investigation may be whether the therapy reduces spasticity and improves function; the final question of which therapy is the best choice for a child, his/her parents, and the clinician needs to be answered.

References

1. Simeonsson RJ, Cooper DH, Scheiner AP: A review and analysis of the effectiveness or early intervention programs. *Pediatrics* 1982;69:635–641.
2. Parette HP Jr, Hourcade JJ: A review of therapeutic intervention research on gross and fine motor progress in young children with cerebral palsy. *Am J Occup Ther* 1984;38:462–468.
3. Harris SR: Early intervention for children with motor handicaps, in Guralnick MJ, Bennett FG (eds): *The Effectiveness of Early Intervention*, Orlando, FL, Academic Press, 1987, pp 175–212.
4. Brown E: Diagnostic and therapeutic technology assessment (DATTA): Dorsal rhizotomy. *JAMA* 1990;264:2569–2574.
5. Evans P, Elliott M, Alberman E, et al: Prevalence and disabilities in 4 to 8 year olds with cerebral palsy. *Arch Dis Child* 1985;60:940–945.
6. Nelson KB, Ellenberg JH: Children who 'outgrew' cerebral palsy. *Pediatrics* 1982;69:529–536.
7. Ashworth B: Preliminary trial of carisoprodol in multiple sclerosis. *Practitioner* 1964;192:540–542.
8. Gage JR, Fabian D, Hicks R, et al: Pre- and postoperative gait analysis in patients with spastic diplegia: A preliminary report. *J Pediatr Orthop* 1984;4: 715–725.
9. Vaughan CL, Berman B, du Toit LL, et al: Gait analysis of spastic children before and after selective lumbar rhizotomy. *Dev Med Child Neurol* 1987;29: 25.
10. Vaughan CL, Berman B, Peacock WJ: Cerebral palsy and rhizotomy: A 3-year follow-up evaluation with gait analysis. *J Neurosurg* 1991;74:178–184.

11. Albright AL, Cervi A, Singletary J: Intrathecal baclofen for spasticity in cerebral palsy. *JAMA* 1991;265:1418–1422.

12. Delwaide P: Oral treatment of spasticity with current muscle relaxants, in Marsden CD (ed): *Treating Spasticity: Pharmacological Advances.* Lewiston, NY, Hogrefe and Huber Publishers, 1989, pp 31–37.

13. Whyte J, Robinson KM: Pharmacologic management, in Glenn MB, Whyte J (eds): *The Practical Management of Spasticity in Children and Adults.* Philadelphia, Lea & Febiger, 1990, pp 201–226.

14. Peacock WJ, Staudt LA: Functional outcomes following selective posterior rhizotomy in children with cerebral palsy. *J Neurosurg* 1991;74:380–385.

15. Goldberg M: Measuring outcomes in cerebral palsy. *J Pediatr Orthop* 1991;11: 682–685.

16. Bayley N: *Bayley Scales of Infant Development.* New York, The Psychological Corporation, 1969.

17. Rosenbaum P, Cadman D, Kirpalani H: Pediatrics: Assessing quality of life, in Spilker B (ed): *Quality of Life Assessments in Clinical Trials.* New York, Raven Press, 1990, pp 205–216.

18. Palmer FB, Shapiro BK, Wachtel RC, et al: The effects of physical therapy on cerebral palsy: A controlled trial in infants with spastic diplegia. *N Engl J Med* 1988;318:803–808.

Chapter 10

Clinically Based Outcomes for Children With Cerebral Palsy: Issues in the Measurement of Function

Peter L. Rosenbaum, MD, FRCP(C)

Measuring clinical function ought to be a straightforward task. In general, clinicians have a clear idea of what they want to know, and can define the domains of behavior they wish to assess. Clinicians are usually aware of gradations in function, and they regularly attempt to quantitate status. For example, they speak of mild, moderate, and severe cerebral palsy, even if these terms are imprecise. When they evaluate change over time, clinicians know what constitutes improvement or deterioration in function and, in fact, usually look specifically for these indicators of change, based on their own knowledge of the clinical conditions with which they work. Finally, clinicians believe they know which qualitative indicators are important, as well as the quantitative changes they wish to promote.

Why, then, do physicians and therapists not do a better job when it comes to measuring function and functional change in children with cerebral palsy? I believe that we have only begun to understand the science and principles of clinical measurement; that is, how to construct an instrument for measuring a specific function, test it, and ensure that the measurements it provides are valid. In the absence of such understanding, several areas of confusion may arise that interfere with the ability to achieve a reliable and valid quantitation of the functional or behavioral phenomena of interest.

This chapter will address four issues in the development and application of clinical measures as they pertain to the evaluation of motor function in cerebral palsy: (1) the structure and functions of measures, (2) the strengths and limitations of norm-referenced and criterion-referenced tests, (3) the ability to recognize whether a measure is used to describe what is being measured or to explain it, and (4) the challenges of assessing qualitative as well as quantitative dimensions of motor function in cerebral palsy.

Structure and Function of Measures

In recent years a number of useful texts,[1-4] reports,[5] and journal articles[6-9] have become available to clinicians interested in the creation and uses of clinical measures. The paper by Kirschner and Guyatt[6] has been of particular use to me and is reviewed briefly here.

Kirschner and Guyatt[6] identify three purposes to which a clinical measure may be put: discrimination, prediction, and evaluation. A discriminative measure may be used to distinguish between people with and without a condition, or with varying degrees of that condition. For example, the Peabody Developmental Motor Scales[10] are used to categorize children's motor function using percentile rank scores, standard scores, or age-equivalent scores. A predictive measure classifies people into categories of expected future status based on current or past functional ability. Bleck's[11] scale predicts ambulation at age 7 in children with cerebral palsy on the basis of specific neuromotor functions in the preschool years. An evaluative measure is used to assess the presence and amount of change in function over time. The Gross Motor Function Measure (GMFM)[12] quantitates change in motor function of children with cerebral palsy.

Clinical measures are generally created and field tested specifically for discrimination, prediction, or evaluation, and a measure intended for one purpose cannot be used for another without clear evidence that it is capable of fulfilling that additional function.[5,8] For example, the Peabody Scales[10] can discriminate children's motor functional abilities, but the Peabody manual provides no evidence that these scales can be used to evaluate change over time. (The existence of earlier information[13] that provides evidence that the Peabody Scales can be put to the latter use only serves as a reminder that it is necessary to obtain the most recent information about the performance characteristics of a clinical measure.) The creation and validation of a clinical measure require clear definition of the domain(s) to be assessed, selection of relevant items, development of a scaling (measuring) system, and establishment of the reliability (consistency) and validity (truth) of the measure in a scientifically credible manner. For evaluative measures, which are particularly needed in clinical cerebral palsy work, the validation step involves establishing that the measure can, indeed, detect clinically meaningful change in function.[8,12]

A simple mechanical example may illustrate the argument about the need to be certain that the measure is equal to the task to which it is being put. In order to undo a screw, one needs a screwdriver. A flat-head screwdriver will work on both conventional and +-shaped screws, while a +-shaped screwdriver will work only on the +-shaped screw, and a Phillips screwdriver will work on neither. All three tools are screwdrivers, but although they have been created to do a similar task (inserting and removing screws), there is a greater or lesser degree of structural specificity to them that makes them more or less capable of working across different tasks.

In summary, it is essential to be precise about what aspect of clinical function is to be measured, and then to find or create instruments capable of making that specific measurement. Several tailor-made evaluative instruments for assessing gross motor function,[12,14] gross motor performance,[15] and upper extremity skills[16] have either recently appeared or will soon be published. These measures illustrate clearly that it is possible to design and evaluate clinically-based instruments for specific populations of interest.

Norm-Referenced and Criterion-Referenced Tests

A fundamentally important issue in clinical measurement concerns the basis on which an individual's performance is judged. Most of the standardized measures of motor function that have been used to assess children with cerebral palsy are norm-referenced tests.[10,17-20] That is, they have been developed and field tested on populations of children, and patterns of response have been established for these populations, which were made up, almost entirely, of children with normal motor function. Generally, the response patterns are subdivided by gender and age, factors recognized as especially important determinants of the level of performance in many dimensions of function, so that a particular child's score can be related to ''norms'' thought to be appropriate as a basis of comparison. The quantified performance of a specific child is usually transformed in some statistically appropriate manner, and may then be presented as an age-equivalent, as a percentile standing, or as a standard score.

Norm-referenced tests can help to identify the presence of a problem, at least insofar as scores outside of the ''normal'' range classify a subject as abnormal. Information from a norm-referenced test can be useful for diagnostic (discriminative) purposes and, thus, potentially for classification, treatment planning, and quantification of degrees of difference from the norm.

There are, however, several limitations to the use of norm-referenced tests for children in special populations.[8,21,22] Most obvious is the fact that the normative population on which the measure is first developed generally includes normal children and often specifically excludes children with problems.[10,17] Thus, use of many of the popular motor assessments of children may result in invidious comparisons between apparently normal and clearly abnormal children. Rarely have norms been developed with and for a special population. (An example of such norms are the growth charts for children with Down Syndrome.[23])

Because cerebral palsy is a heterogeneous group of disorders relative to anatomic distribution and clinical severity, as well as basic clinical dysfunctions, the idea of developing norms for children with this condition is especially daunting. The content of a motor function measure designed for normal children is not likely to be appropriate and applicable to children with cerebral palsy who have dysfunctions in the domain of gross motor function. Furthermore, using norm-referenced tests with children who are substantially different from those on whom the test was developed, presumes that ''normal'' development or function is the only appropriate type of development. This serves to stigmatize and discredit the alternate pathways to achievement so often followed by disabled children.

In addition, many norm-referenced tests of motor function used to evaluate change in motor performance of children with cerebral palsy[10,17–20] have been created as discriminative rather than evaluative measures.[8] This gives rise to a legitimate concern about the validity of judgments made on the basis of score changes in measures that have not been formally shown to be capable of actually measuring change.

An alternative approach to functional assessment of children is the use of criterion-referenced tests. These are measures that have been created to assess individual performance against preset criteria, often performance units of activity. Anastasi[1] believes that criterion-referenced tests are analogous to mastery tests used to evaluate job proficiency in industry. Interest is focused on an individual's capacity to achieve a criterion level of performance rather than on that individual's performance in comparison with others.

According to Anastasi,[1] "A fundamental requirement in constructing this kind of test is a clearly defined domain of knowledge or skills to be assessed by the test. If scores on such a test are to have communicable meaning, the content domain to be sampled must be widely recognized as important." She goes on to point out that comparisons between subjects are much less important than in norm-referenced tests. By implication, change scores of criterion-referenced tests are particularly meaningful when an individual is reassessed on a set of activities previously evaluated, particularly if varying degrees of completion of a task are clearly defined and measurable. Three recent examples of criterion-referenced tests are the Gross Motor Function Measure,[12] the Pediatric Evaluation of Disability Index,[14] and the Quality of Upper Extremity Skills Test.[16] It is clear, however, that there is enormous need for many more such instruments.

Description or Explanation?

Clinical investigators are often eager to both describe and explain clinical phenomena, and these differences of purpose may lead to problems in measurement. Sackett[24] warns against getting caught in what he refers to as the substitution game, whereby what is measured is a surrogate of what really ought to be measured.

For example, if the stated purpose of selective dorsal rhizotomy is to improve gross motor function in the child with cerebral palsy, then simply measuring range of motion at hip, knee, and ankle or assessing spasticity with the Ashworth Scale[25] misses the point. While these clinical phenomena are important and certainly should be evaluated, it is essential that a functional motor measure be used to assess whether selective dorsal rhizotomy actually leads to improved function.

Increased range of motion and/or decreased spasticity may be explanatory factors that contribute to an understanding of how selective dorsal rhizotomy works or how motor function improves. However, changes in either range of motion or spasticity without a clinically relevant change in motor function could not be claimed as evidence of the success of selective dorsal rhizotomy in improving gross motor function in cerebral palsy. The use of these surrogate measures would be an example of the substitution game. Furthermore, it is at least theoretically possible that selective dorsal rhizotomy might improve motor function without altering range of motion or spasticity. This would be important to know, because it would imply that the way in which selective dorsal rhizotomy induces changes is not specifically related to these explanatory variables.

It is obviously important and ethically responsible to measure and evaluate aspects of function that are important to children with cerebral palsy and their parents. Thus, while range of motion may be significant to a clinician investigator, improved gait may be what the child hopes for. Hence the content of clinical measures must include elements relevant to the experiences and expectations of those who are measured.

Clinicians must decide in advance what they want to measure and for what purpose, and they must then be prepared to be honest about the findings. Explanation is important, but it is not a substitute for an assessment of the clinical phenomena under study.

Measuring Quality and Quantity

To date most measures of motor abilities have assessed function quantitatively.[26] Higher scores usually imply that the child does more of that function, with little if any reference to the quality of the performance. This represents a serious limitation in the available measures, because therapeutic endeavors whether treatment is physical, surgical, electrical, or pharmacologic are intended to improve quality as well as amount of function. Because abnormalities in the nature of motor performance are inherent in cerebral palsy, clinicians are always at least implicitly interested in improving the quality of that performance. Physicians and therapists talk of smoother or less awkward gait; they look for better upper limb control; they focus on alignment, weight shift, and coordination among other attributes of motor function. Each of these is at least as much a qualitative as a quantitative feature of motor behavior.

Bertoti[27] explicitly refers to the need for measures that go beyond the strictly quantitative. In discussing the clinical gait analysis results of her study of short leg casting, she notes that "subjectively the therapists in this study observed additional proximal changes exhibited by the casted children *that could not be documented by this measure*" (author's emphasis). Thus, even when an intervention leads to measurable quantitative improvements in motor function, there is a sense that other changes (improvements) are occurring that current clinical measures are unable to capture. A recent study examining both quantitative and qualitative dimensions of motor behavior in the spastic upper extremity is reported by Law and associates.[28] The investigators specifically created a measure[16] to capture aspects of performance they recognized would be missed by existing instruments.

The Motor Measures Group at McMaster University has endeavored for several years to create and validate the Gross Motor Performance Measure (GMPM),[15] a companion instrument to the Gross Motor Function Measure (GMFM),[12] in which the focus was strictly on quantity of change in motor function in children with cerebral palsy. The idea for the GMPM was to take a high-powered view of a selected sample of GMFM items, and to subject them to a systematic assessment of several carefully chosen qualitative attributes that the group believes lend themselves to quantification. If it is indeed possible to measure qualitative changes in motor performance with this and other measures, physicians and therapists may begin to understand what and how changes happen as a result of the many interventions used in treating children with cerebral palsy.

Creation of the GMPM has been an international collaboration by clinical experts,[15] and it illustrates both the complexity of the challenge and the feasibility of using scientifically credible techniques to define, choose, and then apply qualitative attributes of motor function in cerebral palsy to the development of an evaluative measure. In effect, the GMPM quantitates quality, providing a step toward satisfying the enormous need for measures that will enable clinical experts to assess comprehensively all the changes in motor function that they believe can be produced by their interventions in cerebral palsy.

Afterthoughts

Measurement development is usually time-consuming and expensive, and it is rarely as exciting to granting agencies as an intervention study. This consideration, as much as any other, probably contributes to the relative paucity of excellent clinical measures available for assessing change in the complex disorders called cerebral palsy. All clinical investigators in this field must support the need for further creation, development, testing, and dissemination of reliable, valid, and responsive clinical measures of motor function in cerebral palsy. Only with such tools will they be able to evaluate critically whether the many established and new therapies for cerebral palsy actually do more good than harm.

Finally, a word about the ethics of measurement is certainly in order. It is all too easy to measure characteristics, functions, or behaviors, and then forget to inform parents, and children where feasible, of the results. Measuring clinical phenomena can be a powerful and at times frightening process, fraught with implications about how a child measures up and is progressing.

Clinical investigators need to be aware of several obligations. They must use instruments reliably and validly, in the way the instruments were developed, if they intend to apply appropriately the results the measure will provide. They should not use parts of a measure, or apply their own rules to the way they use it, and then expect that measure to perform according to specifications. Finally, they should share their findings with the people they assess, and they should interpret these findings in an honest and compassionate manner. Bald numbers rarely tell a full story and clinical sensitivity in the interpretation of results is vital.

References

1. Anastasi A: *Psychological Testing*, ed 6. New York, MacMillan Publishing, 1988.
2. McDowell I, Newell C: *Measuring Health: A Guide to Rating Scales and Questionnaires*. Oxford, Oxford University Press, 1987.
3. Streiner DL, Norman GR: *Health Measurement Scales: A Practical Guide to Their Development and Use*. Oxford, Oxford University Press, 1989.
4. King-Thomas L, Hacker BJ (eds): *A Therapist's Guide to Pediatric Assessment*. Boston, Little, Brown, 1987.
5. Gowland C, King G, King S, et al: Review of selected measures in neurodevelopmental rehabilitation: A rational approach for selecting clinical measures. *Research Report #91–2*. Hamilton, ON, Neurodevelopmental Clinical Research Unit, 1991.
6. Kirschner B, Guyatt GH: A methodologic framework for assessing health indices. *J Chronic Dis* 1985;38:27–36.
7. Guyatt G, Walter S, Norman G: Measuring change over time: Assessing the usefulness of evaluative instruments. *J Chronic Dis* 1987;40:171–180.
8. Rosenbaum PL, Cadman D, Russell D, et al: Issues in measuring change in motor function in children with cerebral palsy: A special communication. *Phys Ther* 1990;70:125–131.
9. Law M: Criteria for the evaluation of measurement instruments. *Can J Occup Ther* 1987;54:121–127.
10. Folio RM, Fewell RF: *Peabody Developmental Motor Scales*. Allen, TX, DLM Teaching Resources, 1983.
11. Bleck EE: Locomotor prognosis in cerebral palsy. *Dev Med Child Neurol* 1975;17:18–25.
12. Russell DJ, Rosenbaum PL, Cadman DT, et al: The gross motor function measure: A means to evaluate the effects of physical therapy. *Dev Med Child Neurol* 1989;31:341–352.
13. Dubose RF, Folio R: Investigation of short-term gains in motor skill achievement in delayed and non-delayed preschool children. *Peabody J Ed* 1977;54:181–184.
14. Haley SM, Faas RM, Coster WJ, et al: *Pediatric Evaluation of Disability Inventory*. Boston, New England Medical Center, 1989.
15. Boyce W, Gowland C, Hardy S, et al: Development of a quality-of-movement measure for children with cerebral palsy. *Phys Ther* 1991;71:820–832.
16. DeMatteo C, Law M, Russell D, et al: *Quality of Upper Extremity Skill Test Manual*. Hamilton, ON, Neurodevelopmental Clinical Research Unit, 1991.
17. Bayley N: *Bayley Scales of Infant Development*. New York, The Psychological Corporation, 1969.
18. Bruininks RH: *Bruininks-Oseretsky Test of Motor Proficiency: Examiner's Manual*. Circle Pines, MN, American Guidance Service, 1978.
19. Hoskins TA, Squires JE: Developmental assessment: A test for gross motor and reflex development. *Phys Ther* 1973;53:117–126.
20. Frankenburg WK, Dobbs JB, Fandel AW: *Denver Developmental Screening Test*. Denver, University of Colorado Medical Center, 1970.
21. McCauley R J, Swisher L: Use and misuse of norm-referenced tests in clinical assessment: A hypothetical case. *J Sp Hear Dis* 1984;49:338–348.

22. Montgomery PC, Connolly BH: Norm-referenced and criterion-referenced tests. Use in pediatrics and application to task analysis of motor skill. *Phys Ther* 1987;67:1873–1876.

23. Cronk C, Crocker AC, Pueschel SM, et al: Growth charts for children with Down Syndrome: 1 month to 18 years of age. *Pediatrics* 1988;81:102–110.

24. Sackett DL, Haynes RB, Tugwell P: *Clinical Epidemiology. A Basic Science for Clinical Medicine.* Boston, Little, Brown, 1985.

25. Ashworth B: Preliminary trial of carisoprodol in multiple sclerosis. *Practitioner* 1964;192:540–542.

26. Boyce W, Gowland C, Rosenbaum P, et al: Measuring quality of movement in cerebral palsy: A review of instruments. *Phys Ther* 1991;71:813–819.

27. Bertoti DB: Effect of short leg casting on ambulation in children with cerebral palsy. *Phys Ther* 1986;66:1522–1529.

28. Law M, Cadman D, Rosenbaum P, et al: Neurodevelopmental therapy and upper-extremity inhibitive casting for children with cerebral palsy. *Dev Med Child Neurol* 1991;33:379–387.

Chapter 11

Outcome Assessment in Cerebral Palsy: Has Walking Improved?

David H. Sutherland, MD

Introduction

A dominant medical theme of the decade of the nineties is outcome assessment. Funding agencies, governmental bodies, specialty societies, and practicing clinicians are increasingly aware that answers are mandatory regarding outcome of medical treatment. We want to know how our patients differ following treatment and whether or not they are functionally improved. It is well known that ambulatory cerebral palsy patients walk differently following surgical treatment, but whether they are improved can be challenged. Gait analysis has undergone a very great transformation in the last two decades with the development of automated movement measurement systems, improved electromyography and force measuring techniques, and rapid computer processing of the data.[1-4] Improvements in technology have led to an improved understanding of human gait and offer the possibility of obtaining scientific answers to replace subjective evaluations of outcome. This task is so important that every clinical gait laboratory should dedicate substantial effort to it. It is the primary reason for their existence. Clinicians without access to gait laboratories are handicapped as far as contributing in the area of documenting gait abnormalities before and after treatment. However, they should be willing partners, not foes, of the documentative effort, because all will benefit from published information on this crucial subject.

The most important question to be asked in a gait outcome study is: Can the subject walk with less effort after treatment? A related question is: Does the subject actually walk more following treatment? The latter question takes our quest for information outside of the gait laboratory into the home and community and opens avenues for clinicians without access to gait laboratories. A great deal of important information can come from simple studies that document changes in the quantity of daily walking after treatment.

The gait laboratory can offer vital information about the effort of walking.

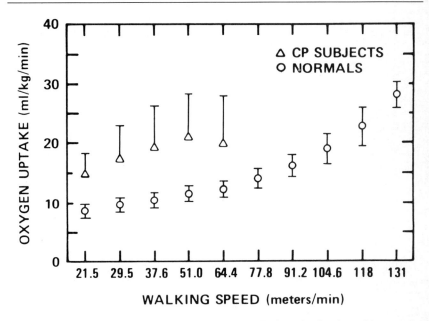

Fig. 1 *Oxygen uptake plotted against walking speed of cerebral palsy subjects and normal controls. (Reproduced with permission from Rose et al.[8])*

Oxygen Consumption and Oxygen Cost

To understand the physiology underlying energy studies of walking it is essential to understand the concepts involved in the analysis of oxygen consumption, which is expressed in ml/kg/minute, and oxygen cost, which is expressed in ml/kg/meter. Both normal subjects and patients with cerebral palsy tend to naturally select a walking speed that maintains an aerobic state of metabolism, minimizing oxygen consumption (Fig. 1). Data on oxygen consumption of normal children between the ages of 6 and 19 years indicate that the mean rate of oxygen uptake for children is significantly greater for teenage subjects than for younger children (Fig. 2). The oxygen cost to walk a unit distance (meter) is also higher in children 6 to 12 than in adolescent subjects from the ages of 13 to 19 (Table 1). It has been proven experimentally that both very slow and fast walking increase energy consumption, and that subjects who are not intent on accomplishing a time-related task will naturally select a walking speed that is most efficient from the standpoint of oxygen consumption.[5-10] Subjects with cerebral palsy walk more slowly than normal subjects to achieve the same end, ie, to avoid the discomfort of anaerobic walking.[8] These simple concepts are fundamental in evaluating walking outcome in the context of energy expended.

The accurate measurement of oxygen consumption, after the subject has achieved steady state (usually 3 minutes), with the subject walking

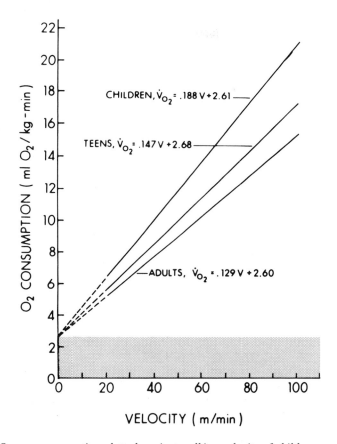

Fig. 2 *Oxygen consumption plotted against walking velocity of children ages 6 to 12 years, adolescents 13 to 19 years, and adults. (Reproduced with permission from Waters et al.[10])*

at a self-selected speed, can be used to calculate both the oxygen consumption rate (ml/kg/minute) and oxygen cost or energy cost (ml/kg/meter). This measurement remains the standard against which other methods for measuring the ease of walking must be compared.[5,7–11] This is the positive side of the application of this measurement technique. The negative side is that the equipment is cumbersome, a large space must be available for achieving the steady state unless a treadmill is used, and many subjects with cerebral palsy have great difficulty in walking on a treadmill and/or in using the mouthpiece. A further drawback is that, because information gained through the measurement of oxygen consumption does not supplant the kinematic and kinetic data required for treatment planning, the cost of gathering oxygen consumption data is added to the already considerable costs of gait analysis. These facts have limited the use of this important scientific technique

Table 1 Energy Expenditure of Customary Normal Walking

	O_2 Cost (ml/kg-m)*	
	Children (6–12 yr)	Teens (13–19 yr)
Female	0.217	0.172
	0.040	0.015
Male	0.224	0.181
	0.030	0.025
Total	0.221	0.176**
	0.035	0.020

(Adapted with permission from Waters et al.[10])
*Mean and 1 SD
**Significant (p < 0.05) difference between preceding value in younger age group

to a small number of centers. Fortunately, there are other methods to approach the problem of measuring energy expenditure in walking.

Energy Expenditure as Measured by the Force Plate

Newton's third law of motion states ''To every action there is always opposed an equal reaction: or, the mutual actions of two bodies upon each other are always equal, and directed to contrary parts.''[12] The extent to which a force plate illustrates the truth of this law can easily be demonstrated. By increasing the gain of the force plate, the heart beat of a subject standing motionless on the plate is recorded as vertical force. The upward surge of blood brought about by ventricular contraction produces a downward reaction detected by the force plate. Because the force plate faithfully records the summation of the interaction of all of the body segments, the output of the force plate can give powerful information about energy expenditure.

Cavagna[13] is credited with adapting the use of force measurements to energy calculations in walking. To do this properly he found it necessary to collect two consecutive steps, and a long force plate was designed for this purpose. Some time ago, in my laboratory, energy output was calculated using a modification of Cavagna's technique.[3] The steps used to calculate energy output were as follows: (1) Convert the vertical force and fore-aft shear output from percentage of body weight to instantaneous acceleration, using data from left and right cycles. (2) Integrate the acceleration curves to obtain velocities in the vertical and horizontal directions. (3) Integrate the vertical velocity curve to obtain the vertical displacement of the center of mass. (4) Calculate the kinetic energy in the vertical and horizontal directions and the potential energy. (5) Total the kinetic and potential energies for each 1% interval of the cycle to obtain instantaneous total energy. (6) Total the positive changes in total energy to find the amount of energy expended by the subject.

My laboratory introduced two major modifications into Cavagna's technique. He used data from two consecutive steps on his long force plate, but we had to use data from two different walk cycles because our single-step force plate was smaller. We also used movie film, instead of photocells and light beams, to measure velocity and cycle-timing events. We temporarily ceased using this method of energy measurement because of the possible inaccuracies that can be introduced by using data from two different walk cycles. The addition of one more force plate or pressure pad to our present complement of two force plates would greatly enhance the use of this measurement technique. The method has appeal because it can be made a routine part of gait analysis, but only for subjects who do not require walking aids. The principles of this method have also been used to give a kinetic analysis of the center of gravity in normal and pathologic gait.[14]

Walking Velocity

Walking velocity has been shown to be closely related to energy consumption in both normal subjects and those with cerebral palsy. As I have already noted, both types of subjects adjust their self-selected walking speed to conserve energy.[8] Walking velocity—routinely measured in all gait laboratories—can easily be measured in a nonlaboratory setting by using a stopwatch to determine the time required for progression over a measured distance.

Heart Rate

Another parameter related to energy expenditure is heart rate. Rose and associates[8] have investigated the relationship of heart rate to oxygen consumption both for children with cerebral palsy and for normal children. They found that oxygen consumption and heart rate were related in a linear fashion throughout a wide range of walking speeds (Fig. 3). They concluded that heart rate, which is easily measured, can be used as an index of energy expenditure. I have no personal experience with the use of this methodology. However, it is appealing because of its simplicity. The limiting condition for use of heart rate as an index of energy expenditure is development of the anaerobic state. If aerobic capacity is exceeded, oxygen debt occurs and the heart rate is no longer an indicator of energy expenditure. Other factors that can produce inaccuracies are anxiety or emotional stress. These conditions can be observed and usually can be prevented by allowing time for familiarization with the laboratory environment.

Dynamic Joint Angles

Kinematic studies of changes in joint angles, which are now routinely used in most fully equipped and staffed gait laboratories, can help to pinpoint the changes in movements between segments and are crucial in obtaining an overall picture of gait symmetry. The dynamic joint angles provide information about function as well as appearance or

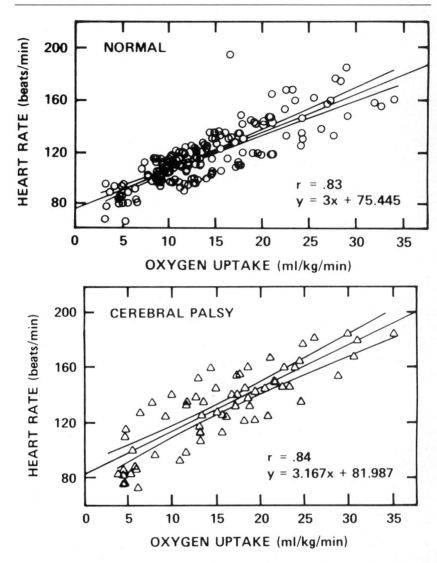

Fig. 3 *Heart rate plotted against oxygen uptake in normal children (**top**) and in patients with cerebral palsy (**bottom**). (Reproduced with permission from Rose et al.[8])*

cosmesis. For example, the individual who maintains exaggerated hip flexion throughout stance (Fig. 4) is likely to have, as a consequence of restricted hip extension, limited stride length as well as unsightly lordosis and increased knee flexion in the stance phase.

Joint Moments and Powers

Joint moment is the product of the forces of gravity and inertia and the lever arm (Fig. 5).[15] Joint moment can be determined by measuring

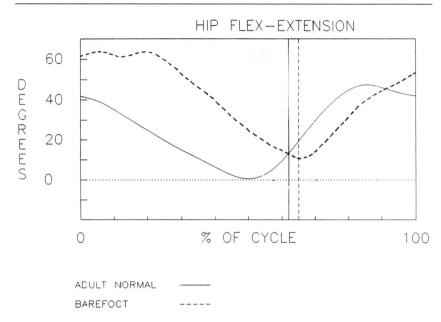

Fig. 4 *Dynamic hip flexion-extension joint angle of patient with cerebral palsy of the spastic diplegic type. Note exaggerated hip flexion throughout the joint cycle. (From San Diego Children's Hospital Motion Analysis Laboratory.)*

the magnitude and direction of the ground-reaction force and calculating its perpendicular distance from the joint center (Fig. 6). Inclusion of the contribution of the centers of inertia of the distal segments, often neglected, has been strongly recommended by Winter.[16] The calculation of joint moments extends the value of force measurements beyond that of giving information about the whole body center of mass. The calculation of joint moments is helpful in the analysis of function at the level of joints. The orthopaedic surgeon planning treatment of a subject with cerebral palsy examines function at individual joints to select intervention measures. It is logical that a calculation of joint moments will aid in this planning, and that a reexamination of the same joint moments should be made after treatment to determine the outcome. In the past, this capability was present largely as a research effort, but software packages are now available that provide moment measurements and power calculations along with dynamic joint angles and force.

Some problems remain. The accurate determination of joint center is still elusive, and small errors in joint center position cause serious errors in joint moment calculations, particularly at the level of the hip joint. Another problem is that the centers of inertia used in the moment calculations are taken from normal values and no consideration is given to disease-induced alterations in segment size or composition. To eliminate this problem it will be necessary to develop an accurate, cost-effective method of estimating the volume of the individual body segments. Work is going forward in this area. While measurement of the

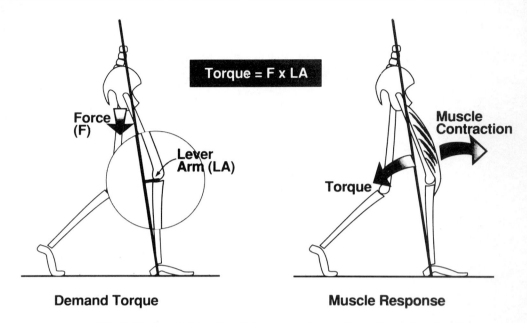

Fig. 5 *Extrinsic joint torque (joint moment) at the knee. (Reproduced with permission from Perry.[15])*

volume will not answer questions about relative composition, it will eliminate a major source of error. Magnetic resonance imaging may provide ultimate answers about volume and composition; however, because of costs and the need for general anesthesia for small children, clinical application is not justified.

Winter[16] has emphasized the importance of joint power, which is defined as the product of angular velocity and joint moment (Fig. 7). The velocity is given a positive or negative sign indicating power absorption or power generation. For example, consider a knee moment tending to increase knee flexion and knee angular velocity directed toward increasing flexion. This indicates a power absorption state with the quadriceps (if active as shown by electromyography) absorbing power and acting eccentrically. While this same information can be gained by separately viewing dynamic joint angle and joint moment graphs, their combination is very helpful in rapidly appreciating eccentric and concentric action of muscles. To complete the analysis, dynamic electromyography is required to verify that the muscle or muscles in question are active.

Summary

There are now multiple methods of objectively determining the outcome of treatment in cerebral palsy. The motion analysis laboratory is

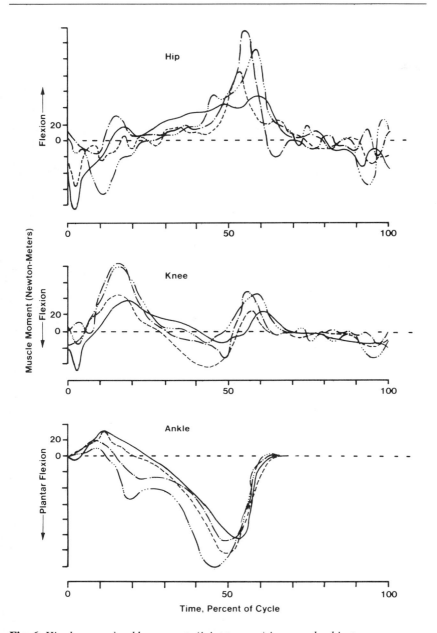

Fig. 6 *Hip, knee, and ankle moments (joint torques) in normal subjects. (Reproduced with permission from Inman et al.[6])*

indispensable in arriving at scientific documentation of walking function before and after treatment. The most frequently used evaluation techniques include kinematic measurements of time/distance parameters and dynamic joint angles. Walking velocity is particularly helpful

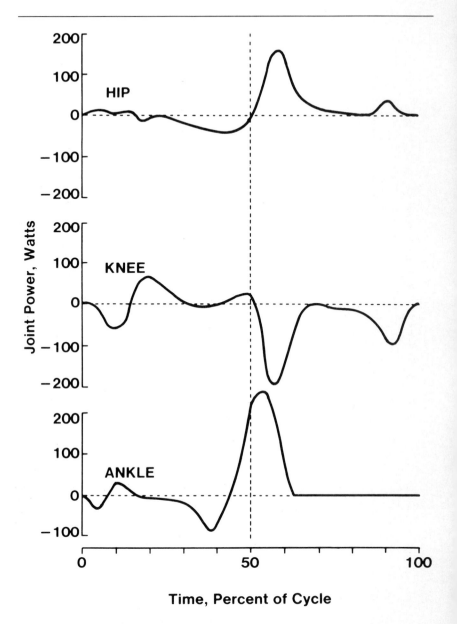

Fig. 7 *Joint powers (moment × angular velocity) of hip, knee, and ankle. (Reproduced with permission from Inman et al.[6])*

in determining outcome because it has been shown to be related to energy requirements. Both normal subjects and those with walking disorders tend to adopt an energy conserving walking speed to maintain a comfortable aerobic level of oxygen metabolism.

The measurement of dynamic joint angles gives invaluable information about function and cosmesis; however, the addition of dynamic electromyography and the calculation of joint moments and joint powers provide insights into the abnormal forces producing alterations of movements. The determination of oxygen consumption and oxygen cost provides the ultimate outcome information because they measure the energy required in walking. The complexity of equipment for measuring oxygen consumption and the difficulties that some patients have experienced in walking on a treadmill have made it necessary for this test to be performed in a relatively large area so that a steady state in level walking can be reached before measurement begins. These difficulties have hindered widespread use of oxygen measurements. Consequently, most of the studies reported have been supported by research funding. Heart rate measurements are easily obtained and there may be sufficient correlation with oxygen consumption to allow the substitution of this technique in routine clinical outcome studies. The work of walking can be calculated by measuring the difference between kinetic and potential energy for each 1% of the cycle after the method of Cavagna.[13]

Further validation of the outcome measures should be carried out, particularly heart rate and work of walking from force plate studies. Each laboratory should adopt the outcome measurements most compatible with their goals, capabilities, and the patient population that they serve.

References

1. Gage JR, Fabian D, Hicks R, et al: Pre- and postoperative gait analysis in patients with spastic diplegia: A preliminary report. *J Pediatr Orthop* 1984;4:715–725.
2. Sutherland DH: Gait analysis in cerebral palsy, review article. *Dev Med Child Neurol* 1978;20:807–813.
3. Sutherland DH, Cooper L, Daniel D: The role of the ankle plantar flexors in normal walking. *J Bone Joint Surg* 1980;62A:354–363.
4. Sutherland DH: *Gait Disorders in Childhood and Adolescence.* Baltimore, Williams & Wilkins, 1984.
5. Bard G, Ralston HJ: Measurement of energy expenditure during ambulation, with special reference to evaluation of assistive devices. *Arch Phys Med Rehabil* 1959;40:415–420.
6. Inman VT, Ralston HJ, Todd F: Energy expenditure, in Lieberman JC (ed): *Human Walking.* Baltimore, Williams & Wilkins, 1981, pp 63–77.
7. Ralston HJ: Energy-speed relation and optimal speed during level walking. *Int Ztschr Angen Physiol* 1958;17:277–283.
8. Rose J, Gamble JG, Medeiros J, et al: Energy cost of walking in normal children and in those with cerebral palsy: Comparison of heart rate and oxygen uptake. *J Pediatr Orthop* 1989;9:276–279.
9. Waters RL, Hyslop HJ, Campbell LT: Energy cost of walking in normal children and teenagers. *Dev Med Child Neurol* 1983;25:184–188.
10. Waters RL, Lunsford BR, Perry J, et al: Energy-speed relationship of walking: Standard tables. *J Orthop Res* 1988;6:215–222.
11. Torburn L, Perry J, Ayyappa E, et al: Below-knee amputee gait study with dynamic elastic response prosthetic feet: A pilot study. *J Rehabil Res Dev* 1990;27:369–384.

12. Newton I: Mathematical principles of natural philosophy, axioms, or laws of motion, in Hutchins RM (ed): *Great Books of the Western World*. Chicago, Britannica, 1952, vol 34, p 14.
13. Cavagna GA: Force platforms as ergometers. *J Appl Physiol* 1975;39:174–179.
14. Iida H, Yamamuro T: Kinetic analysis of the center of gravity of the human body in normal and pathological gaits. *J Biomech* 1987;20:987–995.
15. Perry J: *Gait Analysis: Normal and Pathological Function*. New York, McGraw-Hill, 1992, pp 413–429.
16. Winter DA: *Biomechanics and Motor Control of Human Movement*, ed 2. New York, John Wiley & Sons, 1990.

Consensus

Retrospective analysis of patients who have undergone a specific treatment for orthopaedic problems associated with neuromuscular disease is no longer sufficient. A wide variety of other factors must be brought into the equation before a treatment can be considered effective. In fact, four primary areas need to be addressed when assessing outcome: (1) the technical outcome; (2) the functional outcome; (3) patient satisfaction with the outcome; and (4) the cost of the procedure in the broadest sense.

Technical Outcome

Technical outcome is the usual focus of clinical research papers on evaluation of a treatment modality for children with cerebral palsy. The technical outcome can be assessed by follow-up physical examination, radiographic evaluation, gait analysis studies, and similar methods in which observations are made before and after the treatment. Examples include evaluation of range of motion before and after soft-tissue surgery; evaluation of muscle tone or strength before and after rhizotomy; evaluation of the position of the femoral head before and after surgery to reduce a dislocated hip; and evaluation of the magnitude of a spinal deformity before and after surgical treatment.

The Gait Analysis Laboratory can be used to evaluate the dynamic function of multiple joints within the lower extremities as well as the entire gait pattern before and after treatment. Measurements of technical outcome should also include evaluation before and after medical treatment, pharmacologic treatment, orthotic treatment, and physical therapy. Complications should be noted and the frequency of complications determined for each treatment method.

One problem with determining the technical outcome is knowing when to make the appropriate assessment. For example, the appropriate time to assess the technical outcome varies with the procedure being evaluated. While evaluation of the child at the end of a period of intensive physical therapy would be most appropriate for evaluating this treatment, repeat evaluation in one to two years is necessary. Evaluation of orthopaedic surgical procedures is appropriate at least one year after surgery, and, in the case of rhizotomy or other procedures changing neurophysiologic function, evaluation should be continued for several years after surgery. In addition, serial evaluation should continue as the child grows, taking into account effects of bone and muscle growth as well as the effects of increasing neurophysiologic maturity.

Another problem with evaluating technical outcome in children with cerebral palsy is that multiple procedures are often recommended. Rather than evaluating each operative procedure on an extremity that requires multilevel surgery, the multilevel procedure should be considered as a single package and the entire treatment plan evaluated based on appropriately established preoperative criteria. Finally, for proper evaluation of a treatment, it is important to have clearly established goals for that treatment before undertaking it.

Functional Outcome

Functional outcome is the change in physical, social, and/or intellectual function that occurs as a result of the treatment. The primary changes in functional outcome in children with spastic diplegia involve ambulation. Among children with cerebral palsy it is also appropriate to address changes in the quality of mobility. Examples of functional changes include a decrease in energy needed to walk; improvement in velocity of gait; improvement in dexterity, such as the ability to navigate stairs and reach distances more easily; improvement in participation in certain sports activities; lengthening of distances that a child can walk into the community; and overall improvement in status and cosmesis.

Assessment of improvements in social function includes evaluation of such areas as improvement in activities of daily living and in the ability of the patient to help him/herself. Another example of improvement would include the ability to go to a friend's house that previously was not accessible because of barriers to wheelchair use. This area would also include evaluation of the impact of the neuromuscular disease and limited mobility on family problems and the effect the treatment might have had on function of the overall family unit.

The evaluation of intellectual function is also important. Some believe that rhizotomy and/or use of intrathecal baclofen decreases the spasticity to a degree that allows for improvement in concentration and intellectual function. It has been reported that intellectual function may improve if the child sleeps well at night; this factor may be of some importance if use of night braces does not allow the child comfortable sustained sleep. In the same category, treatment that relieves pain or reduces excessive tone may improve the temperament of the child and, thereby, allow for improved individual social and intellectual development.

Parent Satisfaction

The third area that requires evaluation is the satisfaction of the parents and the child. Obviously, some children with spastic diplegia, either because of age or associated defects, will have difficulty evaluating the outcome of their treatment. All of the previously mentioned functional results will

impact on the family's satisfaction with the treatment used. Questions must be posed in layman's terms, which cover evaluation by the parents and the child of improvement in mobility or social functioning or intellectual achievement. The family and the child must also be happy with the type of treatment given and with the setting in which it was given.

The American Academy of Orthopaedic Surgeons has set the period of one year following completion of surgical treatment as an appropriate time to evaluate patient's and parent's satisfaction regarding the treatment. Satisfaction studies must be able to discern why the parent or patient is or is not pleased and must also evaluate satisfaction in terms of the parents' or the patient's expectations prior to treatment. For example, a child might be doing well from the orthopaedic procedure while having more recent medical problems as a result of a worsening seizure disorder. Evaluation of the parent's satisfaction with the treatment provided should be ongoing.

Treatment Cost

The fourth area that must be addressed in outcome assessment is the cost of the treatment given. The costs of treatment are different from the charges of the hospital, physician, or therapist provided, and, at present, are difficult to determine accurately in most hospitals and doctors offices. The actual cost of treatment includes the cost of pretreatment diagnosis, the cost of treatment both in the hospital and in the physician's or surgeon's office, the cost of therapy and/or bracing, and the family's loss of earnings. Costs related to the specific treatment being evaluated should be compared with costs of other types of treatment possible for the same condition. Establishment of a cost/benefit or cost/utility ratio appears to be a major goal of the government in the years ahead.

Summary

Outcome assessment is a complex undertaking. To allow for appropriate assessment after the treatment has been completed, the studies should be randomized, controlled clinical trials with standardized clinical and possibly laboratory evaluation before initiation of treatment. Multicenter studies may be needed to provide a sufficient volume of patients for evaluation of a specific treatment modality. A protocol is needed and must be followed closely if multicenter studies are to have any chance of success. Investigators must be carefully chosen and questions phrased according to guidelines available from the American Academy of Orthopaedic Surgeons to allow for valid responses. Despite the complexity of outcome assessments, these studies have become an essential part of the clinical management of children with spastic diplegia. Attention needs to be focused on the areas of study design and outcome assessment.

Section Four
Surgical Decision Making

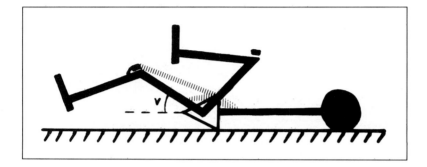

Chapter 12

Clinically Based Decision Making for Surgery

Jørgen Reimers, MD

It is important to expend the energy required to make the best possible decision. As Mercer Rang[1] said, "The decision is more important than the incision."

Many very good books and articles have been written on this subject, therefore I will deal mainly with my experience in Denmark, a country with free medical care in which per capita expenditures are 50% of those in the United States. Twenty-five years' experience has shown me that the following principles are clearly applicable to patients with spasticity.

Principles

The decision for treatment rests on some conditions: First, what is the main objective of intervening into the natural course of cerebral palsy? I think it is to keep a happy individual in an intact family. This requires that the person be free of chronic pain and able to sit well, even if it is necessary to use a special chair. It is important to be able to move around, but it is not absolutely necessary to walk.[2] Therefore, additional steps taken to obtain walking capacity are open to debate.

Everyone knows that children grow, but sometimes people forget that muscles and tendons must also grow to avoid relative shortening of these structures that would limit movements of the affected joints.

Opposing muscles should be in harmony to grow normally relative to the growth of the bones (Fig. 1, *top*). In the case of spasticity, however, the stronger of a pair of muscles will not be stretched by its antagonist (Fig. 1, *bottom*). The result is a shortening of the agonist and a progressive disharmony between the function of the muscles.

For normal function of a muscle group, the opposing muscle group must be sufficiently long and free from spasticity. The apparently paralyzed antagonist may function after elongation and weakening of the spastic agonist, as seen after flexor carpi ulnaris transfer[3] and elongation of the Achilles tendon.[4]

It is tempting to transfer the deforming force to the paralyzed site,

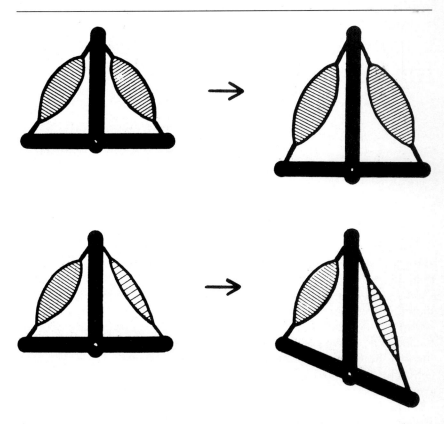

Fig. 1 *Top, When there is harmony between opposite functioning muscle groups, they grow in length, as the bone does.* **Bottom**, *When disharmony is present, the weakest muscle group can't stretch the strongest and perhaps spastic muscles, resulting in a relative shortening of the strongest group in relation to the growing bone.*

but because children are capable of regenerating both nerves and tendons,[5,6] the long-term effect is no better than that accomplished by a simple elongation of the tendon or myotenotomy.

Bones and joints are also affected by the surrounding muscles in children. Examples include valgus in the ankle joint if the soleus is paralyzed[7] or migration of the hip joint if the gluteal muscles are too weak. Therefore, during childhood it is possible to prevent bony deformities by producing harmony between the functions of the surrounding muscles if action is taken soon enough.

Clinical Judgment

Unfortunately it takes years for clinicians to learn to notice all the different deviances in children's motor functions. And it is time-consuming, because it is necessary to see the patient sit; crawl; walk, with or without walking-aids, bandages, and footwear; and spontaneously run after a bouncing ball. A video recording could be a good help in the beginning. Proper clinical judgment also requires a radiograph of the hip joints, because the clinician must establish that the hip joints are sufficiently stable.

Muscle Status

Normal motor function implies that the muscles and tendons are sufficiently long. The organic lengths of these structures are important only for static functions such as sitting and standing. When a person is walking or running, it is the dynamic length of the muscles that is the limiting factor for movement of the joints and for the function of the opposing muscles. Therefore, measurement of the dynamic shortening of the structures is of decisive importance. This measurement, called PMDE (Poor-Man's-Dynamic-Electromyography), is performed by a rapid stretching with about the same strength the person would use when functioning normally. These measurements should be recorded on a form, so that the changes that occur from one examination to the next can be seen easily (Fig. 2).

Some of the measurements need an explanation: Extension deficit of the hip joint, calculated with a straight back, and, if necessary, with elevation of the other leg, is used to determine the organic and spastic shortness of the iliopsoas muscle.

Limited rapid flexion of the knee, with the patient in prone position, is caused by shortening of the rectus muscles. If the greater spasticity is in the proximal part of the quadriceps muscle, the pelvis will rise off of the mattress. If the pelvis does not rise, the spasticity is in the distal part of the quadriceps muscle.

The dorsiflexion of the foot is carried out with the foot in neutral position, with the calcaneal bone placed below the talus—the position in which the foot should function after a possible operation. If, during rapid dorsiflexion with flexed knee, the foot goes beyond 90 degrees, there is no serious involvement of the soleus muscle.

The migration percentages of the hip joints[5] are entered on the same form, because the connection between the abduction of the hip, with the hip and the knee flexed to 90 degrees, and the degree of instability of the hip, serves to indicate the strength of the hip abductors. If the hip joint is subluxated in spite of a good abduction, the abductor muscles will also be weak after myotenotomy of the adductors. A limited abduction of less than 40 degrees and a barely subluxated hip (migration percentages greater than or equal to 33%) indicate that the gluteal muscles, after an operation on the adductors, could regain the strength necessary to make the hip migrate inward.

Static and Dynamic

Motor function depends on the dynamic length and strength of the muscles and the effort expended to compensate for a possible handicap.

LEDSTATUS

den passive bevægelighed

Rigshospitalet

NAVN_____   PERS.NR. _____ 06 08 87

	DATO	6/8 -91													
	SIDE	HØ	VE	HØ	VE	HØ	VE	HØ	VE	HØ	VE	HØ	VE	HØ	VE
MIGRATIONSPROCENT		40	17												
flexionskontraktur		o	o												
flexion bøjet knæ		5	o												
H abduktion 90° i hofte og knæ	langsomt	40	60												
O	hurtigt	25	40												
F abduktion strakt hofte og knæ	langsomt	20	50												
T	hurtigt	10	35												
E indadrotation bugleje	langsomt	90	75												
L	hurtigt														
E udadrotation bugleje	langsomt	40	60												
D	hurtigt														
K flexion bugleje	langsomt														
N	hurtigt														
Æ extensionsdefekt 90° flekteret hofte	langsomt	50	60												
L	hurtigt	90	70												
E															
D extensionsdefekt		o	5												
F dorsal flexion strakt knæ	langsomt	o	5												
O	hurtigt	-30	-10												
D dorsal flexion bøjet knæ	langsomt	10	20												
L	hurtigt	o	5												
E **D**															
A extensionsdefekt															
L supination 90° i albue															
B															
U pronation 90° i albue															
E															
UNDERSØGER		JR													

Fig. 2 *Muscle status. Form used to record Poor-Man's-Dynamic-EMG in Denmark.*

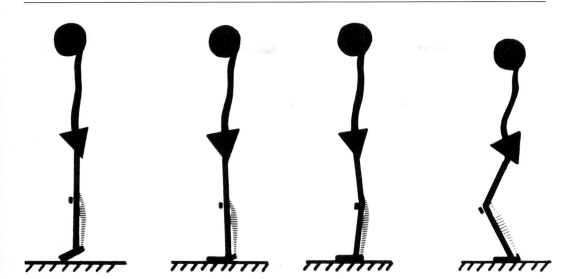

Fig. 3 *Organic or dynamic shortening of triceps surae may produce toe walk (**left**), valgus foot (**left center**), or hyperextension of the knee (**right center**). **Right**, A triceps that is too long after elongation or high heels results in flexed knee and hip and hyperlordosis. (Reproduced with permission from Reimers.[8])*

When spasticity, is accompanied by dyskinesia or athetosis, the problems become even more complex, although the same principles are valid.

If, by a rapid passive movement, the corrected foot can be dorsiflexed to only 5 degrees short of a right angle, a short triceps surae is present. Small children with this problem will be toewalkers. If, however, such children have soft ligaments or get intensive physiotherapy, the foot will turn in a valgus direction. A stable foot or a stiff cavus foot, combined with a short Achilles tendon, will force the knee into extension, or even hyperextension (Fig. 3). The forefoot, pressed flat, will later develop a hallux valgus and will tend to distort, also in a valgus direction.

Shortening of the hamstrings with an extension deficit of more than 30 degrees, when the hip is flexed to 90 degrees, will result in a kyphotic sitting position (Fig. 4), short stride (Fig. 5), increased wear of the shoes, and bruises on the shin because the foot is not lifted high enough up from the ground to avoid stumbling.[6] Eventually, short hamstrings will produce highstanding patellae with grating behind the patella and, in active persons, will also produce tearing of the tuberositas tibiae (Osgood-Schlatter disease) or the distal tip of the patella (Sinding-Larsen-Johansson disease). An extension deficit of 60 degrees or more will prevent the person from achieving full knee extension while walking.

In some cases the rectus muscle becomes so strong and spastic after

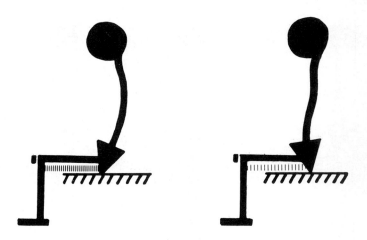

Fig. 4 *When hamstrings are short, lumbar kyphosis might develop because it is tiring to sit with the hip flexed 90 degrees. (Reproduced with permission from Reimers.[8])*

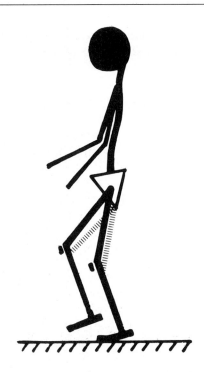

Fig. 5 *Short stride and shambling walk are some of the results when hamstrings are short. (Reproduced with permission from Reimers.[6])*

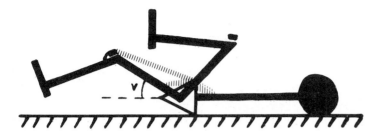

Fig. 6 *The angle v indicates the degree of hip flexion deformity. (Reproduced with permission from Reimers.[6])*

hamstring lengthening that the rectus must also be lengthened and weakened.[9] This can be done proximally or distally, depending on which muscle group is causing the deformation.

If the extension deficiency at the hip caused by a rapid movement is more than 30 degrees (Fig. 6), the iliopsoas muscle is too tight. In such cases, the pelvis is tilted and the abdomen protrudes during standing or walking. This situation causes the knees to be pressed backward into hyperextension. To avoid this hyperextension, most patients will flex their knees (Fig. 7).

In Copenhagen, contrary to data from many other centers, the iliopsoas does not dislocate the hip joint and does not aggravate femoral anteversion. There you may see short hip flexors, a stable hip, and pronounced subluxation without shortening of psoas. Twenty-two isolated lengthenings of the hip-flexors, without myotenotomy of the adductors, did not influence the course of migration of the hips.[5] When the iliopsoas is lengthened and weakened in the absence of marked shortness, there is a risk that the hip extensors will take over with an anterior luxation.

The adductors of the hip should work in harmony with the abductors to keep the hip joint stable. If the abductors are too weak, because of paralysis or because of a steep angle of the femoral neck, the hip will migrate outward, and anteversion will increase whether or not the adductors are short. A radiograph of the hip joint may show that, while standing, stimulation of the abductors may diminish the migration percentages relative to that for the usual supine projection. A series of radiographs taken to measure hip migration across time will determine whether the hip is, in fact, migrating outward. The Migration Index[5] will indicate whether it will be necessary to operate to retain the hip and how long the surgery can be delayed.

A person with hip abductors that are too weak will not be able to stand alone. Such patients may be able to run or walk with support, but not unaided, and there will be a tendency toward scissoring of the legs. If abduction, with flexed hip and knee, is decreased to less than 40

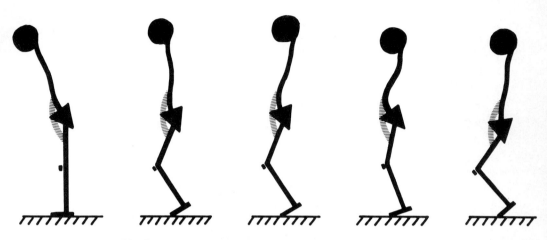

Fig. 7 *Shortness of hip flexors produces various degrees of tilting of the pelvis and flexion of the knee. (Reproduced with permission from Reimers.[8])*

degrees because the adductors are shortened, abductor function will be diminished.

The asymmetric child with a bat-shaped ear opposite to the adducted and outward migrating hip is treated according to the principles mentioned above. When only the affected hip is treated by radical myotenotomy of the short adductors, perhaps including resection of the anterior branch of the obturator nerve, the asymmetry is changed to the opposite side, and the affected hip will migrate inward. Often, in such cases, an adductor operation must be performed on the other side after some time (Fig. 8). If surgery is performed simultaneously on the adductors on both sides, the asymmetry will continue, and the hip will continue to migrate outward.

Among 760 children with cerebral palsy seen last year as outpatients, there were, among the 432 diplegics, 4% with subluxations. Thus, the risk of serious hip problems is not great in that group, provided that the necessary operative prevention and treatment are carried out in time.

Treatment

Muscle Care

If the spastic muscle is not treated and is not stretched by its antagonist, its growth in length will be diminished and it will lose its elasticity. It is therefore obvious that muscle care, consisting of brief stretching of the relaxed muscle for at least one minute every 12 hours, is required.

Muscle care ought to be a precondition for offering an operation. On

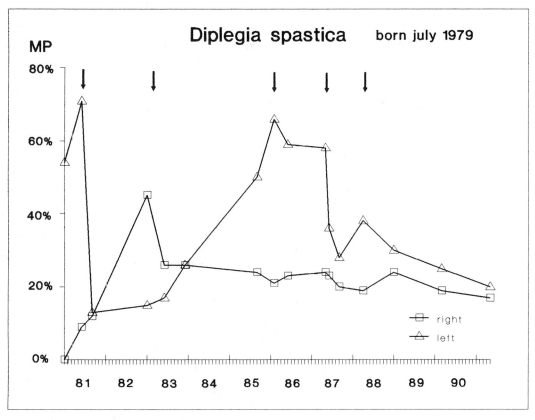

Fig. 8 *Migration percentage in relation to time before and after operations in a squinted diplegia with windswept hip joints. Arrows point to time of each operation. Year of age: 2: left adductor-myotomy (am). 3.04: right am. 6.05: left am. 7.07: left femoral osteotomy. 8.07: left am. 12: stable, symmetrical hip joints. She is able to stand with support.*

the other hand, if the surgeon, as a result of the operation, achieves harmony between the agonist and antagonist, the latter will be able to stretch the surgically corrected muscle, which will then retain or improve its elasticity. Moreover, because children with spastic diplegia have not chosen their parents or the personnel of the institution in which they may reside, they deserve a chance to function better and easier, even in the absence of muscle care.

When to Operate

In principle, surgery should be considered, independent of age, when there is an impediment to the child's progress or ability to function as well as possible. It is advisable, however, to wait until the child is not afraid of strangers.

What to Correct

All the dynamic tendons that are too short should be lengthened in the same procedure; for example, the adductors, hamstrings, rectus, Achilles tendon, toe flexors, and peroneal tendons. Doing this avoids postoperative spasm in the unoperated muscles.

If the child has just begun to walk unaided, it may be necessary to divide the lengthening between two operations in order to make sure that the function is not made worse. In such cases, it is important to correct the most proximal shortness first.[1,8]

If bony deformities are not avoided or corrected with muscle and tendon surgery alone, or if the untreated patient comes from elsewhere, it may be necessary to correct malrotation and a steep femoral neck-shaft angle. Only rarely is it necessary to correct the acetabulum, because as long as growth continues, the acetabular roof can reshape enough to be able to retain the femoral head.[10] If the waiting list is too long, arthrodesis of the feet could wait until growth has finished. An adult should be without orthoses.

The following is an example of the distribution among the operations I performed most frequently for cerebral palsy in 1991: In 133 procedures, I did 87 adductor-tenomyotomies, including 27 resections of the anterior obturator nerve and 13 lengthenings of the psoas; 83 lengthenings of the Achilles tendon and 48 fasciotomies of the gastrocnemius (Vulpius), including 66 lengthenings of the toe flexors and 48 peroneus tenotomies; 126 distal and 14 proximal lengthenings of the hamstrings, and 33 lengthenings of the rectus. Compared with these soft-tissue procedures, I did one tibial and nine femoral osteotomies and nine arthrodeses of the feet.

How to Operate

Use small incisions, subcuticular sutures, and lightweight bandages that can be removed with ease; make the hospitalization as short as possible; and operate so that the children are able to stand on their legs a few days later. These steps should ensure that if a second operation is needed, the child will not fear it.

Summary

The principles for decision-making in spastic diplegia are essentially the same as for other problems in pediatric orthopaedics. Spastic diplegia presents special difficulties because the spasticity aggravates an existing disharmony between the agonist and antagonist. The complications caused by the patient's handicap and the fact that, even after a successful operation, there will still be a diplegia, are also difficult factors.

Motor function depends on the dynamic length of the muscles, which is estimated by a rapid stretching of the muscle in question. This Poor-Man's-Dynamic-Electromyography is most important when assessing the influence of the different muscles on the static and dynamic and deciding to operate.

By doing soft-tissue operations at the right time, it is possible to prevent or treat deformation of bones and joints, because the bones, joints, muscles, etc., continue to grow with the child. These operations can be done with only small discomfort to the child, so the main goal of keeping a happy individual is not forgotten.

References

1. Rang M: Cerebral palsy, in Morrissy RT (ed): *Lovell and Winter's Pediatric Orthopaedics*, ed 3. Philadelphia, JB Lippincott, 1990, pp 465–506.
2. Andrews G, Platt LJ, Quinn PT, et al: An assessment of the status of adults with cerebral palsy. *Dev Med Child Neurol* 1977;19:803–810.
3. Stotz S: *Quantitative elektromyographische Untersuchungen zur Indikation und Beurteilung muskelentspannender Operationen bei der Infantilen Zerebralparese.* Uelzen 1, Med Lit Verlag, 1978, pp 1–47.
4. Reimers J: Functional changes in the antagonists after lengthening the agonists in cerebral palsy: I. Triceps surae lengthening. *Clin Orthop* 1989;253:30–34.
5. Reimers J: The stability of the hip in children: A radiological study of the results of muscle surgery in cerebral palsy. *Acta Orthop Scand* 1980; 184(suppl):1–100.
6. Reimers J: Contracture of the hamstrings in spastic cerebral palsy. A study of three methods of operative correction. *J Bone Joint Surg* 1974;56B:102–109.
7. Dias LS: Valgus deformity of the ankle joint: Pathogenesis of fibular shortening. *J Pediatr Orthop* 1985;5:176–180.
8. Reimers J: Static and dynamic problems in spastic cerebral palsy. *J Bone Joint Surg* 1973;55B:822–827.
9. Reimers J: Functional changes in the antagonist after lengthening the agonists on cerebral palsy: II. Quadriceps strength before and after distal hamstring lengthening. *Clin Orthop* 1989;253:35–37.
10. Reimers J: Acetabular development following femoral osteotomy in cerebral palsy after the age of four years. *J Pediatr Orthop*, in press.

Chapter 13

Limitations of Technologic Assessment

Chester M. Tylkowski, MD

Introduction

Technologic tools for observation are used to extend the senses and register in a more objective manner that which the human senses cannot. Once the technologic tools have registered it, this information can be documented and processed by mathematical techniques. In this light, it is possible to observe a phenomenon with an assortment of senses and to grasp aspects or the essence of it, but not possible to record the event except by reproducing it based on subjective analysis in writing or a drawing. In a similar sense, because of the limitations of human sensors, it may not be possible to see certain phenomena that occur, such as electromyographic activity and moments and powers about joints.

The ability to measure and mathematically represent a recorded event is the advantage of technologic tools. Further analysis and comparisons can be performed to define the data set that has been generated. Similar events or patterns may be compared and grouped to further delineate the mechanism of action of the process. In this review, I will discuss the current limits of these new technologic systems, and whether they represent the phenomenon of walking in a factual and useful manner.

There are many different methods for recording function or activity. Examples are electrogoniometers; oximeters; accelerometers; video imaging; and kinematic, electromyographic, and kinetic analysis. This discussion is limited to methods currently used in most clinical gait analysis facilities to assess walking disorders in children with spastic diplegia. Systems used for recording other functional activities are not discussed.

Problems With Measurement Techniques

Problems with the system of measurement may be grouped into several categories. These include subject observation, subject definition, recording equipment, and software methods used in tracking or digitizing the event as well as for mathematical processing.

Subject Observation

When an activity is viewed on command in isolation, the person doing that activity may react differently than when doing the same activity spontaneously and not under conditions of critical observation. When asked to walk along a defined path where observers are ready to record the event so they can assess, critique, and possibly offer therapeutic modifications for improvement, the patient may modify the walk to an expected norm, which deviates from the spontaneously occurring activity, the so-called "clinic walk." This may be less of a problem with children who have impaired motor control because of their limited ability to modify the pathologic pattern. However, the milder the deficit, the more likely it is that the pattern will be modified. This "clinic walk" may also occur with nontechnical methods; it is not unique to instrumented observation. This phenomenon must be kept in mind during an instrumented study, and the personnel conducting the study should attempt to minimize it.

During instrumented analysis, the subject is often burdened with devices to define body segments, electromyographic electrodes, preamplifiers, transmitters, tape, straps, etc. This may cause an altered stance or pattern to avoid rubbing, moving, or damaging the equipment. Circumferential materials may constrict the limb, impede joint motion, and alter the feedback encountered during limb movement in walking (Fig. 1).

It is crucial that the above impediments be kept in mind when designing and applying the equipment used to monitor walking. An ideal system would be able to follow the body through space without markers. The techniques for imaging and recording body motion in four dimensions (3 spatial dimensions and time) with the ability to perform all the calculations on the body segments, joint centers, and so forth are just in their infancy.[1-3] The computer power necessary to handle the data and computations exceeds the budgets of clinical gait analysis laboratories.

There is no current method that allows the recording of muscle electrical activity without direct contact. Most preamplifiers, transmitters, or trailing cable devices are bulky and require adhesive devices to be secured to the body. Design of smaller devices, although costly to manufacture, would greatly diminish the problems associated with applied devices.

Although they are less of an encumbrance to movement, force plates mounted in the floor often become apparent to subjects who then intentionally change their gait pattern to strike the force plate. The data thus generated, which are used to calculate ground-reaction forces (GRF), moments, and powers, may not be representative of the usual walking pattern. If the person is cooperative and walks repeatedly without an attempt to strike the plate, but fails to perform a satisfactory foot strike, fatigue may affect the pattern.

Force plates cannot be used to assess individuals who have more severe impairments and who require assistance from devices such as

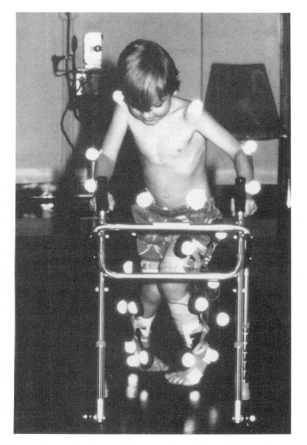

Fig. 1 *A child wearing reflective markers, surface electrodes, and preamplifiers preparing to walk for his gait study.*

walkers or crutches unless those individuals are able to cross the sensor without contact from the device. The GRF and center of application of force are distributed to the upper and lower limbs because of the assistive device. The advantages that could be gained from moment and power computations for these individuals are lost.

Subject Definition

As has been noted above, techniques are not yet available to easily record a body in space using computer video imaging alone. Therefore, body segments must be marked so their positions may be defined for computation. The segments are then combined to define joints.[4] The limited number of markers recorded by camera, identified by video processor, or hand digitized on a frame-by-frame basis can be listed in a computer file. This limited list of numbers can be handled by current lower-cost computing equipment, allowing affordable clinical systems.

The price paid for this low-cost solution to body segment imaging is noise.[5] The markers are placed on skin. Depending on anatomic location and the subject's body fat distribution, considerable motion is added to the marker that is not related to the motion of the body segment. The motion expected of a solid and rigid body segment is affected by the motion of skin over fat, muscle, and bone, as well as motion caused by the muscle contracting and changing shape.[6] This additional motion changes the angular relationship of the segments and leads to errors in the calculation of joint angular motion.

Markers imbedded within the body skeleton or cine radiography would allow more accurate tracking, but are not clinically relevant solutions. It is desirable to select anatomic locations for marker application in which skin is near bone, but this is not always possible. The noise generated must then be filtered, usually mathematically.[7] Problems associated with mathematical filtering will be discussed later.

Recording Equipment

Kinematics The state-of-the-art for video imaging is apparently quite satisfactory for the recording of markers attached to an individual.[8] The use of 50 Hz to 200 Hz shuttered cameras is satisfactory, even for higher speed events such as running. Cinematography, although requiring hand digitization, is quite satisfactory in allowing markers to be identified. However, an adequate number of cameras is required to record obscured or hidden markers with either technique. Methods for seeing markers by reflected light or pulsed light-emitting diodes have been in use for many years, and perform satisfactorily. Marker shapes and sizes have been customized to fit the particular observation.

Video Processing Commercially available systems to capture the video information and record the path of markers perform satisfactorily. There has been continual improvement in methods of acquiring the data contained in a frame of the recorded event. The precision and accuracy of some systems have been reported, and can be acquired for others using standard techniques.[9,10]

At present, the limitations that are imposed on the recording of human gait by the need to use markers is the greatest problem. Although all information contained in the entire recorded scene is digitally accessible, to capture all the information in each frame of the recorded event would require a vast amount of computer memory. Also, computational speed and time would be significant factors, requiring computer capabilities quite beyond the clinically-affordable range. The development of computer software to process the data, record the motion of body segments, and make it clinically relevant is in its infancy.[3]

Force Plates Precision force transducers combined to produce force plates are an industry standard. The transducer sensitivities, construction of the platform, and limitations for applied forces are delineated in the biomechanics literature.[5,8] Methods of calibration, standard amplification techniques, and limitations based on type of transducer are carefully covered by the force systems available commercially for gait analyses. The position of the force plate may be obscured by various techniques to prevent the patient from aiming for the device during a recorded walk.

The greatest limitation is recording the forces of individuals when assistive devices are used. Crutches or walkers allow upper extremity weightbearing, which can be recorded only if transducers are placed into the weightbearing ends of the devices. This force information then is available for analysis.

Electromyography (EMG) EMG has been reasonably well standardized to meet the need for recording of comparable data.[11] Electrode application and positioning have been described in the literature and are fairly standard in most laboratories (Fig. 2).[12]

The discussion of surface versus fine wire inserted electrodes continues to help delineate the advantages and disadvantages of each method.[8,13] The problem of cross-talk recording of near muscle groups is recognized, and discussion of muscle group activity and careful assessment of signals are used to exclude data not representative of the group monitored. This problem is more serious in children because they have smaller limbs.

Fine wire electrodes will record the electrical activity within a small area of a single muscle; therefore, multiple sets of electrodes may be needed to adequately represent the activity of the entire muscle. Limited patient tolerance to insertion of the wires, which is the main disadvantage of this method, limits the ability to define critically what each specific muscle is doing through a gait cycle during a routine clinical study of an individual with pathologic gait.

The ability to get the signal to the recording devices is another problem of recording gait EMG. Trailing cables may impede walking, but they result in a less noisy signal. The need to attach preamplifiers to a common cable junction adds bulk and may alter the subject's gait. Telemetry systems add size to the unit. Unless custom-made devices are used, commercial preamplifier/transmitter units tend to be larger for ease and decreased cost of manufacture (Fig. 3). Telemetry eliminates the trailing cable, but may add significant noise and interference to the signal, requiring hardware or software filtering to restore the information sought from the muscles.

Software Most of the software available at present requires that a fairly sophisticated computer user interact with the system to prepare it, record the event, and process the data. Although some systems are becoming easier to use, they certainly have not yet become the turnkey, push-button systems most clinicians would prefer.

Substantial controversies still exist concerning methods of tracking data, means of estimating obscured or merged markers, and best methods to filter data mathematically to eliminate noise. The filter options that exist within most systems require an intelligent decision on the best mathematical filter to apply to the event recorded. Blindly looking

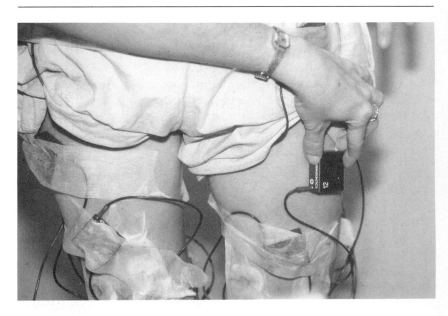

Fig. 2 *Surface electrode applied over quadriceps group of muscles. Proximity of other muscles may result in cross talk.*

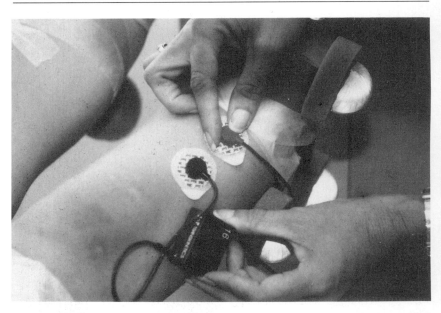

Fig. 3 *Size of preamplifiers and transmitters may make placement on the limbs of a small child difficult.*

at data generated by a system in which filters were selected as a compromise by the designer can cause errors in interpretation of the data. The use of these data, which may not reflect the true motion, can lead to significant errors in clinical decision-making and theorization of gait patterns. The greatest technical limitation in this area is the uninformed user. Much basic work has been done in this area, and assumptions accepted in the users' system must be understood.[5,7]

The mathematical methodology used to calculate angular motion and attach to it a certain joint motion is dependent on conventions of the sequence of calculations.[8,14–16] Most clinically-based systems use the calculation of Eularian angles. Depending on the order of calculations, quite different joint angles may ensue. This method should be well defined when looking at the joint motion output data.

Methods for calculating true joint motion are not well established. Joints vary, and most do not fit the simple hinge model generally applied. The difference between joints can result in the description of motion using a mathematical model of the joint that does not fully take into account the unique anatomic characteristics of that joint. The link segment model assumed by many systems may be adequate for clinical applications, but its limitation in representing anatomic motion must be understood.[5,7]

Methods used to locate joint centers, for example the hip, are not precisely defined. Assumptions are made based on standard skeletal anthropometric measurements that may not apply across all ages, populations, and races. Methods for locating hip joint centers from patient data are still in the development stage. Different methods of calculation result in the plotting of different joint angles.[14,17]

As advanced methods of mathematical analysis of walking become more accessible to the clinical user, further limitation of the data generated must be noted. Winter,[18] Burdett and associates,[19] and Zarrugm[20] have used calculations on joint angles, GRF, and limb segment definitions to produce moments, power, and energy plots. Controversy still exists on the best methods of calculation for four-dimensional data (I. Stokes, personal communication, 1991). Norms for anthropometric data do not exist for the patients most likely to be seen in the clinical laboratory.[21] The output of these calculations must be interpreted very cautiously, because it will probably change when different norms or the patients'[2] own anthropometric data are applied.

Software or hardware processing of electromyographic data also requires several levels of decision-making that can alter the output. Best methods in these areas are still being defined.[22,23] Do individual walks or a summation of many walks offer the best information? At what signal level is a muscle active or not active? How does a level of electrical activity relate to the work output of the muscle and its subsequent effect on body segment motion? How does this relate to the clinical grade of muscle strength? These questions are being explored in the research arena,[24–26] but no clear recommendations have as yet emerged that will allow unquestioned clinical usefulness.

Conclusion

The previous description of technologic limitations can be viewed in two ways. One view would suggest that the limitations are significant and gait analysis is not practical. This would be a harmful assumption. Techniques are evolving that will continue to enhance the ability to analyze and understand the data generated. The other view offers the hope that by taking a tool and using it, the users can refine that tool to a state in which its usefulness is enhanced and that in its current state the tool can provide useful information, which must be assessed with recognition of the technical limitations. Certainly, the definition of clinical problems acts as a superb catalyst to create a technology that can enhance patient care.

References

1. Huang TS: Motion analysis, in Shapiro S (ed): *Artificial Intelligence Encylopedia*. New York, John Wiley & Sons, 1987, pp 620–632.
2. Huang TS: Modeling, analysis, and visualization of non-rigid motion. Presented at the International Conference of Pattern Recognition, Atlantic City, June 1990.
3. Huang TS: Motion estimation in computer vision. Presented at the International Symposium on 3-D Analysis of Human Movement, Montreal, Quebec, July 1991.
4. Apkarian J, Nauman S, Cairns B: A three dimensional kinematic and dynamic model of the lower limb. *J Biomech* 1989;22:143–155.
5. Winter D: *Biomechanics and Motor Control of Human Movement*. New York, John Wiley & Sons, 1990, pp 33–36.
6. Bryant JT, Small CF: Error reductions in data capture: A review of three papers. Presented at the International Symposium on 3-D Analysis of Human Movement, Montreal, Quebec, July 1991.
7. Winter D: *Biomechanics and Motor Control of Human Movement*. New York, John Wiley & Sons, 1990, pp 36–47.
8. Tylkowski CM: Assessment of gait in children and adolescents, in Morrissy R (ed): *Pediatric Orthopedics*, ed 3. Philadelphia, JB Lippincott, 1990, pp 57–90.
9. Greaves JOB: Stage of the art in automated motion tracking and analysis systems, in Ponseggi BG(ed): *High Speed Photography, Videography, and Photonics IV*: Proceedings SPIE 1986;693:277–281.
10. Wilson SR: Software for automatic tracking of moving targets in three dimensions, in Ponseggi BG (ed): *High Speed Photography, Videography, and Photonics IV*: Proceedings SPIE 1986;693:269–276.
11. Winter D: Units, terms and standards in the reporting of EMG research. Report by the Ad Hoc Committee of the International Society of Electrophysiological Kinesiology, August 1980. Distributed by the International Society of Electrophysological Kinesiology, 1980.
12. Delagi EF, Perrotto A: *Anatomic Guide for the Electromyographer: The Limbs*, ed 2. Springfield, IL, Charles C. Thomas, 1982, p 136.
13. Komi PV, Buskirk ER: Reproducibility of electromyographic measures with inserted wire electrodes and surface electrodes. *Electromyography* 1970;10: 357–367.
14. Tylkowski CM, Simon SR, Mansour JM: Internal rotation gait in spastic cerebral palsy, in *The Hip: Proceedings of the Tenth Open Scientific Meeting of the Hip Society*. St. Louis, CV Mosby, 1982.

15. Woltring HJ: Definition and calculus of attitude angles, instantaneous helical axes and instantaneous centres of rotation from noisy position and attitude data. Presented at the International Symposium on 3-D Analysis of Human Movement. Montreal, Quebec, July 1991.

16. Davis RB, Ounpuu S, Tyburski DJ, et al: A comparison of two dimensional and three dimensional techniques for the determination of joint rotation angles. Presented at the International Symposium on 3-D Analysis of Human Movement. Montreal, Quebec, July 1991.

17. Stivers K, Tylkowski C, Howell V: Prediction of the hip joint center location from the relative motion between thigh and pelvis: A pilot study. Presented at the International Symposium on 3-D Analysis of Human Movement, Montreal, Quebec, July 1991.

18. Winter D: *Biomechanics and Motor Control of Human Movement.* New York, John Wiley & Sons, 1990, pp 75–138.

19. Burdett RG, Skrinar GS, Simon SR: Comparison of mechanical work and metabolic energy consumption during gait. *J Orthop Res* 1983;1:63–72.

20. Zarrugm MY: Kinematic prediction of intersegment loads and power at the joints of the leg in walking. *J Biomech* 1981;14:713–725.

21. Winter D: *Biomechanics and Motor Control of Human Movement.* New York, John Wiley & Sons, 1990, pp 51–73.

22. Wotten ME, Kadaba MP, Cochran GVB: Dynamic electromyography: I. Numerical representation using principle component analysis. *J Orthop Res* 1990;8:247–258.

23. Wotten ME, Kadaba MP, Cochran GVB: Dynamic electromyography. II. Normal patterns during gait. *J Orthop Res* 1990;8:259–265.

24. Milner-Brown HS, Stein RB, Yemm R: The contractile properties of human motor units during voluntary isometric contractions. *J Physiol* 1973;228:285–306.

25. Milner-Brown HS, Stein RB, Yemm R: The orderly recruitment of human motor units during voluntary isometric contractions. *J Physiol* 1976;228:359–370.

26. Milner-Brown HS, Stein RB: The relation between the surface electromyogram and muscular force. *J Physiol* 1975;246:549–569.

Chapter 14

Gait Analysis and Its Automated Interpretation in Cerebral Palsy

Sheldon R. Simon, MD
Michael Weintraub, PhD
Tom Bylander, PhD

Within the past decade gait analysis laboratories have been developed which hold the promise of providing standardized, accurate measurements of the various parameters of a patient's gait. These laboratories have been most useful and significant in the evaluation of children with cerebral palsy. A prime goal of treatment in this population group is to improve the child's gait or to prevent it from getting worse. A variety of nonsurgical as well as surgical approaches are used to achieve this goal.[1]

Gait analysis laboratories can further this effort by providing objective data relating to measurements of the patient's time-distance parameters, motion of limb segments and joints, activity of muscle groups, and force plate data, as well as derived kinetic and kinematic features of gait such as torque and muscle work and effort. These data, in combination with the patient's history and physical examination, provide extensive information for use in patient evaluation and treatment selection.

While many clinicians are trained and experienced in the interpretation of data obtained through physical examination and patient history, interpretation of data provided by the gait laboratory is less commonly understood, is a difficult skill to learn, and is a time-consuming activity. As a result, because only a few experts interpret gait laboratory data, its availability to gait-impaired patients is limited.

Interpretation of gait, especially in the child with cerebral palsy, is a difficult task because the neurologic control often is not normal. The result of interaction between abnormally controlled muscles is a disordered gait that often is not isolated to a single joint or limb segment but involves multiple limbs and joints, which are affected in various phases of the gait cycle. In addition, overactivity or underactivity of muscles must be considered in conjunction with muscle weakness, tightness, or joint contracture and related to previous surgical procedures as well as the underlying neurologic problem. The number of possible interpretations and the complexity of musculoskeletal interactions, thus, make gait analysis a very complex task. Another complicating factor in gait analysis is that the amount of data available to the analyst is limited. For example, because electromyographic activity of every muscle is not monitored, the analyst must infer some muscle activities, even for gait reports.

The large amount of data collected during a gait study can be overwhelming and can compromise the clinician's ability to assess all the important data. Moreover, the number of clinicians who are well-trained experts in gait analysis currently is limited, and training individuals for this task is a very costly and time consuming operation, making such training a long-term possibility at best. An alternative solution is the development and use of expert computer systems to assist the clinician in interpreting gait. Such systems will insure standardized, high-quality analysis, will decrease the time required to perform this analysis, and will serve as a tool for instruction in gait interpretation.

Advances in artificial intelligence computer programming have provided methods that can be used to develop an expert system to interpret gait-study data. With such a system, the computer could be used not only to provide information for use in subjective clinical decision making, but also to assist in interpreting that information. If we knew exactly how clinicians interpret gait data, we could use existing computational techniques to organize this material so it could be used to identify, with a great chance of likelihood, the abnormalities existing in a gait pattern of a child with cerebral palsy and to suggest the possible causes of those abnormalities. The success of such a program depends not only on engineering knowledge and skill in artificial intelligence programming, but also on the expertise of the clinician who is consistently and knowledgeably organizing an interpretation scheme that takes into account identification of each gait abnormality and its causes. This necessary first step is, interestingly, one that cannot be gleaned from the literature. Although reports of various studies have described the success of certain procedures for the correction of cerebral palsy gait abnormalities, and many physiologic and biomechanical descriptions of normal gait have been written, no well-defined report and no uniformity in clinical interpretation/decision-making has been established. In an attempt to develop such a program over the last six years, Simon has had to formalize his concepts with regard to interpretation of motion abnormalities and their causes in cerebral palsy.

This chapter describes the considerations involved in determining gait abnormalities and the causes thereof that can be and have been used to develop an artificial intelligence program,[2,3] and that may be helpful for the subjective clinical interpretation of gait data obtained from gait laboratories. The beauty of this attempt to develop an expert system for use in interpretation of gait analysis data is that it mandates a very detailed organizational framework, a consistent approach to information that is well known, and uniform interpretation of information that is less well known. In this sense, it cannot be theoretical but must be practical.

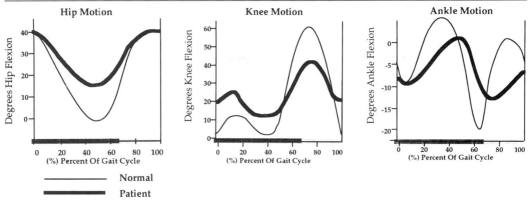

Fig. 1 *Graphs of sagittal plane hip, knee, and ankle motion obtained from data derived from a gait laboratory comparing motion of a child with cerebral palsy to that of a normal child. Motion data in time is expressed (normalized) as a percentage of the gait cycle. Stance phase is indicated by thickened bar on axis.*

Identification of Motion Deviations

Normal gait is efficient, adaptable, pain-free, and requires no assistive devices. The normal neurologic system controls the muscles through coordinated commands to rotate limbs at every joint in a very repeatable fashion, providing body propulsion and stability for walking. The process is repeatable from step to step, and, in any given gait cycle, different demands are placed on the leg at the initiation of stance, during single limb stance, during weight release as swing is initiated, and as swing phase occurs. Therefore, it is appropriate not only to examine the gait cycle in such overall performance parameters as velocity, cadence, and stride length and in the motions produced at each joint but also to view such motions as they are produced by particular muscles as well as their interaction with body weight and momentum at different times during the gait cycle.

Gait analysis laboratories graphically display the subject's joint motion in several planes, along with normal data for each joint. Gait data from subjects having a normal gait pattern but different walking speeds can be compared by displaying motion data for each joint as a percent of the gait cycle time. This format is currently used in most gait laboratories to compare subjects with abnormal gait to those with normal gait. On graphs with two lines, one depicting normal and the other patient data, it is easy to see what differences exist and at what phase in the gait cycle they occur (Fig. 1).

From these graphs, the clinician infers which sections of each joint motion differ from normal motion. It has, however, been shown that variations in joint motion occur from gait cycle to gait cycle and between individuals. Therefore, a normal motion pattern must be considered not as a single angle at each instant in the gait cycle, but as a

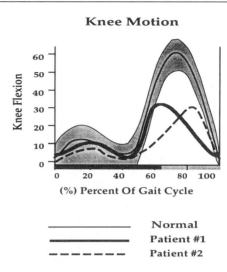

Knee Motion

Normal
Patient #1
Patient #2

Fig. 2 *Graph of knee flexion/extension of two children who have the same amount of reduced flexion in swing phase that occurs at two different times from two different causes. The normal range of knee motion for children of similar age is included.*

series of angles within a range. The exact nature of this range of normal motion in children and how it varies as the child grows has not been fully elucidated, but has been reported for children 1 to 7 years of age.[4] Therefore, the first consideration in defining abnormality is to define this range.

But, should any angle outside this normal range of motion be considered clinically significant? For example, the knee joint rotates from 10 degrees of flexion at the initiation of swing to up to 60 degrees by mid swing. Variations of 10 degrees here would not be very significant. In contrast, 10 degrees would constitute over 100% of the total arc of motion that occurs at the ankle joint (excluding plantarflexion in weight release) during weight acceptance, single limb stance, and swing phase. This variation leads to the question of how much of a deviation outside the normal range at any instant in time in any plane of motion constitutes an abnormality warranting attention.

Regardless of the magnitude of the deviation that is considered abnormal, a second question that needs to be asked is, how long should an abnormal motion continue before it is considered to be abnormal? Clearly abnormal motions at the knee that last for 5% of the gait cycle during the initiation of swing may not be significant because they go on such a short period of time that, given our current treatment techniques, we could not isolate a correction for them. However, a single incident of deviation such as a peak maximum or minimum of a curve could be considered to represent the summation of a series of previous events and be a significant degree of abnormality that might be very important. For example, if the knee only flexes to 35 degrees in swing,

Knee Motion

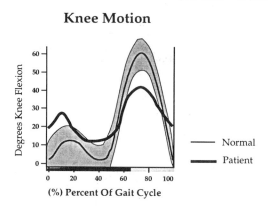

Fig. 3 *Graph of knee flexion/extension of child who has a limitation in knee flexion of 15 degrees below the maximum (as well as excessive flexion at the end of swing, beginning of stance). In swing, the limitation is only minimally less than the normal range, but it is preceded by a change in the rate of rise of knee flexion.*

the deviation is large and definitely abnormal (Fig. 2). Even here, one incident in time does not properly reflect the motion deviation present. For example, the low value of peak flexion could arise from either of two causes: (1) A normal rise of flexion in early swing that then abruptly halts might be related to activity of the quadriceps mechanism. (2) A delay in initiation of swing or a low rate of rise of swing throughout the swing period both might be related more to the leg's momentum and the inability of the hip flexors to initiate swing than to any sudden abnormal activity of the quadriceps mechanism. It is clear that physicians trained to interpret gait analysis data look at when the motion abnormalities occur as well as the preceding and subsequent pattern over time rather than at an abnormality seen at a single point of motion. Therefore, the issue of how much of the gait cycle should be looked at and consistently described could be addressed by establishing a rule that takes into account the mean value of abnormal motion over a given period of time.

Data analyzed according to this rule still might not accurately reflect the existence of an abnormal motion. In the example of knee flexion in swing phase, it is possible that a slightly more rapid rise in knee flexion initiates swing phase followed by a sudden decrease in the rate of rise of flexion such that by the time peak flexion is reached, the motion deviation may be as much as 15 degrees below the normal value (Fig. 3). It would seem that this abnormality should be described and that it would be related to prevention of further knee flexion by a sudden increase in quadriceps activity. However, this abnormality would not be detected if, over the given time period, we measured the magnitude of abnormality at each instant in the gait cycle. Even if we averaged the deviations over this total time, the abnormality still would not be detected. Furthermore, even if an abnormality exists over a time period during which it could be detected, we must examine whether or not its detection is significant, and if leg clearance is not a problem one might not want to clinically address the abnormality. Finally, despite the fact that current gait analysis techniques provide a reasonably accurate assessment of data, there still are times when this information is in error and apparent abnormalities for short periods of time during the gait cycle relate to technical errors rather than true deviations from normal.

In all cases, the purpose of defining motion deviations is to relate them to causes that are associated with cerebral palsy and are physiologic in their origin. For these reasons, we have selected several criteria other than a 10-degree deviation from normal at any instant in the cycle to define a motion abnormality.

First, the magnitudes of the joint motion patterns are normalized to the time of the individual phases of gait rather than to the entire gait cycle. This allows a better understanding of the demands on the joint from both the external moments and the muscle forces themselves. For example, normal weight release is approximately 0.12 to 0.15 seconds in duration, and during this time knee flexion rises 20 degrees. Suppose that a patient's actual weight acceptance runs 0.08 seconds and the rise of knee flexion during this period is only 15 degrees. Normalizing the magnitude to this particular phase of gait makes it clear that the knee has not accomplished its degree of flexion in the time provided for initiation of swing. Although the magnitude for this absolute time for this percentage of the gait cycle would be normal, the motion deviation for the purpose of that phase would be abnormal.

Second, because it is assumed that joint rotational forces generated by muscles and body weight affect joint motions for discrete time periods that are shorter than a routine phase of gait, the time interval over which a motion deviation is considered abnormal depends on the phase of gait and the joint in which the motion occurs. The general rule we use is to divide the gait cycle phases into units based on the number of sample data points collected within that phase. A typical interval is divided into halves for short phases and quarters for long phases; in essence the cycle is divided into a total of 12 phases. This division is more detailed than that previously described by Perry for observational gait (Fig. 4).[5] However, this division is not included at all joints and in all planes of motion because the function of muscles and forces in given phases often has a single purpose throughout the phase. An example is that of abduction/adduction at the hip during single-limb stance in which the entire phase is considered as one.

Third, in developing a formalized comprehensive definition of abnormalities related to changes in motion patterns having a mean value over time that may not be outside the bounds of a normal range (10 degrees), we generalize a notion of an abnormality as a set of rules that consider velocities and accelerations as well as average joint displacements. This information usually is not displayed in reports but is currently available with most gait analysis programs.

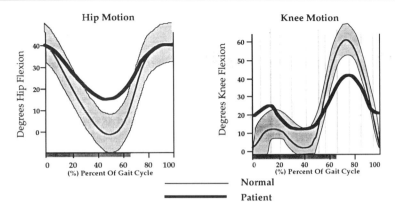

Fig. 4 *Graphs of sagittal plane hip and knee flexion/extension, which demonstrate curves normalized to individual intervals of the gait cycle rather than to the entire gait cycle.*

Defining Clinically Significant Motion Abnormalities

It is clear that gait analysis motion data interpreted by the above technique would define a significant number of motion deviations about each of the joints in children with cerebral palsy. Often a listing of these deviations would fill at least a full page and would be more than an expert kinesiology clinician would state in his/her report. Clearly, when interpreting motion data a clinician must perform a filtering procedure to eliminate from this large number of defined deviations any that are not clinically important. In such considerations, the clinician might not only observe the magnitude and time of the deviation but might also view it in relation to a preceding phase of the cycle or in light of deviations that are occurring simultaneously at the joints above and below.

In this way, the clinician is considering that although a deviation exists, it may not have been caused at that particular point or time in the gait cycle at that joint, but instead is the result of what has preceded it at that joint or what is happening simultaneously at another joint. For example, in stance phase the ankle could be in persistent dorsiflexion of approximately 10 degrees with the knee above it flexed approximately 60 degrees (Fig. 5). The clinician interpreting this information with the knowledge that the hamstrings are tight and the gastrocnemius is spastic, could attribute this pattern to spastic hamstrings creating significant knee flexion and relaxing the gastrocnemius, thereby causing a relative weakness of this muscle and resulting in dorsiflexion at the ankle. The clinician's report could, therefore, merely state abnormality of the knee, because this is the predominant motion deviation, confirmed by physical examination. However, it is possible that if the hamstring deviation were corrected, stance phase ankle dorsiflexion might persist as a result of poor excitation of the gastrocnemius-soleus,

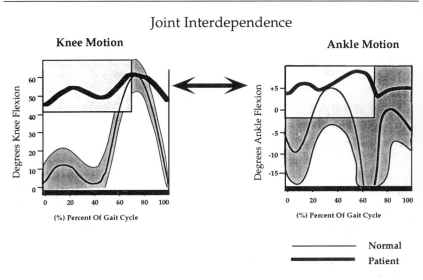

Joint Interdependence

Knee Motion   **Ankle Motion**

——————— Normal
━━━━━━━ Patient

Fig. 5 *Graphs of sagittal plane flexion/extension for the knee and ankle of a child with marked hamstring spasticity. Note the marked knee flexion of 45 to 60 degrees throughout the gait cycle and the calcaneal position (dorsiflexion) of the ankle in stance.*

even though passive physical examination did not reveal this abnormality.

A second example to illustrate the need to view each isolated gait deviation in the context of the entire gait pattern relates to a common motion deviation seen in swing phase at the knee. Not infrequently, in subjects with a low velocity of gait, during the first half of swing phase knee flexion increases slowly, reaching a peak far below the normal, followed during the second half of swing phase by slow knee extension, and never achieving full knee extension by the end of swing phase (Fig. 6). In association with this, a slow increase in hip flexion early in swing could be noted, with full flexion never being achieved by the end of swing phase. A subjective interpretation of these motion deviations based on physical examination knowledge that the hamstrings and quadriceps are spastic and that the patient walks slowly might list only those deviations at the knee and assume that the ones at the hip are related to it. An alternative explanation for this situation might relate to the inability of the hip flexors to develop sufficient force for hip flexion, subsequently affecting the knee and overall velocity. Not identifying hip flexion as less than normal in early swing would then be a significant omission. Because of the nature and amount of data available from gait studies, as well as the time it takes an individual to evaluate this information, errors of omission can arise with subjective interpretation.

To properly define the motion deviations during gait, with the knowl-

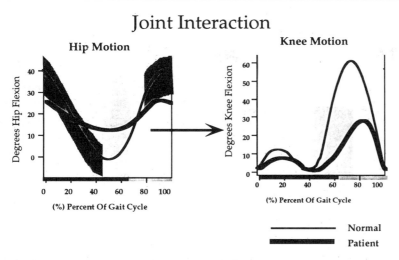

Fig. 6 *Graphs of sagittal plane hip and knee flexion/extension of a child with cerebral palsy. Note the lack of full extension of the hip at the end of single-limb stance (50% of the cycle), the lack of initiation of hip flexion until 65% of the cycle, and the slow rate of rise of hip flexion thereafter (in swing). Associated with these hip motions is a slow rate of rise of knee flexion from 50% to 70% of the cycle and a lack of normal knee flexion at any part of swing.*

edge that computational systems can identify and report as many deviations as necessary within a short period of time, no deviation should be excluded from the report. In addition, actual deviations noted should be separated from causes of those deviations, to ensure that all abnormalities that could be treated are properly identified. Computational techniques are rapid; therefore, separation of these two features of the overall interpretation can be maintained with all motion deviations included.

Interpretation of Muscle Activity Causing Motion Deviations

After identifying the areas of motion deviations, the clinician developing a treatment program must determine the causes of the problems. Features in the history of the child with cerebral palsy that must be taken into account include such obvious things as previous surgical procedures, effectiveness of braces or physical therapy, and the degree of severity of the neurologic involvement. During the physical examination, the clinician takes note of the degree of spasticity, whether contractures are present, etc. Ultimately all these features are brought into play as they relate to abnormalities in the muscle function causing the deviations seen. In interpreting gait analysis data in order to determine a treatment program, it is necessary, therefore, not only to define the motion deviations but also to explain the causes of these deviations in terms of muscle forces produced.

At some time during the gait cycle, many of the approximately 39 muscles in the lower extremity are active. When we wish to consider the causes of motion deviation based on data from gait studies and clinical examination, we must decide on how many muscles we wish to think about and which muscles we can truly identify. In general, the physician considers muscle groups, such as the quadriceps and the medial hamstrings, rather than individual muscles. At times, however, specific muscles are considered, such as the posterior tibialis and the rectus femoris. Neither physical examination nor gait study can provide the amount of information about all the muscles in the lower extremity that is needed for interpretation of the causes of motion deviations. The clinician attempting to interpret the results must make some assumptions and must consider the possibility that some muscles from which data are not obtained may play a role in the motion deviations seen.

Children with cerebral palsy have disordered neurologic control of gait. In normal gait there is a set pattern for the activity of specific muscles in the lower extremity, which cannot be assumed to exist in children with cerebral palsy. Therefore, dynamic electromyographic (EMG) studies, usually obtained via surface electrodes in gait analysis laboratories, are extremely valuable.

Surface electrodes have their limitations, however. They cannot separate rectus femoris activity from that of the remaining quadriceps muscle group, and often they cannot distinguish between the gastrocnemius and soleus. Because surface electrodes may not be specific enough, in certain situations wire electrodes are used that will monitor the activity of specific muscles such as the posterior tibialis and the rectus femoris. For example, if knee flexion early in swing phase is normal, and a sudden cessation occurs and knee motion reverses towards extension with good hip flexion and good velocity of walking, there is a reasonable chance that the rectus femoris alone, or in combination with the quadriceps muscle, could be the primary factor. At the ankle, if relatively minor equinus exists during stance phase but significant inversion and plantarflexion exist during both stance and swing, continuous activity of the posterior tibialis and toe flexors might be the leading cause of this problem rather than the gastrocnemius-soleus complex.

In the absence of concrete evidence, the clinician must make certain assumptions. By combining knowledge as to which actions of specific muscles create motion deviations that may be different in stance than in swing with knowledge of the relative contribution of each muscle to the total load sharing that could produce such deviation within a muscle group, it is possible to assess the cause of the deviation with a specific scale of certainty. Clearly the more information that is available about a muscle's activity, for example, a fine-wire EMG recording demonstrating its activity, the greater the probability of determining whether that specific muscle is the cause of the motion deviation.

Other features of the physical examination and gait analysis study can provide additional information and increase the likelihood of identifying the specific cause of the disorder. Identification of an equinus contracture suggests a high probability that overactivity of the gastrocnemius or soleus or both is sufficient, whether or not the muscle is in its proper phase of gait, to yield the motion deviation seen. Gait studies could further refine this conclusion by revealing a sudden change in motion. An example, in the case of an equinus, is dorsiflexion at or near the point where physical examination suggested the limitation of the contracture. Here it is possible to state that the passive elements rather than muscle activity could be the major cause of the problem.

Sometimes it is difficult to determine whether a problem is created by the weakness of an antagonist or by overactivity or dysphasic activity of an agonist. Two simple examples are (1) ankle plantarflexion in swing phase, and (2) eversion of the ankle during swing phase. Physical examination alone often cannot discriminate whether lack of dorsiflexion in swing is created by absence of tibialis activity or by abnormal activity of the gastrocnemius-soleus complex or whether eversion of the ankle is caused by overactivity of the peroneals, underactivity of the posterior tibialis, or a combination of both. However, physical examination may provide a significant amount of diagnostic information. Observation of voluntary activity of the anterior tibialis during the physical examination and of prominence of its tendon during gait when the child walks barefoot, as well as the absence of any inversion or eversion, would suggest that the gastrocnemius-soleus is abnormally active in swing phase. An Achilles tendon lengthening in the patient's history, dorsiflexion of 5 degrees on physical examination, and a lack of prominence of the tibialis anterior tendon at the ankle joint during a request for voluntary dorsiflexion, as well as during gait, would suggest that lack of activity of this muscle is the prime culprit for the equinus position of the ankle during swing phase. Noting marked prominence or even dislocation of the peroneal tendons during physical examination, as well as a high arch to the lateral aspect of the foot with pronation of the forefoot during standing and a lack of ability to invert the foot voluntarily, might suggest that eversion was caused by a spastic abnormal response of the peroneals during gait. Confirming these facts with EMG recordings during gait can provide an additional level of certainty regarding the cause of the problem.

All these features, therefore, combine to provide a certain degree of probability as to the cause of the motion deviation. When the complexity of this task is considered, it is clear that a clinician subjectively interpreting gait data must know a great deal about muscle physiology and kinematics as well as the effects of cerebral palsy on muscle control. Expert clinicians perform this task almost unconsciously; those with less knowledge or experience do not do it as well. The thoroughness with which even experts are able to assess motion deviations may not be optimal at all times.

Therefore, the first step in demonstrating the possible causes of a motion deviation is to list all the possibilities. Whether this is done subjectively by a clinician or analytically by a computer, a long list will be produced. On a subjectively produced list, some possibilities may be missed. The program we have established lists all of the possibilities first. Each additional piece of information pertinent to the probability of a specific cause is automatically included. If information is available, it is appropriately weighted as a percentage of probability. Where a specific piece of information is missing, the possibility that that muscle may still be the cause of the problem is maintained throughout the interpretation. In this way, the system develops a degree of certainty as to the cause of the problem.

We have incorporated all these features into a knowledge base of our expert (artificial intelligence) system for gait interpretation. Just as the clinician has knowledge with which to interpret the gait data, the interpretation program has knowledge stored in the computer, which it may call on. Actions are included of all major muscle groups and individual muscles that act in the lower extremity, including the quadriceps, hamstrings, iliopsoas, gluteus maximus, gluteus medius, adductors, gastrocnemius-soleus, peroneals, posterior tibialis, anterior tibialis, and rectus femoris. The muscles are considered as both two-joint and one-joint muscles for their actions, and the time in a normal gait cycle serves as a baseline showing when each muscle is or is not active. When demographic information about a particular patient is entered, and the history shows previous surgery or the use of a brace, the knowledge base in the computer states that the muscle is considered weaker than if there had been no previous treatment. The knowledge base can understand the difference between muscle contractures and joint contractures, and also knows how a spastic muscle behaves (increased force and abnormal timing) when such data as presence of excessive tone or clonic movements are entered for a particular subject. The presence or absence of activity of the muscle during a particular time of gait is then considered as additional information obtained from dynamic EMG studies for the interpretation portion of the program. Where motion deviations about a joint in more than one plane or between two joints suggests a specific muscle rather than a muscle group, the program can understand that information from wire electrodes, if provided, provides an additional degree of certainty. Having already stored knowledge of the overall mass of the muscle as well as its normal demands during gait, the computer program can then consider differentiating further between two possible causes of a problem. For example, during swing phase of gait if the ankle is in equinus and no contracture exists at the ankle, and EMG activity suggests activity of the anterior tibialis, toe extensors, and gastrocnemius-soleus complex, then the deviation would be attributed to the gastrocnemius-soleus complex.

Kinetics as Related to Muscle Cause Identification

When considering the causes of motion deviations, it is important to realize that in addition to determining the contribution of a specific muscle or group of muscles, body weight and momentum as well as the position and forces occurring at other joints need to be taken into account. If a major contracture or severe rigidity of a muscle is present at a specific joint, that contracture or rigidity will be a major factor, contributing to the motion about that joint. Many situations, however, are more complex, and in these cases the conditions at the other joints must be taken into account. Additionally, although deviation from normal motion is present and can be related to a specific muscle or muscles, it may not be considered an abnormality but rather a compensation for what is occurring at another joint. Therefore, a thorough interpretation of gait, either analytically (by computer) or subjectively (clinically) determined, must include forces that are arising at other joints and the external torques created by body weight and momentum.

Without gait analysis data it is difficult to obtain data on forces at other joints and on external torques, but these data often can be obtained in a clinical setting. A 60-degree hamstring contracture easily seen during gait in combination with calcaneus at the ankle, without previous heel cord surgery and spasticity noted in the gastrocnemius-soleus complex on physical examination, could indicate that the cause of the problem both at the knee and the ankle is related to the hamstrings. Gait analysis data could further refine and clarify the situation, but not alter the overall conclusion. What is needed for interpretation, regardless of whether the information is provided from gait analysis data or from clinical evaluation, is knowledge, on the part of the interpreter, of the kinetics and kinematics of normal and abnormal gait.

For data derived from gait studies, we have expressed this knowledge in a qualitative model of gait. The model is defined in a set of qualitative equations for each joint in each plane. The forces modeled in these equations include the effects of other joints on the joint in question and the effect of preceding phases on the current phase. In any given plane, each equation specifies possible muscles and indirect forces that effect a given rotation. In addition, each term in the equation is augmented with information describing its strength relative to the other terms. For example, in equations for the ankle in stance, the gastrocnemius-soleus complex is much more powerful than the other muscles that affect ankle dorsiflexion/plantarflexion. In this way, a qualitative model provided with gait analysis data can better define how all these other factors contribute to the cause of the motion deviation.

Summary

It is important to differentiate between the interpretation of information provided about the gait of a child with cerebral palsy and the identification of the motion abnormalities that exist. The first step is to identify clearly the abnormalities that exist. Without gait study data, it is difficult to see motion deviations at all joints and to pinpoint them to specific times in the gait cycle. While knowledge of the timing of specific muscle activity can be appropriately determined from clinical examination in some cases, it may not be easy to determine in others. Adding gait analysis data to the identification process improves the ability to properly describe abnormalities. However, other problems arise when these data are interpreted subjectively. Conclusions vary from individual to individual, and this lack of uniformity limits understanding of the pathophysiology and its treatment. By creating a clear understanding of the nature of the problem and its causes, an analytical approach mediated through computer programs could be of significant assistance to individuals interested in this field.

References

1. Bleck EE: *Orthopaedic Management of Cerebral Palsy.* Philadelphia, WB Saunders, 1979.
2. Hirsch D, Simon SR, Bylander T, et al: Using causal reasoning in gait analysis. *AAI* 1989;3:253–272.
3. Weintraub MA, Bylander T, Simon SR,: QUAWDS: A composite diagnostic system for gait analysis. *Comput Methods Programs Biomed* 1990;32:91–106.
4. Sutherland D, Olshen R, Biden E, et al: *The Development of Mature Walking.* London, MacKeith Press, 1988.
5. Perry J: *Gait Analysis: Normal and Pathological Function.* New York, McGraw-Hill, 1992.

Chapter 15

Computer Based Decision Making

James R. Gage, MD

Introduction

Computer-based decision making has only recently entered the clinical arena, and it is being met with a great deal of skepticism from those who are still unfamiliar with its current uses and its future potential. In actuality, it constitutes just one of the three types of examinations that are necessary to accurately assess a patient with cerebral palsy. The other two are the standard clinical examination and the examination under anesthesia that takes place just before corrective surgery begins. Each of these three examinations provides the examiner with some unique pieces of information that cannot be gleaned from the other two. Thus, each has a very important role to play. In addition, computer-based decision making fulfills a useful function after surgery in that it accurately and objectively documents the outcome, which, in turn, allows meaningful comparison between the pre- and postoperative status of the patient. In order to understand why three separate types of examination are necessary in the treatment of cerebral palsy, it is necessary to understand the cerebral palsy lesion and its clinical ramifications. Therefore, before I can begin a discussion on the usefulness of a particular treatment modality, it is necessary to briefly review the nature of the cerebral palsy lesion as well as the state-of-the-art with respect to treatment.

The Pathophysiology of Cerebral Palsy

A simple schematic of cerebral control is illustrated in Figure 1. Because of the damage to the central nervous system, a patient with spastic cerebral palsy will demonstrate some or all of the following features: (1) loss of selective muscle control; (2) dependence on primitive reflex patterns for ambulation; (3) abnormal muscle tone; (4) relative imbalance between muscle agonists and antagonists across joints, which, with time and growth, leads to muscle contracture and bony deformity; and (5) deficient equilibrium reactions.

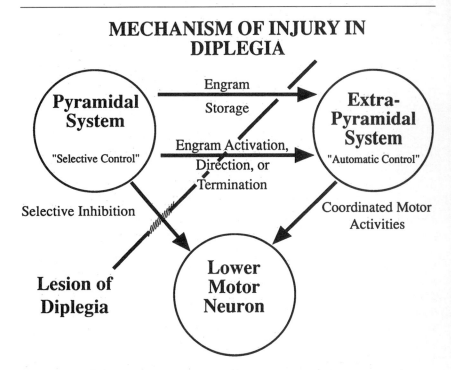

Fig. 1 *A simple schematic diagram of the motor control system of the brain. The pyramidal system initiates voluntary motor activities (engrams) and supervises or oversees the extrapyramidal system in which the engrams are stored. The pyramidal system also prevents excessive tone through its inhibitory action on the spinal cord neurons. A lesion in the region of the internal capsule (represented by the slashed line) can disrupt the pyramidal system's connections to both the extrapyramidal system and the lower motor neurons in the spinal cord. The result of such a disruption would produce abnormal muscle tone, relative imbalance between muscle agonists and antagonists, loss of selective motor control, dependence on primitive reflex patterns for ambulation, and deficient equilibrium reactions. (Reproduced with permission from Gage JR:* Gait Analysis in Cerebral Palsy. *Oxford, MacKeith Press, 1991, p 56.)*

Loss of Selective Control and Dependence Upon Primitive Reflex Patterns

Loss of selective muscle control is a primary problem, ie, it is a direct result of injury to the central nervous system. Fortunately, many of the movement patterns required for walking are preprogrammed in lower brain centers. With injury to the motor cortex, these primitive reflex patterns, which are located mainly in the basal ganglia, become the means by which ambulation is accomplished. Thus, the emergence of primitive locomotor reflex patterns, which result from central nervous system injury, constitutes the means by which the individual with cerebral palsy manages to walk in spite of the loss of selective motor control. The simplest example of this is the typical hemiplegic stroke patient who may have great difficulty in moving his/her paralyzed extremity, but can still walk quite well by reciprocating two primitive reflex patterns. Limb advancement in swing is accomplished by using a mass flexion reflex that produces hip flexion, knee flexion, and ankle dorsiflexion. The body is advanced in stance on the affected side via a mass extension reflex that features hip and knee extension in conjunction with ankle plantarflexion. Thus, loss of selective motor control can be thought of as a primary abnormality as it comes directly from the brain injury.

The predominance of primitive reflex patterns, although also a direct result of injury to the central nervous system, is nevertheless useful because without them the individual would not be able to walk at all. In addition, however, the individual alters gait patterns to compensate for the primary problem. An example of this is circumduction of the lower extremity when the knee cannot be adequately flexed for clearance. In this example, the primary problem is at the knee, and the compensation is hip abduction with forward flexion in swing phase. Because these compensations require voluntary control and because the more proximal joints are under better voluntary control than the distal, these compensatory or coping responses usually occur at the hip or pelvis; or, in other words, proximal compensations are used for distal deviations. The point is that pathologic gait is a mixture of primary abnormalities imposed by the loss of selective control, primitive patterns of gait, which emerge after injury to the higher centers, and compensatory responses that are under voluntary control. There is no way to adequately separate out all of these deformities without computerized gait analysis.

Abnormal Muscle Tone

The extent of damage to the pyramidal system determines the amount of selective control remaining. Because the corticospinal tracts act to inhibit and balance the tone enhancement emanating from muscle spindles, maintenance of normal muscle tone is also dependent upon the integrity of this system. The amount of spasticity present depends in part upon the aggregate damage to the pyramidal system. When there is damage to the extrapyramidal system, muscle tone is not spastic, but dystonic. This may vary greatly in degree from decreased tone (hypotonia) to markedly increased tone (rigidity or tension athetosis). In mixed cerebral palsy, both patterns of abnormal tone are present, and the patient will exhibit a mixture of spasticity and dystonia.

Relative Agonist/Antagonist Imbalance Across Joints

In spastic diplegia, spasticity is most prominent in the hip adductors, flexors, and internal rotators; knee flexors (hamstrings); ankle plantarflexors; and peroneals. This produces a walking posture of hip flexion, adduction, and internal rotation; knee flexion; and ankle equinus with pes planovalgus. Interestingly, when these muscles are studied with dynamic electromyography (EMG) in a spastic patient, they tend to be overactive, that is, they have prolonged activity during the gait cycle.

Their antagonists, on the other hand, often show relatively normal electromyographic activity. When spasticity occurs, only dynamic muscle contractures are present initially, but with time and growth they become fixed.

Long bones grow at the level of the epiphyseal plates by the process of endochondral ossification. Muscles grow by adding sarcomeres at the musculotendinous junction. The stimuli for this growth are somatotropin (growth hormone) and stretch.[1] Thus, as the normally growing child runs and plays each day, the child's muscles are stretched over the continually growing bone. If a muscle agonist is dominant over its antagonist, the latter will receive excessive stretch, whereas the former will be stretched inadequately. This combination produces excessive growth of the antagonist and insufficient growth of the agonist muscle, which will ultimately lead to contracture. It is probably the consistent spastic tone in certain muscle groups that produces the relative agonist-antagonist imbalance across joints, leading to contracture, because joint contracture is not a feature of athetoid cerebral palsy, in which dystonia is present rather than spasticity.

Deficient Equilibrium Reactions

The vestibular system is the seat of balance and equilibrium. It consists of receptors located in the inner ear, peripheral nerve fibers to mediate information from the vestibular nuclei in the midbrain, and ascending and descending pathways from these nuclei. The vestibular system reinforces the tone of the extensor muscles of the trunk and limbs, enabling the muscles to support the body against gravity and maintain an upright posture. In an animal whose brain is transected at a midbrain level, a condition develops that is known as decerebrate rigidity. In humans this condition is characterized by extension of all the limbs with the arms adducted and internally rotated. Sherrington[2] showed that decerebrate rigidity is dependent on intact reflex arcs and the vestibular system. Therefore, it can be abolished by transection of the dorsal spinal cord roots and/or lesions of the central nervous system that interrupt the descending vestibular and reticular pathways.

Ascending pathways from the vestibular system synapse on the somatic motor nuclei of the cranial nerves that supply the extra-ocular muscles. The vestibular system is extremely important in controlling conjugate eye movements in response to head movement and to the position of the head in space. Without the vestibular system, the eyes could not remain fixed on stationary objects while the head and/or body are moving.

Primitive reflexes that involve the vestibular system may become prominent when an injury to the cerebral cortex unmasks the suppressive effect of the higher centers. Examples of these are the tonic reflexes. Tonic reflexes are those that maintain reflex contractions, which are the basis of posture and attitude. The control of body position in space and the maintenance of balance are heavily dependent on these reflexes. The principle tonic reflexes are the symmetrical and asymmetrical tonic neck reflexes and the tonic labyrinthine prone and supine reflexes.[3]

Now that I have discussed the abnormalities seen in cerebral palsy, it should be apparent that, of all the items on the list, only abnormal muscle tone and relative imbalance between muscle agonists and antagonists across joints are amenable to current surgical treatment. Furthermore, it should be evident that the abnormalities of gait that occur as a result of the cerebral palsy lesion are complex and cannot be adequately elucidated without sophisticated methods of analysis.

What's Wrong With Depending Solely Upon Clinical Parameters?

The necessity for the routine use of gait analysis in the management of gait problems is most easily defended by looking at the current situation with respect to the treatment of children with cerebral palsy.

What is the Current Status of Treatment?

The treatment available to most children is far from ideal. To begin with, many surgeons who treat cerebral palsy lack a good understanding of the pathophysiology of the condition. Instead, the decision as to what surgery needs to be done is based almost entirely upon clinical examination and watching the child walk. Unfortunately, the observer of gait usually has inadequate knowledge of the mechanisms of normal walking and even less of pathologic gait. Once surgery is undertaken, it is frequently staged with correction of one muscle group at a time and with long periods of immobilization after each intervention. Thus, the golden period of childhood is reduced to a series of operations and recoveries, a phenomenon that Mercer Rang has termed "the birthday syndrome."[4] Finally, the critical parameters of evaluation at Gillette Children's Hospital, such as oxygen consumption and gait analysis, indicate that many children treated in this way may be iatrogenically injured rather than helped by their surgery. In my mind, making surgical decisions for children with cerebral palsy with only clinical assessment is much akin to attempting to make accurate decisions regarding coronary artery surgery using no diagnostic tools other than a stethoscope.

What Type of Information Can We Gather From Gait Analysis?

In general, gait analysis involves three types of studies, each of which provides us with a different type of information.

Kinematics   Kinematics is the subdivision of mechanics that deals with the geometry of motion, without regard to forces. Kinematic analysis relates further to the study of relative motion between rigid bodies, called links, and finds application in analysis of gait and other body movements where each limb segment is considered a link. It provides information about parameters, such as joint angles, displacements, velocities, and accelerations, that are used to describe locomotion.

Kinetics Kinetics is the subdivision of mechanics that deals with variables, such as ground-reaction forces (GRF), joint moments, and joint powers, that are the cause of locomotion. Kinetics is becoming very important because it provides information that is one step closer to the source of pathology. The two types of kinetic assessments commonly used in modern gait analysis are joint moments and joint powers.

A moment is defined as a force couple, that is, a force acting at a distance about an axis of rotation to cause an angular acceleration about that axis. Mathematically, moments are equal to force times distance from the center of rotation and, as such, usually have units of Newton·meters (N·m). When comparing moments between individuals, it is necessary to standardize them by dividing them by the subject's body weight in kilograms (N·m/kg) and to normalize them according to when they occur in the gait cycle. The external moments around the joints are produced by the GRF. The internal moments, which balance the GRF, are produced by muscle action. Joint-moment graphs provide information as to which muscle groups are dominant.

Joint power is defined as the product of the net joint moment and joint angular velocity. The unit of measurement is watts/kilogram (W/ kg). Joint-power graphs indicate which muscles are generating or absorbing energy. Because work equals power times time, integration of power curves enables estimation of the net work that is being produced at each joint during one gait cycle (Fig. 2). Thus, by integrating sagittal-plane power graphs of the hip, knee, and ankle, it has been estimated that in normal walking, 54% of the total energy required comes from the hip, 10% comes from the knee, and 36% comes from the ankle (Fig. 3). Power curves provide extremely useful information because knowledge of which muscle groups are the source of power generation is critical to surgical decision making. If the sources of propulsive power in pathologic gait can be identified, then surgical intervention on those muscle groups that are critical to power generation can be reduced to a minimum, and surgical procedures can be chosen with respect to their potential for minimizing loss of the muscle strength needed for propulsion.

Dynamic EMG EMG is the recording and study of the electrical activity of muscle. Dynamic EMG is used in most gait laboratories to determine when a muscle or muscle group is active; however, it cannot accurately measure the magnitude of that activity. In the treatment of cerebral palsy, EMG can provide several very useful pieces of information.

Dynamic EMG is used to determine which muscle is responsible for dysfunction in situations where there are several possibilities. Two situations in which EMG may help to discriminate are varus deformities of the foot and/or flexion deformities at the hip.[5] In order to isolate the activity to a specific muscle, many investigators feel that insertion of fine-wire electrodes is necessary. Using fine-wire EMG, Perry[6] has shown that in patients with cerebral palsy many of the two-joint muscle stretch tests are invalid, because they invoke a response from both mono- and biarticulate muscles.

THE ANKLE

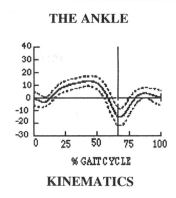

KINEMATICS

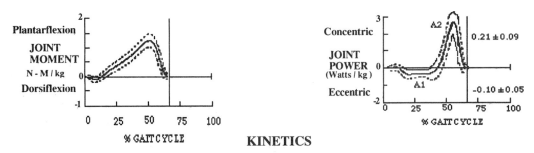

KINETICS

Fig. 2 *An illustration of normal ankle kinematics and kinetics. The solid line represents the mean and the dotted line one standard deviation. Notice that during first rocker there is a small dorsiflexor moment. At the end of loading response a plantarflexor moment begins, which reaches its peak at terminal stance and then rapidly falls to zero during preswing (double support). Power is obtained by multiplying the moment times the joint angular velocity. The sign convention is such that a negative power indicates negative work, ie, that the muscle is contracting eccentrically and absorbing energy. Positive power indicates that the muscle is contracting and performing positive work, ie, producing an acceleration. Using Winter's convention, each burst of ankle power begins with A and is numbered successively from left to right. The numbers at the right of the graph are an integration of all positive and negative powers plus or minus one standard deviation and represent the total work done in joules. Hence the total positive work done during one gait cycle is 0.21 ± 0.09 joules/kg. (Reproduced with permission from Gage JR:* Gait Analysis in Cerebral Palsy. *Oxford, MacKeith Press, 1991, p 84.)*

By comparing the timing on the patient's EMG to that of a normal standard, inferences can be made regarding whether or not the muscle or muscle group being studied is behaving appropriately or pathologically (Fig. 4). However, if EMG and kinetic moment data are used in conjunction with each other, much more specific information can be obtained. Because the external moments produced by the GRF are balanced by the internal muscle moments, their onsets and cessation should be simultaneous. Thus, a muscle may be assumed to be under voluntary control even if its EMG signal is prolonged, provided the duration of the GRF that requires the muscle action is prolonged by the same amount (Fig. 5).

POWER GRAPHS

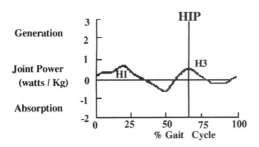

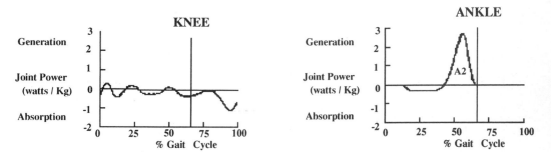

Fig. 3 *Power graphs of the hip, knee, and ankle. Gait cycle is on the axis, and power in watts is on the abscissa. Positive power indicates generation, negative power indicates absorption. The major power bursts for propulsion are generated by the ankle plantarflexors (A2), the hip extensors (H1), and the hip flexors (H3). These represent about 36%, 32%, and 22%, respectively, of the total. The remaining 10% is generated by the knee extensors. (Reproduced with permission from Gage JR:* Gait Analysis in Cerebral Palsy. *Oxford, MacKeith Press, 1991, p 31.)*

In addition to these parameters, an increasing amount of emphasis is being placed on estimating the amount of energy expended during gait. Currently, the most common and accepted way of doing this is by measurement of oxygen consumption.

An Example

Orthopaedic treatment must address five major areas of deficit to improve ambulation. These are: (1) Restoration of stance phase stability, (2) improvement of clearance on the swing side, (3) appropriate prepositioning of the foot in terminal swing, (4) enablement of an adequate step length, and (5) reduction of energy expenditure.

A child with type III hemiplegia shown in Figure 6 is a good example.[7] Before surgery, he had stance phase instability, ie, he couldn't get his right foot down flat on the floor. In addition, he had cospasticity of

PRE-OPERATIVE EMG

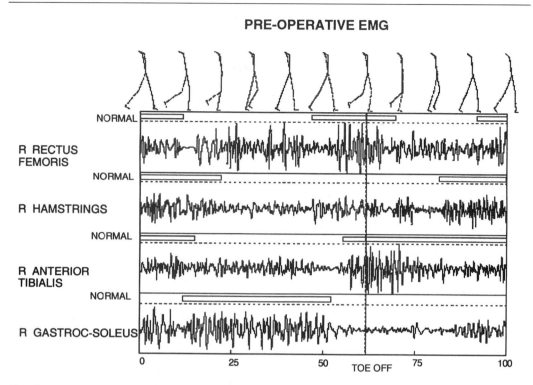

Fig. 4 *EMG display. Electromyographic (EMG) data is brought through electronic filters to remove as much of the underlying electronic noise as possible. On the left is the EMG format that is in use at Newington and Gillette Children's Hospitals. (Reproduced with permission from Gage JR:* Gait Analysis in Cerebral Palsy. *Oxford, MacKeith Press, 1991, p 25.)*

his rectus femoris and hamstrings on the affected side so that he had difficulty clearing his foot in swing. He had a shortened stride and poor preposition of his foot in terminal swing. Finally, he had excessive energy consumption.

A year after surgery (Fig. 7), the child is walking at the same speed with excellent stance phase stability and good swing phase clearance. He has a longer stride length because his leaf-spring ankle-foot orthosis maintains his foot in the appropriate position in terminal swing. Because his clonus has been eliminated, energy consumption across the ankle, as measured by integration of ankle power curves, has been reduced by half.

Postoperative Assessment

Postoperative gait analysis enables precise analysis of outcomes, discovery of treatment errors, collective study of results, and gain of additional insight into the pathology and the results of treatment. Figure 8 provides preoperative and postoperative kinematic sagittal plane data

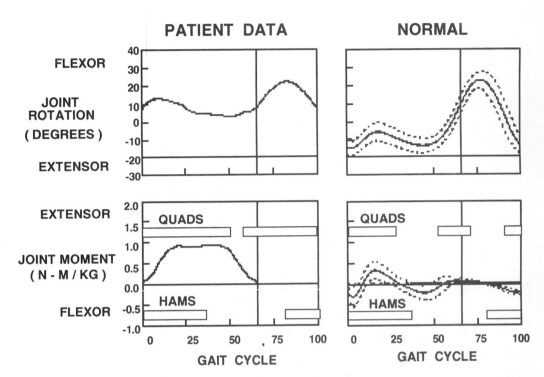

Fig. 5 *Combined EMG and moments. Patient data are on the left, and normal data are on the right. The kinematic graph of the patient (**top left**) shows that the knee is continuously in flexion during the stance phase of gait. Consequently, the moment graph of the patient's knee (**bottom left**) indicates a persistent extensor moment of the muscle, which is necessary to balance the flexor moment created by the GRF. Because the quadriceps are the principle extensors of the knee, they must remain active throughout stance and, hence, the EMG of the quadriceps, although abnormal, in this case is clearly responding to an abnormal moment. Thus, this muscle group may still be under good voluntary control. Modern gait analysis provides the surgeon with the ability to look at the EMG signal of a muscle "in the light of the moment" and, thus, provides objective evidence of whether the muscle signal is abnormal as a result of the central nervous system injury or whether it is under voluntary control and is merely responding to an abnormal moment. (Reproduced with permission from Gage JR: Gait Analysis in Cerebral Palsy. Oxford, MacKeith Press, 1991, p 82.)*

on the ankle, knee, hip, and pelvis of the patient compared to a normal file. Figure 9 presents preoperative and postoperative kinetic sagittal plane data on the ankle compared to a normal file. Even without an understanding of normal gait mechanics and gait analysis, an astute observer should see that the solid line more closely mirrors the normal. In addition, it is possible to see exactly what the surgery has accomplished at the ankle.

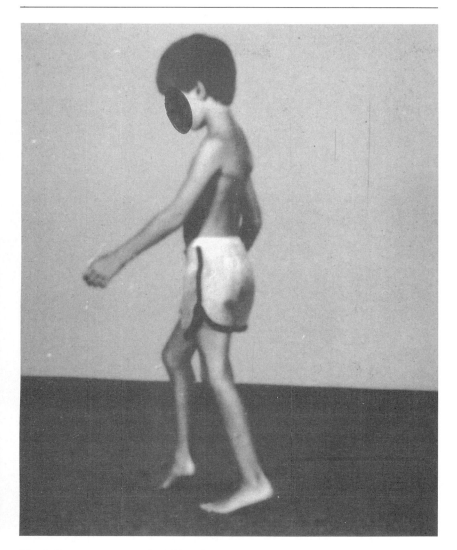

Fig. 6 *Preoperative gait. A child with type III hemiplegia on the right side prior to orthopaedic intervention. On the right side he is missing all of the normal prerequisites of gait, ie, stability in stance, clearance in swing, pre-position of the foot in swing, and adequate step length. (Reproduced with permission Gage JR:* Gait Analysis in Cerebral Palsy. *Oxford, MacKeith Press, 1991, p 142.)*

Why Should Computerized Gait Analysis Be Used?

I feel that computerized gait analysis offers many advantages: (1) It provides a dynamic assessment of the pretreatment status with the child in an upright position, thus avoiding the changes in tone that are present on the static, recumbent examination. (2) Motion analysis allows precise evaluation of the gait deviations imposed by the child's cerebral palsy (the primary problems) as well as separation of these primary

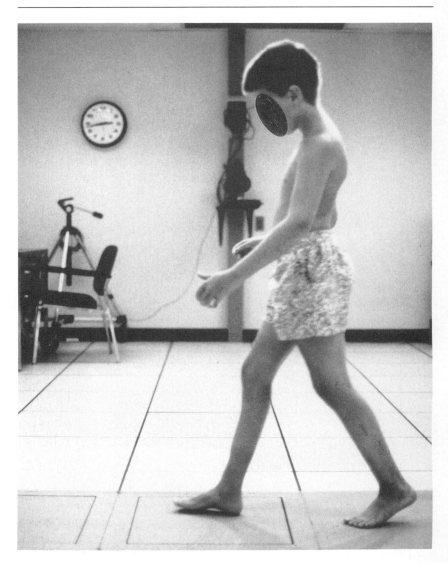

Fig. 7 *Postoperative gait. The same child a year postsurgery. The right foot is now in the line of progression and is stable in stance. Knee flexion during swing on the hemiplegic side now approximates normal. Finally, the knee shows better extension and the foot is more appropriately pre-positioned in terminal stance. In other words, the normal prerequisites of gait have been largely restored. (Reproduced with permission from Gage JR:* Gait Analysis in Cerebral Palsy. *Oxford, MacKeith Press, 1991, p 146.)*

problems from the secondary gait adaptations that essentially are coping mechanisms. (3) Once the abnormalities of gait can be isolated, specific treatment can be directed to each of the primary abnormalities while avoiding the coping mechanisms. Thus, staging of surgery can be avoided with less fear of error or iatrogenic injury. (4) There is an

SAGITTAL PLANE KINEMATICS

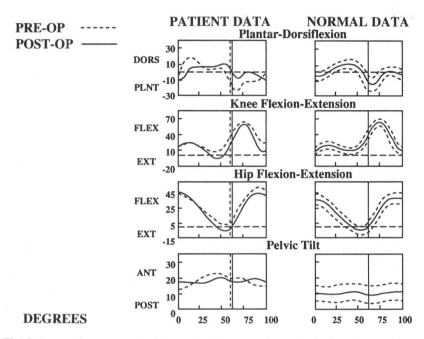

Fig. 8 *Pre- and postoperative kinematics. Postoperative sagittal plane kinematics demonstrate functional improvements at the ankle, knee, hip, and pelvis when compared to those taken preoperatively. The knee, hip, and pelvic tilt graphs are all essentially within normal limits postoperatively. The ankle graph demonstrates a mild drop foot in terminal swing and at initial contact. On the basis of these graphs, the patient would now be classified as a type I. (Reproduced with permission from Gage JR: Gait Analysis in Cerebral Palsy. Oxford, MacKeith Press, 1991, p 147.)*

objective, accurate record of the patient's gait both before and after treatment, which permits a valid assessment of the surgical outcome. (5) Objective evaluation of surgical outcomes and understanding of gait mechanics increases understanding of movement patterns, which in turn leads to better decision making.

Summary

Gait analysis allows practical application of the scientific method, which is the accumulation of facts, organization of these facts into principles or laws, postulation of hypotheses to account for the facts and laws, and comparison of the hypothetical deduction with the experimental result. Before computer-based gait analysis was available, surgeons would start with a spastic child who walked abnormally and end with a spastic child who walked differently, but it was very difficult to tell exactly what the surgery had accomplished. Today, it is possible to

ANKLE KINEMATICS & KINETICS

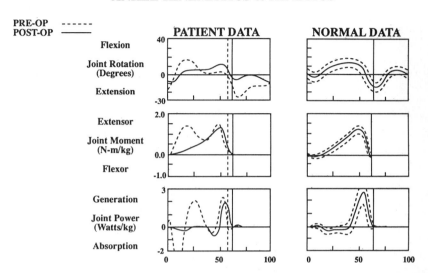

Fig. 9 *The pre- and postoperative sagittal plane kinematics and kinetics of the ankle in the subject shown in Fig. 8. Note that all of the preoperative graphs more closely approximate the normal, and that the double burst of power that was present preoperatively, as a result of the patients gastrocnemius clonus, has been eliminated. (Reproduced with permission from Gage JR:* Gait Analysis in Cerebral Palsy. *Oxford MacKeith Press, p 148.)*

critique surgery accurately. Gait analysis has been used to do this for 10 years at Newington Children's Hospital and for 4 years at Gillette. As a result of gait analysis, children with cerebral palsy have a brighter future, because as therapists learn from the past, they can avoid perpetuating errors into the future.

In the past few years, I have reached the point where, after performing gait analysis, I can sit down with the parents, demonstrate their child's gait abnormalities with the data, and then show them the pre- and postoperative videotape of a child who was affected similarly. Following this I can say, "This is what you have a right to expect." It took a long time to get this far, but it was well worth the effort. Therefore, because preoperative evaluation and outcome measures can be done easily with the new methodology, and computerized gait analysis is now commercially available at reasonable cost, the benefits are obvious. I feel that the reasons for clinging to old methods of treatment in the face of the suboptimal outcomes of the past are neither apparent nor logical. Therefore, the burden of proof rests not with those who wish to take up better ways, but rather with those who are unable or unwilling to lay down the old.

References

1. Ziv I, Blackburn N, Rang M, et al: Muscle growth in normal and spastic mice. *Dev Med Child Neurol* 1984;26:94–99.
2. Denny-Brown D: *Selected Writings of Sir Charles Sherrington*. New York, Paul B. Hoeber, 1940, pp 314–396.
3. Bleck EE: *Orthopaedic Management in Cerebral Palsy*. Oxford, MacKeith Press, 1987, pp 24–28.
4. Rang M, Silver R, de la Garza J: Cerebral palsy, in Morrissy RT (ed): *Lovell and Winter's Pediatric Orthopaedics*, ed 3. Philadelphia, JB Lippincott, 1990, p 402.
5. Perry J, Hoffer MM: Preoperative and postoperative dynamic electromyography as an aid in planning tendon transfers in children with cerebral palsy. *J Bone Joint Surg* 1977;59A:531–537.
6. Perry J, Hoffer MM, Antonelli D, et al: Electromyography before and after surgery for hip deformity in children with cerebral palsy. A comparison of clinical and electromyographic findings. *J Bone Joint Surg* 1976;58A:201–208.
7. Winters TF Jr, Gage JR, Hicks R: Gait patterns in spastic hemiplegia in children and young adults. *J Bone Joint Surg* 1987;69A:437–441.

Consensus

Making orthopaedic surgical decisions for children with spastic diplegia can be extraordinarily difficult (as contrasted with most children with spastic hemiplegia or total body cerebral palsy) and requires every effort to gather adequate data and to evaluate these data with caution.

Appropriate Goal Setting

The patient's (or family's) chief complaint must be clearly delineated. The goals of the patient or the parents may be different from and may even conflict with those of the orthopaedic surgeon and others involved in the child's care. Whatever the goals may be, it is important that they are attainable within the child's neurologic limits.

The orthopaedic surgeon's goal is to make the child as normal as possible within a happy family. Within this broad statement, the priority of goals is first to prevent deformity or future problems. For people with spastic diplegia, particular attention must be paid to those aspects that can become problems in later childhood, such as hip subluxation, and in adulthood, such as patellofemoral, foot, and lumbar spine difficulties, and hip arthritis. While contractures are a particular problem during the growing years, they may also progress after maturity. However, there is a paucity of good data on the problems that plague the adult with spastic diplegia. Further study is needed.

A second goal is to improve present and anticipated future function, as estimated by kinetics, kinematics, energy consumption, and functional abilities. The third goal is to improve appearance. There is difference of opinion as to the degree to which surgery should be done solely to improve appearance. While some feel this is seldom warranted, the general feeling is that there are definitely times when an improvement in appearance can lead to an enhanced sense of self worth with improved overall function in society. Many feel this decision should be left to the patient and parents.

History

General information, beyond the usual medical history, should focus on the psychosocial aspects of the child's setting in the family. Birth history is important when deciding about selective posterior rhizotomy. Detailed information should be sought regarding previous management of the patient's cerebral palsy, including any previous surgeries and how the child and family responded, as well as how they responded to bracing or other treatments.

The child's cognitive level should be evaluated in respect to its impact on rehabilitation potential. There is uncertainty as to the degree to which children who are cognitively deficient should be restricted from undergoing surgery. Because some surgeries require postoperative "training" to optimize outcome, a child's ability to cooperate can make a significant difference to the postsurgical result. However, for conditions where the postoperative changes in function are automatic as compared to trained, surgery can be undertaken without concern for a child's decreased cognitive level or for the presence of an attention deficit. The child's ability to perform must be considered for

(1) operations that require prolonged immobilization (especially where the use of a hip spica cast is contemplated) and may require postoperative physical therapy; (2) surgery to correct crouched gait, which requires more active physical therapy; (3) multiple surgeries at one sitting in which the child sustains a large physiologic insult and may require training; and (4) reverse phase muscle tendon transfer, which may require tendon transfer training. An older child whose IQ is particularly high may be more confused by the postoperative posture changes and require more extensive training than children with lower IQs. Data should be obtained to clarify the importance of cognition on postoperative management.

The motivation of both patient and parents must be evaluated. Parental motivation should be within the bounds of realistic goals for the child. There are no clinically useful measures of motivation in children with cerebral palsy to guide the clinicians. Such tests should be developed to make this as objective as possible.

Physical Examination

Evaluation of Posture The examiner must evaluate the patient's general standing and sitting alignment (the head and trunk; the hips, knees, ankles, and feet) in both the frontal and sagittal planes.

Evaluation of Static Joint Ranges
Range of motion for the hips should include the degree of hip flexion and extension and the extension deficit, making certain that the lumbosacral spine is flat on the examining table; abduction both with the hips and knees extended and with them flexed 90 degrees; adduction with the hip and knee extended; and prone internal and external rotation. Many orthopaedic surgeons feel that palpation of the greater trochanter throughout the rotation range is an important measure of anteversion.

Range-of-motion testing for the knee should include flexion (prone); the extension deficit with the hip fully extended (the knee flexion contracture) and with the hip flexed 90 degrees (the popliteal angle). The position of the patella should be carefully checked to establish the presence or absence of patella alta.

Range-of-motion testing for the ankles should include dorsiflexion with the ipsilateral knee extended and flexed and plantarflexion, as well as measures of alignment (the thigh/foot angle and the bimalleolar axis). These tests should also be performed with the patient upright so that the influence of the vestibular and primitive contact systems are included. Range-of-motion testing for the feet should include inversion and eversion as well as measures of fixed hindfoot valgus position (using Coleman's test with blocks under the heel) and measures of position of the midfoot (adductus or abductus).

All of these measures should be done with a goniometer. However, there is little objective data as to the measurement error (both interobserver and intraobserver) of such evaluations. The moderate body of information on the measurement errors of clinical evaluation of ranges of motion is scattered throughout the orthopaedic and physical therapy literature. This information should be collated and evaluated to see what new measurement error information is needed.

Evaluation of Dynamic Joint Ranges
This evaluation seeks to find the impact of the child's spasticity on passive motion. Ashworth's measure of muscle tonicity is not felt to be useful by most. Each of the ranges described above should be done both slowly to determine the joint range of motion and quickly to incite a spastic response.

The presence of clonus, which is repeated joint motion, that lasts for two or more seconds following the reflex stimulus, as a measure of spasticity should be noted. Presence of clonus persisting for more than one minute should warn the surgeon that there may be intraspinal pathology.

Evaluation of Motor Control Children with better motor control can be expected to have better surgical results. The central nervous system damage in a child with spastic diplegia may include the inability to process the sensory information as well as an inability to control the peripheral muscles to achieve the desired motor result. Children with spastic diplegia who lack normal selective control may substitute mass primitive patterns (simultaneous activity of the hip, knee, and ankle). This basic synergy, particularly between the knee and ankle, can be defined clinically, using upright motor control testing. A general assessment of a patient's voluntary control of single joint movement in response to verbal commands is used as a general measure of motor control; however, the reliability of this measure needs assessment. Motor control evaluation can be extended by observing the child sitting, standing, and stair climbing.

A child's ability to balance while sitting and standing should be determined. No clear objective tests for balance using simple clinical tools are available. Interpretation of a child's inability to balance while standing should be made with caution, because the test may represent a small support area rather than a central lack of control. Estimating the degree of force a child places on the examiner's hands during a check of standing balance may enhance the estimation of balance and also help predict how much aid/support may be needed postoperatively for the child to walk.

The presence of athetosis (or dystonia, though rare) should be assessed, and if either of these patterns predominate, surgery may be contraindicated.

Assessment of Gait

Evaluation of the abnormal gait of children with spastic diplegia (as differing from those with spastic hemiplegia) can be difficult for even the most experienced clinicians, and becomes a daunting task for those less experienced. If we are to improve our understanding of the outcomes of surgery for spastic diplegia, careful documentation of gait is needed both before and after surgery.

There should be more teaching of the fundamentals of gait, both normal and abnormal, to residents and fellows in orthopaedic surgery, especially those anticipating treating children with cerebral palsy.

While the complexity of surgical decision making for these patients is recognized, there is consensus that the establishment of special credentials for treating children with cerebral palsy is not appropriate. However, it should be recognized that the treatment of a child with cerebral palsy who requires orthopaedic surgery should not be done by everyone.

Observational Evaluation of Gait
Observational evaluation of gait is fundamental to any examination of the child with spastic diplegia; therefore, all orthopaedic surgeons should be better trained to do this. This evaluation must be done systematically, and should be repeated on different days on at least three occasions if a surgical decision is to be made. Videotape recording (especially with rapid, stop frame capabilities) can be a useful aid to the observational evaluation of gait.

There are no good data on the "representativeness" of this examination. Many feel that asking the parents whether the gait being observed is representative of the child's usual gait at home is an important part of the testing. Data should be gathered to help answer this question.

The stride length, cadence, and velocity of gait can be calculated by determining the number of steps and the time taken to walk a marked distance. The child needs to be able to come up to speed before starting the measured interval. Ten meters is an adequate distance for testing. Children need enough distance beyond the test interval so that they can slow down without fear of bumping into a wall (and thereby not slow down over the latter part of their test run).

Changes in a child's pulse rate can be used as a measure of energy consumption. This test requires a long run (50 m) for a child to reach a steady state. However, this tool has not been validated sufficiently for clinical use at this time.

Gait Analysis Laboratory The gait analysis (motion analysis) laboratory allows for the objective and quantitative documentation of certain parameters of gait both before and after surgery. These data permit objective assessment of the benefit of surgery and will be helpful in the development of treatment algorithms. Preoperative surgical decision making may be augmented by a knowledgeable clinician using the facilities of a gait analysis laboratory to assess motion using three-dimensional techniques, to assess forces using a force plate and calculations of moments and power, and to assess the extent of cocontractions and out-of-phase firing of muscle using dynamic electromyograms. Energy consumption studies, especially if they can be associated with specific motion or muscular deviations, may be very useful in predicting which children will benefit from surgery. The exact methods used will vary with the severity of the motion deficit, the skills and expertise of the observer, and the availability of specific equipment and technologic support.

The number of motion analysis laboratories currently available is not adequate to evaluate all children with spastic diplegia for whom surgery is being considered. The sprouting of a plethora of mini gait labs run by people who are not particularly competent could be worse than no information at all. Regional Diagnostic Centers should be established to which orthopaedic surgeons could send a child for gait laboratory evaluation and consultation when needed.

Section Five
Nonsurgical Interventions

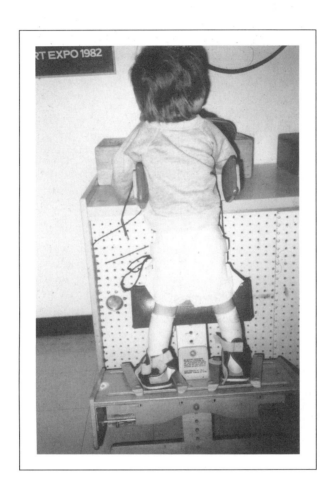

Chapter 16

Rationale for Physical Therapy in the Management of Children With Spastic Diplegia

Susan Harryman, MS, RPT

Introduction

At a conference sponsored by the American Physical Therapy Association in 1990 on "The Efficacy of Physical Therapy in the Management of Cerebral Palsy" the consensus was established that no definitive support for the efficacy of physical therapy, or the lack thereof, in the management of cerebral palsy exists in the research literature.[1] Only one reviewed report specifically addressed physical therapy related to children with spastic diplegia,[2] and it concluded that physical therapy has not been shown to be an effective early intervention approach for promoting motor milestone attainment in infants with spastic diplegia.[2] Existing evidence suggests that physical therapy has a number of effects in the areas of motor and neurologic development and posture in cerebral palsy and that it lacks others,[1] but each of these areas must be documented further before definitive conclusions can be reached. All other potential effects of physical therapy lack supporting research evidence.

The executive summary of the conference concludes that, based on the currently available evidence, therapists should not make claims regarding the therapeutic effects of physical therapy in children with cerebral palsy.[1] However, at some time in their lives, physical therapy is provided for the majority of children with spastic diplegia. Children are referred by physicians, and parents request and participate in therapy programs. Physical therapy is an integral part of many educational programs, and providing early intervention has been recently intensified by the advent of Public Law 99–457,[3] which mandates that early intervention services be implemented for infants and toddlers from birth to age two, inclusive, who are experiencing developmental delays, who have a diagnosed condition that has a high probability of resulting in developmental delay, or who demonstrate atypical development that is likely to result in subsequent delay.

The prevalence of physical therapy intervention programs in the absence of definitive clinical research support for efficacy points to the need for further clinical investigation to examine the rationale upon which these programs are based. Currently, clinical beliefs and opinions based on history, experience, and empirical evidence appear to be the primary rationale for the provision of physical therapy services to children with spastic diplegia.

Early Intervention Programs

The frequent association of spastic diplegia with prematurity provides part of the rationale for the presence of a physical therapist in neonatal intensive care units and follow-up clinics. As reported by Piper,[4] physical therapy intervention in this high-risk group of infants has not led to a decreased incidence of cerebral palsy. However, therapists are often primary care providers in long-term management of children with cerebral palsy and are able to provide support and guidance to parents.[4] Resnick[5] has reported that developmental interventions have a positive effect on the quality of caregiver-infant interactions and suggests that parents need to be educated as soon as possible to learn to respond to cues of the infant and to provide appropriate stimulation. Therapists working in neonatal care units agree with Wilson[6] that optimal positioning of infants in the nursery may lead to the prevention of secondary postural deformities and, thereby, provide the opportunity for the infants to produce the most normal quality of movement.

Screening programs for neuromotor dysfunction, held in conjunction with clinics for high-risk infants, are often able to provide the first level of intervention for children with possible or identified neuromotor problems. Although initial screening is usually done by a pediatrician or nurse, a physical therapist present during screening may be able to provide more specific assessment of motor behaviors. A pediatric physical therapist has specific expertise in evaluating the quality of motor skills or patterns of movement in children, as well as the development of automatic movement reactions. In the neurodevelopmental approach to physical therapy, these reactions are considered a group of normal postural reactions integrated at subcortical levels to maintain a background of normal posture for coordinated movement.[7]

The automatic movement reactions of righting and equilibrium appear in developmental sequence in the normal child and are used as a measure of the level of central maturation. The development of components of these reactions serves as a marker for the emergence of motor skills and is an essential part of the neuromotor profile. Equilibrium reactions are assessed in the context of weight shift in the child's center of gravity in prone, supine, sitting, or standing positions and do not require the child's cooperation because the weight shift may be imposed by the examiner. Controlled weight shift through the shoulder and pelvic girdles is intrinsic to the expression of equilibrium reactions. Additional components of equilibrium include stability on the downward side and countermovements on the upward side. The countermovements are lateral flexion and rotation of the head, lateral flexion of the trunk, and abduction of the extremities toward the upward side.

In infants with spastic diplegia, the presence of increased tone in the lower extremities may delay the initiation of active movement as well as decrease the range of spontaneous movement. In the presence of spastic diplegia, the component parts of equilibrium reactions thus are likely to differ in quality as well as the timeliness of expression. Although an infant may show clearly defined countermovements against gravity in the head, shoulder girdle, and trunk, the weight shift through the pelvis and the countermovements of the hips may be absent, delayed, or limited in comparison to the response elsewhere, indicating possible neuromotor dysfunction. As an astute observer of spontaneous motor behavior, the physical therapist who is familiar with infant assessment is able to provide ongoing analysis of the expression of components of equilibrium during facilitation of developmental activities. For example, during facilitation of rolling to and from prone, in conjunction with handling procedures to optimize posture or muscle tone, the physical therapist is able to isolate specific components of equilibrium reactions that have developed but are not available for spontaneous motor behavior because increased muscle tone is interfering with their expression. Such ongoing analysis results in more complete and objective neuromotor findings, provides a baseline for continued monitoring of sequential motor development, and may lead to a recommendation for intervention.

The presence of milder degrees of involvement which will later manifest as spastic diplegia is difficult to detect in infancy. However, families of children with minor abnormalities in muscle tone, which are frequently seen in the premature population, may be offered access to ongoing monitoring and to management suggestions based on that monitoring. Specific management suggestions related to handling, positioning, and environmental adaptations should be tailored to each parent and infant through direct and intimate observation and careful interview by skilled and knowledgeable therapists. In my experience, such management permits the child to experience more flexibility in patterns of posture and movement, to take advantage of other developmental strengths, and to fulfill his/her developmental potential. Guralnick[8] strongly considers that this, in turn, will have a positive impact on parent-infant interaction and will foster and reinforce parental competence.

A management and monitoring program for infants at risk for neuromotor dysfunction usually can be provided by a physical therapist in a setting in which children are already gathered for screening purposes. A program can also be provided for a child referred to a therapist for in-depth assessment of suspected motor dysfunction. In this management/monitoring framework, children need not have a diagnosis of motor disability, and neither the source of referral nor the child's family need be concerned that referral will automatically result in enrollment in a specific ongoing therapy program or inappropriate diagnostic label.

Because the most rapid motor development occurs in the first year of life, physical therapy screening and intervention programs may help establish normal posture and movement to serve as a foundation for later developmental tasks. However, therapists must remain cognizant of the range of normal motor development and that they may be providing intervention for an apparent dysfunction that will spontaneously improve. On the other hand, there may be a risk in waiting to provide intervention until motor abnormality is more definitive, although this risk has not yet been substantiated through clinical investigation.

Intervention for Preschool Children

Direct services are most often recommended when the diagnosis of spastic diplegia is more clinically evident. Postural control to establish sitting and some means of mobility are frequently short-term objectives for children enrolled in therapy programs during the first 18 months of life. The child with more severe involvement is usually referred to therapy earlier than the child with mild involvement as a result of the more significant increase in lower extremity muscle tone and/or clinically abnormal patterns of movement and posture. The increase of extensor tone across the pelvis and hips in the child with significant involvement may lead to referral because of the child's inability to maintain a sitting position. A child with less involvement and more distally increased tone may not be referred until a delay or abnormality in walking is evident.

The goal of physical therapy intervention for individuals with spastic diplegia should be to optimize motor performance, enabling optimal interactions with the environment in the most efficient manner. In the young preschool population, there also is an opportunity to promote more normal motor development before abnormal patterns become firmly established. Through analysis of current motor patterns and of the maturation of automatic movement reactions, a therapist is able to develop an individualized treatment program that will allow the child to function at his/her neuromotor potential. In some situations, handling and positioning techniques to optimize muscle tone, used in conjunction with facilitation of more normal motor patterns, will result in the relatively rapid acquisition of more diverse motor behavior. In other situations, facilitation techniques provide sensorimotor experience in optimal postures and movement transitions until neuromotor maturation is achieved, which will allow continued development of the motor system.

Successful intervention programs in the preschool population demand activities integrated into daily management with the cooperation of the family and/or other caregivers. To initiate realistic home management programs, the therapist must be responsive to needs of the family and what they desire for their child. Strategies must be designed within the context of the family environment if the program is to be realistic and successful.

Harris[9] found no study in which measurements of family functioning were used as outcome criteria to evaluate the effectiveness of physical therapy. However, Guralnick[8] proposed that building and strengthening the ability of a family to nurture their child confidently and competently are essential ingredients of an intervention program, and that instructional activities, when properly placed in this context, may add an additional dimension to intervention effectiveness.

If independent sitting with optimal posture cannot be maintained at a developmentally appropriate age, a secure means of supported sitting should be established with the family to be used for meals and toy play. The simplest solution is adaptation of the high chair and/or stroller. Any supported seating system for a child with spastic diplegia must start by stabilizing the pelvis in a neutral position, perpendicular to the seating surface. Increased extensor tone in young children with spastic diplegia usually contributes to posterior pelvic tilt in sitting, which leads to compensatory forward flexion of the trunk. The pelvis must be stabilized in a neutral position for optimal trunk extension over the pelvis and for the arms to be free to engage in a wide range of activity. If asymmetry is present, lateral trunk supports may be added for optimal postural control. Increased extensor tone across the pelvis may also result in knee flexion and, over a period of time, shortening of the hamstrings. A seating system that addresses maintenance of hamstring length may minimize this process.

If the need is indicated by the neuromotor profile of the child, an active intervention program should be established with the family towards the goal of maintaining an independent sitting position. Indications of readiness for sitting include the presence of equilibrium in a prone position including weight shift through the pelvis, some ability to maintain the trunk extended over the pelvis in sitting, emerging countermovements of the extremities in sitting, and the presence of lateral protective extension reactions in the upper extremities. Such a program will require parental or other caregiver involvement in learning handling techniques for preparatory tone reduction, facilitated trunk extension, and optimal pelvic control, as well as learning how to structure sitting opportunities into daily management activities. Once a stable midline sitting position can be maintained in structured play, weight shifting activities should be introduced because the ability to shift weight through the pelvis while engaging the hands in activity is necessary for activities such as dressing and play. The ability to access the countermovement of hip abduction is important for function in the sitting position and may be a difficult or impossible task for children with significant spastic diplegia. The facilitation of transitions into sitting encourage the child to actively move against increased extensor tone, to combine components of flexion and extension, to use rotation between the trunk and pelvis, to weight shift through the pelvis, to disassociate the lower extremities, and to countermove in hip abduction with extension.

When caregivers are familiar with the rationale for intervention and are able to integrate activities into daily management, the potential exists to establish alternatives to the W-sitting position used by many children with spastic diplegia (Fig. 1). In this position, the legs are maintained in a flexed position by the weight of the body. Although

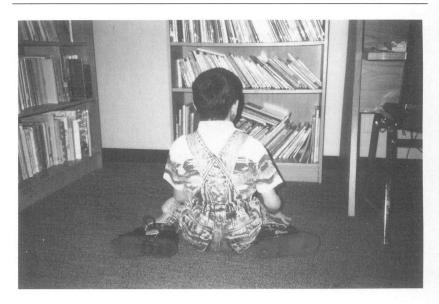

Fig. 1 *Child in W-sitting position.*

W-sitting is often a stable and functional posture for children with spastic diplegia, it limits the use of the pelvis and precludes the use of the lower extremities to assist in maintenance of balance within sitting as well as during transitions in and out of sitting. Although W-sitting by the spastic diplegic cannot be completely eliminated, early intervention in the area of sitting may facilitate the use of other positions and can provide the child and family with alternatives to W-sitting for prolonged periods of activity in a sitting position.

Self-initiated mobility, such as rolling and creeping, is a primary means of exploring the environment and attaining desired objects. These skills may be limited in children with more severe spastic diplegia. These children usually learn to roll prone to supine but, as a result of increased extensor tone in the lower extremities, may have difficulty in initiating hip flexion to roll from supine to prone or in accessing components of the final weight shift into prone. Facilitation of rolling during daily management, for children who have developed equilibrium in prone, will usually result in fairly rapid acquisition of this skill. Children who do not spontaneously roll to prone usually spend limited time, other than during sleep, in the prone position. The daily structured use of prone play, with desired objects in proximity, is often sufficient to encourage reaching and weight shift activities that will lead to creeping in the prone position.

A program to establish standing and walking activities is probably the most frequent physical therapy intervention for children with spastic diplegia. For those children with significant involvement who are diag-

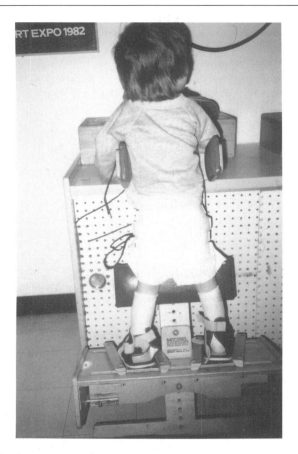

Fig. 2 *Child using prone stander.*

nosed relatively early as a result of increased extensor tone in the lower extremities, the use of a prone stander is frequently recommended (Fig. 2). Use of the prone stander on a daily basis with hips abducted, hips and knees extended, and feet flat, has the potential to assist in maintenance of lower extremity range of movement.

Daily use of the long sitting position, with the pelvis in neutral and the knees extended, will also assist in maintenance of hamstring length. The introduction of weight shifting activities in long sitting may lead to improved sitting equilibrium, including the countermovements of hip abduction and extension in preparation for standing and walking activities.

Because all parents want to help their children stand and want to play with them in the standing position, parents should be given early instruction in facilitation of optimal lower extremity posture. If caregivers understand the rationale for optimal positions, they may provide alternative sensorimotor experiences and avoid the familiar adduction, internal rotation, equinus standing posture of the child with significant spastic diplegia. Therapeutic standing activities should be introduced with the child standing at a support with the pelvis and trunk free from the support to allow weight bearing primarily through the lower extremities. Cruising with the pelvis free from and parallel to the support should be promoted in order to encourage weight shift through the pelvis and hips, to reinforce maintenance of hip abduction and extension of the stance leg, and to initiate movement with hip abduction in an extended position. Facilitation of pulling to stand through half kneel further encourages weight shift through the pelvis and disassociation between the lower extremities. Reaching while standing may promote weight shift through the pelvis, maintenance of hip extension on the weight-bearing side, and use of hip abduction in extension on the unweighted side. These activities to optimize hip control, in addition to activities such as movement from sitting to standing to facilitate hip and knee extension in an abducted position, make it easier for the child to use the components of movement necessary for walking.

If the child does not continue to progress towards independent walking, the use of assistive devices (walker, canes) for functional ambulation should be considered. The specific device chosen should provide sufficient support for optimal posture while demanding active use of hip musculature to promote improvement in hip stability.

Intervention During School Years

As the child with spastic diplegia approaches school age, the primary focus should be on education and not motor disability. Although there may be specific goals for therapeutic intervention, frequently on a periodic short-term basis, long-term direct therapy services during school hours are usually limited. The physical therapist should, however, be available for regular reassessment and consultation to assist in establishing optimal function in the environment. It is important for therapists to remember that integration of children with handicaps with their normally developing peers provides an important avenue for stimulation and subsequent learning.[10] The part time use of powered mobility, such as a scooter, should be considered for optimal peer and environmental interaction of children who are not free ambulators, have difficulty with speed or endurance, or are unable to efficiently move within their environment. Children with limited mobility have often been deprived of experiences afforded preschool children, such as self-initiated interaction and the freedom to explore their neighborhood.[11] The use of powered mobility not only expands interactional possibilities but also provides the opportunity for the child to begin to assume lifetime responsibility for such activities as safe practices and the limits of exploration and behavior.

Intervention in Conjunction With Orthopaedic Surgery

At some point, many children with spastic diplegia will undergo orthopaedic surgery. In the past few years, several reports have appeared related to physical therapy programs in conjunction with orthopaedic intervention at the hips and knees.[12–16] Although the most obvious expectation of orthopaedic surgery is to improve musculo-skeletal alignment, improved quality of movement and functional abilities may also be anticipated. Presurgical assessment by the physical therapist should be planned with the expectation that there will be potential for change following surgery. In addition to the familiar evaluation techniques related to orthopaedics, physical therapy assessment should include analysis of patterns of posture and movement during developmental activities, prewalking as well as walking, to delineate factors interfering with function. The physical therapy assessment of the potential for improved function following surgery should assist in timing and selection of procedures as well as planning of optimal post-surgical management. Children with spastic diplegia often stabilize in abnormal patterns using increased tone before surgery, and they need to establish a new means of postural control and coordinated movement following surgery. Children exhibiting compromised expression of the equilibrium reactions of hip abduction and extension, combined with abnormal postural alignment secondary to increased tone and muscle shortening, are particularly amenable to physical therapy intervention immediately following surgery. Girolami and Hertz[13] report that physical therapy programs providing immediate postsurgical mobilization of the lower extremities after soft-tissue procedures allow more rapid return of function with less pain, stiffness, and muscle weakness.

Surgical intervention to the adductor muscles and/or psoas muscles gives the therapist an opportunity to promote more normal patterns of posture and movement at the pelvis and hips. With postoperative treatment, the achievement of a more neutral position of the pelvis, increased mobility of the pelvis on the trunk and the femur on pelvis, improved access to hip abduction, and the ability to combine hip abduction with hip extension may lead to functional improvement in sitting stability, sitting transitions, and lower extremity weightbearing.

Following surgical lengthening of the hamstrings, it is possible to achieve and maintain a neutral position of the pelvis in sitting, with the trunk extended over the pelvis. The lower extremities now have more freedom to move separately from the pelvis with increased range at both the hips and knees. With postsurgical physical therapy, children frequently have a dramatic qualitative improvement in sitting posture, leading to increased stability and function in the first 2 to 3 weeks following surgery.[13] Lengthening of the hamstrings, combined with surgical intervention for the rectus femoris and/or psoas if necessary, provides the therapist the opportunity to promote more normal standing posture with hip and knee extension. This, in turn, leads to improved stability, function, and efficiency in standing and walking.

The opportunity to facilitate improved posture and function following orthopedic surgery must be continually addressed to be sure the child does not revert to previously used abnormal patterns as means of stabilization. For example, children need considerable structured experience in sitting following surgery to develop optimal midline trunk control in contrast to the habitual trunk flexion that they have used as a compensation for posterior pelvic tilt. Children who have been ambulatory before hamstring lengthening often have a hard time adapting to a weightbearing posture with the knees extended. Hip flexion has frequently been a compensatory posture before surgery, and following surgery it may be attempted as a stabilizing posture in combination with knee extension and increased lumbar lordosis. Treatment activities, therefore, focus on achieving and maintaining hip extension in combination with hip abduction and knee extension, use of the abdominals to support the pelvis, and midrange control of the knee.

The proposed rationale for physical therapy in the immediate postsurgical period is, therefore, to establish new improved postures and patterns of movement and, as also reported by Girolami and Hertz,[13] to allow the child to acquire strength and functional skills in a relatively short period of time while avoiding the joint stiffness, muscle atrophy, and muscle weakness commonly associated with surgical intervention.

Intervention for Adolescents and Adults

As individuals with spastic diplegia approach adolescence and adulthood, independence in functional activity and decrease in dependence on family members are primary needs to be addressed. Ongoing consultation with a physical therapist may help the individual achieve optimal function in specified situations over a period of time. Individuals should be instructed in activities required to maintain range and flexibility and taught to self-monitor functional abilities and movements. Fitness programs and recreation activities in the community may be recommended not only to maintain optimal function but also, as in the nondisabled population, to support physical and mental well-being. Adaptations to kitchens, bathrooms, and workplaces can improve efficiency in movement and function. The ability to access computer technology may assist individuals with learning disabilities or fine motor, accuracy, or speed problems to complete school or work activities in a more timely and capable manner. According to Lundberg,[17] decrease in net efficiency of movement over time in individuals with spastic diplegia points to the need for anticipatory guidance and long-term monitoring, with intervention and environmental adjustment as appropriate to maintain optimal function and quality of life for those individuals.

Summary

In conclusion, although no definitive support for the efficacy of physical therapy in the management of cerebral palsy exists in the research literature, current physical therapy contributions include screening, motor assessment, and direct service as well as consultation for monitoring, management, caregiver education, and environmental adaptations. Participants in the consensus conference[1] believed that expected effects of physical therapy include improved efficiency of movement, increased endurance for physical activity, prevention of disability, greater functional independence in activities requiring mobility, and improved family functioning and comprehension of the effects and management of disability. Previous research on the efficacy of physical therapy in the management of cerebral palsy has concentrated on study of its effects on rate of motor milestone acquisition, an outcome that is an important but not a primary concern of physical therapy. Future research should emphasize evaluation of treatment outcomes that are of more central concern, including prevention of contracture and deformity and improvements in posture; functional motor skills; family interactions; and functional independence in the home, school, and community.[1]

Physical therapists providing intervention for children with spastic diplegia have an obligation to assist in establishing the most effective management for these individuals. Detailed evaluations, established baselines, well-defined treatment strategies, and objective monitoring of progress are necessary for critical assessment of therapeutic intervention. In addition to this systematic collection of objective data, therapists must be willing to share and report results of therapeutic interventions in order to establish the efficacy of physical therapy for children with motor impairments.

References

1. Campbell SK: Proceedings of the consensus conference on the efficacy of physical therapy in the management of cerebral palsy. *Pediatr Phys Ther* 1990; 2:125,176.
2. Palmer FB, Shapiro BK, Wachtel RC, et al: The effects of physical therapy on cerebral palsy: A controlled trial in infants with spastic diplegia. *N Engl J Med* 1988;318:803–808.
3. PL 99–457, Education of the Handicapped Act, Amendments of 1986, 100 Stat 1145–1177.
4. Piper MC, Kunos VI, Willis DM, et al: Early physical therapy effects on the high risk infant: A randomized controlled trial. *Pediatrics* 1986;78:216–224.
5. Resnick MB, Armstrong S, Carter RL: Developmental intervention program for high-risk premature infants: Effects on development and parent-infant interactions. *J Dev Behav Pediatr* 1988;9:73–78.
6. Wilson JM: Cerebral palsy, in Campbell SK (ed): *Pediatric Neurologic Physical Therapy*. New York, Churchill Livingstone, 1991.
7. Bobath B: *Abnormal Postural Activity Caused by Brain Lesions*. Rockville, MD, Aspen Systems Corp, 1985.
8. Guralnick MJ: Recent developments in early intervention efficacy research: Implications for family involvement. *Top Early Child Spec Educ* 1989;9:1–17.
9. Harris SR: Efficacy of physical therapy in promoting family functioning and functional independence for children with cerebral palsy. *Pediatr Phys Ther* 1990;2:160–164.
10. Adam SL, McEvoy MA: Integration of young children with handicaps and normally developing children, in Adam SL, Kumes MB (eds): *Early Intervention for Infants and Children with Handicaps*. Baltimore, Paul H. Brooks, 1988.
11. Breed AL, Ibler I: The motorized wheelchair: New freedom, new responsibility and new problems. *Dev Med Child Neurol* 1982;24:366–371.

12. Okuawa A, Kajiura I, Hiroshima K: Physical therapeutic and surgical management of spastic diplegia: A Japanese experience. *Clin Orthop* 1990; 253:38–44.

13. Girolami GI, Hertz K: Early mobilization and post surgical management after hamstring or gracilis muscle release in children with cerebral palsy, in *Topics in Pediatrics*. Alexandria, VA, American Physical Therapy Association, 1990, pp 1–14.

14. Atkins EM, Harryman SE, Silberstein CE: Potential for change following orthopedic surgery. Instructional Course, American Academy for Cerebral Palsy and Developmental Medicine, Orlando, FL, October 5, 1990.

15. Sussman M: Orthopedic management of cerebral palsy. Instructional Course, American Academy for Cerebral Palsy and Developmental Medicine, Boston, MA, October 9, 1987.

16. Harryman SE: Lower extremity surgery for children with cerebral palsy: Physical therapy management. *Phys Ther* 1992;72:16–24.

17. Lundberg A: Longitudinal study of physical working capacity of young people with cerebral palsy. *Dev Med Child Neurol* 1984;26:328–334.

Chapter 17

Expected Outcomes of Physical Therapy for Children With Cerebral Palsy: The Evidence and the Challenge

Suzann K. Campbell, PhD, PT

In order to demonstrate accountability to physical therapy clients and to the public, increased efforts must be made to show the efficacy and effectiveness of physical therapy in the management of movement dysfunction in children with cerebral palsy. In this chapter, I will summarize the evidence for treatment efficacy and issue a challenge for future research. The evidence includes: (1) the results of survey research on the expected outcomes of physical therapy for children with cerebral palsy; and (2) the results of clinical research studies on those outcomes. The challenge that remains is to thoroughly study the outcomes clinicians expect that have not yet been subjected to experimental research. Finally, it is important to study the processes by which physical therapy improves function, ie, prevention of secondary impairment and disability, rehabilitation of underlying neuromuscular impairment, and/or development of compensatory strategies for improving function and preventing disability. Physicians believe that outcomes are based primarily on use of compensatory strategies, such as adaptive equipment. Physical therapists, on the other hand, expect improvement both in underlying impairment and in functional performance based on provision of compensatory strategies, as well as prevention of secondary impairment and disability.

The Evidence for Effectiveness of Physical Therapy

Physicians' Beliefs

Based on a survey of 197 randomly selected physician members of the American Academy of Pediatrics and the American Academy of Cerebral Palsy and Developmental Medicine, which included orthopaedists, neurologists, physiatrists, and pediatricians, the expected outcomes of physical therapy for children with cerebral palsy were found to be: (1) improvement of parental capability to manage disability (82%) and to cope emotionally (76%), (2) prevention of contractures and deformities (69%), and (3) functional improvement.[1,2] Some neg-

Table 1 Physician's expectations of physical therapy effects on impairment in cerebral palsy (N = 197)

Effect	Percentage*
Primary	
Decreased influence of primitive reflexes	34
Improved selective control of movement	33
Improved muscle tone	28
Enhanced sensory integrative function	21
Decreased irritability	18
Improved physical growth	9
Secondary	
Prevention of contractures and deformities	69
Increased endurance for physical activities	63
Improved postural alignment	49
Prevention of need for orthopaedic surgery	19
Correction of contractures and deformities	18

*Percent of respondents who believed outcome to be likely or highly likely. (Based on data from Campbell SK, Anderson J, Gardner HG, unpublished data, 1991; Campbell et al[1]; Campbell.[2])

ative effects on the family, primarily financial strain (35%) and time demands (65%), were also anticipated; other negative expectations regarding childrens' outcomes, such as harm from being labeled, were expressed by less than 8% of the respondents, with the exception of 17% of physicians who believed that physical therapy would not improve motor skills beyond natural maturation. I have categorized the expected outcomes of physical therapy by this group of physicians according to the conceptual framework of Nagi[3] in Tables 1–3. This framework for describing the disabling process stresses the effects of disabling conditions on organ systems (impairment), body functions (functional limitations), and performance of life roles in the context of the family and community (disability).[3] The data show that physicians expect that physical therapy will reduce functional limitations and prevent disability rather than improve underlying impairment produced by central nervous system dysfunction.

Review of the Research Literature

Which of the outcomes that physicians expect to be likely or highly likely effects of physical therapy have been documented by clinical research? The results of a consensus conference on the effects of physical therapy on the management of movement dysfunction in cerebral palsy sponsored by the Section on Pediatrics of the American Physical Therapy Association suggest that very few of the expected outcomes have been thoroughly studied with highly valid experimental methods. Many of the outcomes that physicians and therapists believe to be most likely have not been studied at all.[4]

The outcomes that have received the most attention in the scientific literature include achievement of developmental motor milestones, postural control and alignment, and reduction of abnormal reflexes and tone. The evidence in each of these areas will be summarized briefly.

Motor Milestones   The evidence showing the effects of physical

Table 2 Physician's expectations of physical therapy effects on functional limitations in cerebral palsy (N = 197)

Effect	Percentage*
Maintenance of functional abilities	69
Improvement in functional abilities	65
Improved feeding	50
Increased rate of motor milestone attainment	32
Improved fine motor skills	30
Improved communication ability	27
Improved cognitive development	17

*Percent of respondents who believed outcome to be likely or highly likely. (Based on data from Campbell SK, Anderson J, Gardner HG, unpublished data, 1991; Campbell et al[1]; Campbell.[2])

therapy on motor milestone development is modest at best. A 1986 meta-analysis of nine existing studies demonstrated that the average child receiving physical therapy scored better than 62.5% of children not receiving intervention.[5,6] This is the best cumulative statistical evidence available regarding the efficacy of physical therapy. Piper's review[7] for the consensus conference, however, indicated that only three studies of therapeutic efficacy reported in the literature used a randomized trial with high statistical power. Each of these studies randomly assigned children to a neurodevelopmental treatment group or an alternative treatment strategy; none employed an untreated control group, so these studies do not demonstrate the efficacy of physical or occupational therapy per se. A study by Palmer and associates[8] demonstrated that in children with spastic diplegia, intervention after age one year in the form of six months of parental training in facilitation of multiple aspects of development followed by six months of neurodevelopmental treatment was more effective than 12 months of neurodevelopmental treatment only. The other two studies reported that neurodevelopmental treatment in the form of physical or occupational therapy was more effective in promoting motor milestone development than other forms of therapy.[9,10] Only one child with spastic diplegia was included in these two trials, and children were generally entered at an earlier age so they are not directly comparable to the study of Palmer and associates.[8] Another difference is treatment frequency. Both of the studies reporting positive effects of neurodevelopmental treatment provided therapy two times per week; the trial reporting negative results provided therapy only once every two weeks.

A thorough review of the evidence from these and other studies led Piper to conclude that the evidence supporting the efficacy of physical therapy in promoting the acquisition of motor milestones is limited, in agreement with the report that only 32% of physicians surveyed believe that physical therapy can increase the rate of motor development.[7] It should be noted, however, that there currently is not enough evidence to say that physical therapy does not have an effect, although that effect is not likely to be large. When all of the extant literature was considered, Piper concluded that further study of a number of important treatment variables was warranted. These include frequency of treatment, age of

Table 3 Physician's expectations of physical therapy effects on disability in cerebral palsy (N = 197)

Effect	Percentage*
Increased independence through use of assistive devices/special seating/ mobility aides	86
Improved parental ability to manage the physical aspects of disability	82
Improved parental ability to cope with the social/emotional aspects of disability	76
Improved ability to profit from educational experiences in school	61
Increased cost of health insurance	35
Excessive time demands on parents	32
Improved ability to test cognition	28
Excessive cost/financial burden on family	21
Excessively elevated parental expectations of cure or improvement	16

*Percent of respondents who believed outcome to be likely or highly likely. (Based on data from Campbell SK, Anderson J, Gardner HG, unpublished data, 1991; Campbell et al[1]; Campbell.[2])

initiation of treatment, and type of cerebral palsy. For example, the effect of patient intelligence on treatment efficacy and whether patients with spasticity derive more benefit from treatment than those with dyskinetic types of cerebral palsy (with spastic diplegia treated after age one as a possible exception) needs elucidation. The complexity of the possible permutations of cerebral palsy type, patient intelligence and age, treatment frequency, and type of treatment suggest that a large, multicenter study would be most productive.

Postural Control and Alignment   There are a number of studies involving research on posture, including range of motion, postural reactions, stability, control, and equilibrium.[11] Positive results have been reported from a variety of interventions,[11] including casting, adaptive seating, augmented sensory feedback, electrical stimulation, and therapeutic exercise based on neurodevelopmental treatment or Vojta treatment. Of concern, however, is the fact that no randomized clinical trial has been conducted in this area, so while the results are strongly suggestive that therapy and other modalities can improve several aspects of posture, including range of motion, they must be considered inconclusive. Measurement is a major problem in this area because of the variety of nonvalidated assessment methods that have been reported and the failure to link improved posture to changes in functional performance.

Kanda and associates,[12] one of the few groups to link postural stability improvement produced by Vojta treatment with functional aspects of gait, show the power of an approach that links impairment with functional performance. Their research demonstrated that children in an early-treated group (before 9 months of age) walked an average of 8 months earlier than children treated after 9 months of age, and had better postural stability during gait. Sixty-three percent of the early-treated group of children with spastic diplegia in Kanda's study could walk steadily for 30 minutes, compared with only 33.3% of the late-treated group. It is postulated that early treatment was more effective because it prevented the development of abnormal neck and pelvic postures, which, if used by untreated children when creeping began, were retained when they learned to walk. Although the reliability of their early diagnosis might be questioned because of the absence of an untreated control group, the researchers did report that similar proportions of children in each group were able to walk/not walk.

To promote more productive future research efforts, a consensus by investigators is needed on which measures are most appropriate and valid, as well as on the way to measure the prevention of secondary impairment and disability and the resulting facilitation of improved functional performance. Generation of clinical hypotheses along the lines of those suggested by Kanda and associates,[12] which link reduction of impairments to expected improvements in functional performance, would also be helpful in guiding more theoretically-based research on the processes whereby treatment affects function.

Reflexes and Tone   Five studies using therapy based on neurodevelopmental treatment theory have examined whether abnormal primary reflexes can be inhibited by physical therapy, and five studies have directly addressed the possibility of reducing spasticity.[11] No evidence exists to support the conclusion that neurodevelopmental treatment decreases the influence of abnormal primary reflexes. Problems with assessment of these reflexes[8,13] in the existing reports suggest that further research on the effects of neurodevelopmental treatment using improved measures would be useful; however, I believe that therapy is not likely to affect reflex behavior.

Decreased spasticity has been reported as a result of therapeutic horseback riding,[14] casting,[15] and biofeedback.[16] A second casting study demonstrated no tone reduction[17] while the treatment comparison study of Palmer and associates[8] reported increased tone in subjects receiving neurodevelopmental treatment exclusively. Most of these studies did not provide sufficient quantitative information to judge the reliability and validity of their findings. Further research on effects of therapy on tone reduction are needed; however, any such effects should be clearly related to functional improvement, prevention of secondary impairment, or other important outcomes.

To summarize, modest effects have been reported on improvement of functional outcomes, and inconclusive results have been reported in the area of primary impairment. However, virtually no studies have been reported in the literature on those outcomes clinicians believe to be most likely, namely functional performance and independence in daily life, prevention of secondary impairment and disability, endurance and efficiency of movement, and parental ability to manage functional limitations and prevent disability and handicap while maintaining a semblance of normal family life.

The Challenge: Functional Outcomes Research

The challenge remains to demonstrate the efficacy and effectiveness of physical therapy in improving the quality of life of children with cerebral palsy and their families. Identification of appropriate outcome variables, defined with reliable and valid measures that link impairment, functional limitations, and disability at the theoretical level, is needed. I will use gait as an example of the specification of one model that might be used in a controlled clinical trial.

Locomotion has been documented to be mechanically inefficient in children with cerebral palsy because of jerky motion, inappropriate presence of cocontraction and isometric contractions, and generation of energy at one joint that is nonproductively absorbed at another.[18] Rigidity and contracture of muscle also creates restraint of movement during locomotion.[19] These impairments result in gait that is slow, cosmetically unattractive, and metabolically costly, thus potentially limiting endurance and independence in community mobility. Disabilities can result from inability to participate with peers in age-appropriate activity and other limitations of normal activity. Secondary impairments, such as contractures and deformities, can result from prolonged sitting and overuse of certain muscles in abnormal patterns, leading to the need for orthopaedic surgery or further limiting participation in normal daily activities. Each of these levels of dysfunction can be defined and studied both in controlled clinical trials and in longitudinal studies of the impact of cerebral palsy on quality of life. Variables measuring the effects on the family system in terms of costs, time demands, and limitations on activities and other outcomes could also be studied.

The results of studies employing variables such as these could answer a number of important questions: (1) Does early therapy make a difference? (2) How early and how frequently should therapy be provided for maximum benefit and cost effectiveness? (3) Can primary impairment be decreased? (4) Can secondary impairment be prevented? (5) Can functional limitations be decreased and disability prevented? (6) Can quality of life for the whole family be improved, whether or not children with cerebral palsy benefit directly? (7) What are the costs of any demonstrated benefits?

Summary

A significant degree of belief in the value of physical therapy in the management of movement dysfunction in children with cerebral palsy exists in the clinical community and among the families of children with disabilities. Most of the important outcomes, however, have not been adequately studied. Conceptually-based clinical research that links treatment effects to dysfunction at a number of levels of analysis is needed in order to document the costs as well as the benefits of physical therapeutic intervention on the child and the child's family.

Acknowledgments

The work summarized in this chapter was partially supported by the Agency for Health Care Policy and Research and by the Section on Pediatrics of the American Physical Therapy Association.

References

1. Campbell SK, Anderson J, Gardner HG: Physicians' beliefs in the efficacy of physical therapy in the management of cerebral palsy. *Pediatr Phys Ther* 1990; 2:169–173.
2. Campbell SK: Measurement of motor performance in cerebral palsy. *Med Sport Sci*, in press.
3. Nagi SZ: Disability concepts revisited: Implications for prevention, in Pope AN, Tarlov AR (eds): *Disability in America: Toward a National Agenda for Prevention*. Washington, DC, National Academy Press, 1991, pp 309–327.
4. Campbell SK: Proceedings of the consensus conference on the efficacy of physical therapy in the management of movement dysfunction in cerebral palsy. *Pediatr Phys Ther* 1990;2:121–176.
5. Ottenbacher K, Biocca Z, De Cremer G, et al: Quantitative analysis of the effectiveness of pediatric therapy: Emphasis on the neurodevelopmental treatment approach. *Phys Ther* 1986;66:1095–1101.
6. Ottenbacher KJ: Response to Piper: Efficacy of physical therapy: Rate of motor development in children with cerebral palsy. *Pediatr Phys Ther* 1990;2: 131–134.
7. Piper MC: Efficacy of physical therapy: Rate of motor development in children with cerebral palsy. *Pediatr Phys Ther* 1990;2:126–130.
8. Palmer FB, Shapiro BK, Wachtel RC, et al: The effects of physical therapy on cerebral palsy: A controlled trial in infants with spastic diplegia. *N Engl J Med* 1988;318:803–808.
9. Carlsen PN: Comparison of two occupational therapy approaches for treating the young cerebral-palsied child. *Am J Occup Ther* 1975;29:267–272.
10. Scherzer AL, Mike V, Ilson J: Physical therapy as a determinant of change in the cerebral palsied infant. *Pediatrics* 1976;58:47–52.
11. Campbell SK: Efficacy of physical therapy in improving postural control in cerebral palsy. *Pediatr Phys Ther* 1990;2:135–140.
12. Kanda T, Yuge M, Yamori Y, et al: Early physiotherapy in the treatment of spastic diplegia. *Dev Med Child Neurol* 1984;26:438–444.
13. Sommerfeld D, Fraser BA, Hensinger RN, et al: Evaluation of physical therapy service for severely mentally impaired students with cerebral palsy. *Phys Ther* 1981;61:338–344.
14. Bertoti DB: Effects of therapeutic horseback riding on posture in children with cerebral palsy. *Phys Ther* 1988;68:1505–1512.
15. Bertoti DB: Effect of short leg casting on ambulation in children with cerebral palsy. *Phys Ther* 1986;66:1522–1529.
16. Skrotsky K: Gait analysis in cerebral palsied and nonhandicapped children. *Arch Phys Med Rehab* 1983;64:291–295.
17. Watt J, Sims D, Harckham F, et al: A prospective study of inhibitive casting as an adjunct to physiotherapy for cerebral-palsied children. *Dev Med Child Neurol* 1986;28:480–488.
18. Olney SJ: Efficacy of physical therapy in improving mechanical and metabolic efficiency of movement in cerebral palsy. *Pediatr Phys Ther* 1990;2:145–154.
19. Berger W, Quintern J, Dietz V: Pathophysiology of gait in children with cerebral palsy. *Electroencephalogr Clin Neurohysiol* 1982;53:538–548.

Chapter 18

Muscle Relaxant Drugs for Children With Cerebral Palsy

James A. Blackman, MD, MPH
Michael D. Reed, PharmD, FCCP, FCP
Cathleen D. Roberts, DO

There are roughly 100,000 children with spastic cerebral palsy in the United States. Although the understanding of the causes of spasticity has improved, progress in the development of new, effective treatment modalities has been limited. The major nonsurgical advances have been in the area of adaptive equipment, which serves to compensate for limitations in mobility, communication, and feeding. Nevertheless, there remains a strong interest in treating the underlying pathophysiologic mechanisms in spasticity. The two most promising approaches are posterior rhizotomy, a neurosurgical method of reducing spinal reflex activity by selectively cutting the incoming sensory-feedback fibers to the spinal cord, and pharmacologic dampening of excessive motor activity. Evaluation of muscle relaxant drugs for spastic cerebral palsy in children is the focus of this chapter.

Background

Cerebral palsy is defined as a disorder of movement and posture that results from a cerebral insult during the early developmental period. This insult may result either from an injury to an otherwise normally developing brain or from anomalous brain development. Diagnostic criteria for cerebral palsy include: (1) delayed motor milestones; (2) abnormal neurologic findings; (3) aberrant primitive reflexes and postural reactions; (4) history of risk or evidence of cerebral insult; (5) no clinical progression by history or by repeat examination; and (6) age of insult in early childhood.[1]

Because different types of brain injury affect different parts of the brain, muscle control problems vary and can include spasticity (60% of cases), dyskinesia (20%), and ataxia (1%). In about 20% of cases, affected individuals will have a combination of two or more types, but one will predominate.[2] Besides motor impairment, there may be associated problems with sensory input, such as hearing or visual deficits; central processing, such as communication, intellectual, or perceptual deficits; and physiologic health, such as constipation or seizures.[3–5]

The spastic type of cerebral palsy is characterized by a velocity-dependent increase in tonic stretch reflexes, with exaggerated tendon jerks resulting from hyperexcitability of the stretch reflex.[6] Important clinical signs of spasticity have been enumerated by Nathan:[7] (1) Stretch reflexes that are normally latent become obvious. (2) Tendon reflexes have a lowered threshold to tap. (3) The response of the tapped muscle is increased. (4) Muscles, other than the one tapped, usually respond. (5) Tonic stretch reflexes (ie, resistance to passive movement) are similarly affected. (6) Clonus may be induced.

Spasticity is very disabling for the individual child. It produces hypertonicity, uncoordinated movements, weakness, loss of dexterity, abnormal posture, joint contractures, difficulties with chewing and swallowing, and discomfort.

The specific pathophysiologic mechanisms for spasticity are gradually being elucidated, but are still incompletely understood. Although the site of injury in cerebral palsy is in the brain, spasticity appears to be related to an increased excitatory state at the spinal level.[8] In the spinal cords of patients with spasticity, the abnormal reflexes are initiated by proprioceptive and exteroceptive afferent inputs and produced by the altered activity of alpha and gamma motoneurons and excitatory and inhibitory interneurons participating in the pertinent reflex arcs.[9] Modification of descending inhibitory and/or excitatory controls of the spinal reflex apparatus and modifications of the circuitry and connectivity of spinal reflex arcs appear to be most responsible for the clinical features of spasticity. According to current theory, excessive muscle contraction in response to rapid and sudden stretch of the muscle is caused by lack of inhibitory influence from the damaged brain.

Normally, when a muscle or its associated tendon is passively stretched, as when deep tendon reflexes are elicited with a hammer, impulses from sensory organs (eg, muscle spindles, Golgi tendon organs) travel up afferent nerve fibers that synapse with efferent motor fibers in the spinal cord. In a monosynaptic reflex response, the muscle contracts with passive stretch to prevent overstretching. This feedback loop is monitored and coordinated by extrapyramidal structures (eg, basal ganglia). With damage to these as well as pyramidal tract structures, autoregulation is disturbed. The result, with active and passive movement, is a state of increased tone and unmodulated muscle control. The lack of inhibition also results in cocontraction of antagonistic muscles. Thus, if the intent is flexion of the forearm by contraction of the biceps, concurrent contraction of the triceps occurs as well, resulting in ineffective movement. In more severely affected patients, spasticity results in poor posture, leading to joint contractures and scoliosis. The hypertonia interferes with physical therapy and proper positioning in seating devices.

Muscle Relaxant Drugs

One objective of medical treatment of spasticity is to dampen afferent inputs, inhibit or block excitation of intraspinal neurons, reduce motoneuron output, and ultimately lessen muscle contraction.[9] Three drugs have been used for adjunctive treatment of spasticity: diazepam, dantrolene, and baclofen. These compounds are widely used in children despite very limited investigation of their efficacy and safety in children, cautions in the *Physicians' Desk Reference*[10] about their use in children, and such statements by experts as, "Over the years, a wide variety of so-called myorelaxants or antispastic drugs have proven to be useless despite temporary fads supporting them."[8] However, other experts have expressed the opposite opinion: "Antispasticity agents are an essential part of the management of patients with cerebral palsy."[9] Many experienced clinicians believe these medications are useful and prescribe them liberally despite the lack of scientific evidence to support their claims. These diverse opinions must be interpreted in light of the complete lack of dose-response evaluations of these drugs in children. Furthermore, it is assumed, although not proven, that drug therapy, which reduces muscle hypertonia and normalizes reflex abnormalities, can diminish the clinical disabilities of spastic patients.

Mechanisms of Action for Muscle Relaxant Drugs

One approach to modification of reflex alterations in spasticity is to use agents that inhibit the release of excitatory neurotransmitters from the terminals of primary afferent fibers that synapse on motoneurons and interneurons. Gamma-aminobutyric acid (GABA) mediates such inhibition by suppressing transmission of sensory impulses from muscle to interneurons and motoneurons at the presynaptic level. There are two types of GABA receptors: $GABA_A$ mediates presynaptic inhibition by increasing chloride conductance of terminals, thereby maintaining them in a state of depolarization (ie, inactivity); $GABA_B$ by depressing voltage-sensitive calcium conductances.

Commonly Used Muscle Relaxant Drugs

Diazepam Introduced in the 1960s as an antianxiety agent, diazepam is a benzodiazepine derivative that is insoluble in water and has a molecular weight of 287.74. Tests in animals indicated that it possessed muscle relaxant and spinal reflex-blocking properties. The spinal actions of this drug appear to result from potentiation of the presynaptic inhibitory effects of GABA at $GABA_A$ receptors on spinal afferent presynaptic terminals. In addition to actions at the spinal cord level, benzodiazepines act centrally in the brainstem reticular formation, producing a sedative effect.[9,11] Some patients with cerebral palsy develop increased spasticity when they are anxious, and for them this tranquilizing action of diazepam can be an advantage. Degrees of tolerance to the sedative effect can develop. Addiction and serious withdrawal symptoms have been described in patients receiving long-term diazepam therapy. This potentially serious complication of diazepam is avoided by slowly tapering (ie, weaning) patients off the drug if they have received diazepam for longer than one year.[9,11]

The limited pharmacokinetic data for diazepam in children are derived primarily from its use as an anticonvulsant.[12–14] Diazepam is rapidly and almost completely absorbed following oral, rectal, or intramuscular administration. The elimination half-life in children 3 to 8 years old is reported to average 18 hours as compared to 30 to 60 hours in adults.[12] It is important to note that these data are derived from a pharmacokinetic study that involved only four children. The drug's apparent volume of distribution is large, averaging 0.8 to 2 + 1/kg body weight, reflecting its extensive tissue penetration within the body. Diazepam is metabolized by the liver to pharmacologically active nordiazepam, which on long-term dosing accumulates and undergoes further hydroxylation to another pharmacologically active metabolite, oxazepam (half-life = 5 to 10 hours).[15] As a result of the varying degrees of pharmacologic activity of diazepam and its metabolites, the pharmacologic effect of this drug in the four children studied reflects a summation of the concentrations of each compound. Needless to say, data on drug metabolism in children with spastic disorders are unavailable .

A secondary peak plasma concentration, occurring 6 to 12 hours after administration, probably results from enterohepatic circulation or possibly from redistribution of the drug from tissue stores. Diazepam and its metabolites are excreted from the body by the kidney. The prominent side effects are drowsiness, fatigue, and ataxia. The usual dose in children is 1 to 2.5 mg, two or three times a day initially, with increases as needed and tolerated.[9,11] Clearly, these clinically-used dosing regimens do not take into account the known pharmacokinetic behavior outlined above.

Dantrolene   This drug, available since the early 1970s, differs from baclofen and diazepam in that it exerts its muscle-relaxant effects by direct actions on skeletal muscle. Cardiac and smooth muscle are not as sensitive to dantrolene as skeletal muscle. Because it acts upon, and therefore weakens, normal as well as spastic muscles, dantrolene may reduce rather than increase muscle function. A hydantoin derivative, it is slightly soluble in water and has a molecular weight of 399. Dantrolene acts on the process of excitation-contraction coupling to inhibit the release from the sarcoplasmatic reticulum of calcium ions needed for activation of the contractile apparatus.[16] Most pharmacologic data are derived from its use for the treatment/prevention of an unrelated medical syndrome, malignant hyperthermia.

The drug is believed to be rapidly and extensively absorbed; however, insufficient data on its absorption in children or adults are available to confirm this belief.[17] Peak drug effect often occurs about 3 hours after an oral dose. Seventy-five percent to 85% appears to be metabolized by the liver to predominantly 5-hydroxydantrolene, which is approximately 50% as active as the parent compound. The drug's elimination half-life ranges between 6 and 9 hours; the apparent volume of distribution for dantrolene averages 0.54 1/kg; and its extent of protein binding is unknown.[18] There are no complete pharmacokinetic studies in children receiving dantrolene for spasticity.[19] Unmetabolized dantrolene and its metabolite are excreted from the body by the kidney. The chief potential for toxicity involves the liver. Fatal dantrolene-induced hepatitis has been reported in adults at various dose levels, although the incidence is greatest at higher doses, especially when given for prolonged periods. Transient mild abnormalities in liver function tests occur in 10% of patients in the first few weeks of treatment, but these tests usually return to normal despite continued administration. The other most frequently reported side-effects are drowsiness, dizziness, weakness, general malaise and fatigue, and diarrhea.

The usual starting dose for dantrolene is 0.5 mg/kg body weight twice daily; this is increased to 0.5 mg/kg three or four times daily, and then, by increments of 0.5 mg/kg, up to as high as 3.0 mg/kg two, three, or four times daily. Doses higher than 100 mg four times daily are not used in children, but the rationale for this arbitrary dose ceiling is unknown. Each dosage level is usually maintained for 4 to 7 days to determine patient response. Therapy is usually discontinued if no benefits are observed within 45 days of the start of therapy. Similar to diazepam, no objective clinical aids are available to guide the clinician in discriminating between those children who may respond to dantrolene therapy and those who will not. At the start of dantrolene therapy, liver function tests (aspartate aminotransferase, alanine aminotransferase, alkaline phosphatase, total bilirubin) are performed for baseline data and to determine whether there is underlying liver disease. Previous concerns about accentuation of pre-existing epilepsy have not been substantiated in a double-blind study in which the frequency of seizures was not altered by administration of dantrolene,[20] nor have they been substantiated by clinical experience.

Baclofen   A GABA analog introduced in the mid-1970s, baclofen appears to act as a GABA agonist at the GABA$_B$ receptors. The drug used clinically is a racemate.[21] Pharmacokinetic or dynamic differences that may exist for the individual isomers have not been studied. Baclofen inhibits transmitter release by competitive inhibition of excitatory neurotransmitters at the spinal level. Actions at levels above the spinal cord may occur and contribute to its clinical effects. According to the *Physicians' Desk Reference*[10] the efficacy of baclofen in cerebral palsy has not been established and it, therefore, is not recommended for patients with this disorder. Furthermore, it states that baclofen is not recommended in children because its safety has not been established for those younger than 12 years of age. Nevertheless, this drug is used commonly in children under the age of 12 who have cerebral palsy. Pharmacokinetic data are derived from adults; none are available for children.

Baclofen is rapidly absorbed from the gastrointestinal tract. Absorption may be dose-dependent; it is reduced with increasing doses. In adults, the drug's elimination half-life ranges from 3.6 to 7 hours, with an apparent volume of distribution of 0.8 1/kg body weight. The drug's body clearance approximates the endogenous creatinine clearance.[22,23] The most common side effect associated with baclofen administration is transient drowsiness. Other common adverse reactions include dizziness, weakness, and fatigue. Based on the only reported trial of baclofen in children,[24] the starting dose for children aged 2 to 7 years should be 5 to 10 mg daily, preferably in three divided doses, increasing gradually over a period of two weeks to a maximum daily dose of 30 to 40 mg. The lower doses suggested are often applied to younger children. For children over the age of 8 years, a starting dose of 60 mg daily has been the maximum recommended dose. Because hallucinations and seizures have occurred following abrupt withdrawal of baclofen, the dose should be reduced slowly when the drug is discontinued.

The data provided above for baclofen, diazepam, and dantrolene underscore the extremely limited database available describing the pharmacokinetic-pharmacodynamic interactions of these drugs in children, and more specifically, in children with increased spasticity. From the limited published studies of these drugs, it is virtually impossible to determine whether these agents alone or in combination are efficacious in cerebral palsy, or how best to use them and to monitor patients for efficacy and toxicity.

Previous Clinical Studies

Much of the literature on the use of muscle relaxants for spasticity appeared in the early 1980s or before. Since that time a hiatus in further clinical study has occurred despite the continued common use of these agents and the paucity of information regarding indications, dose, pharmacokinetics, and functional outcomes, especially in children. Most studies have included subjects with multiple causes of spasticity including spinal cord injury, multiple sclerosis, and cerebral palsy. It remains very difficult to draw conclusions from such heterogeneous studies. While some of these studies have included children, they are predominantly focused on adults, describe experiences in small groups of study patients (see below), lack consistent long-term follow-up, and have employed insensitive methods to assess patient response.

Diazepam   All benzodiazepines have muscle relaxant properties. Traditionally, diazepam is the benzodiazepine most often used for muscle relaxation. Lossius and associates[25] found that diazepam serum concentrations needed to reduce spasticity in adults, 300 to 2,200 mg/l, were so high that drowsiness occurred. Thus, Wuis[26] has indicated that, for long term administration in spasticity, diazepam is usually not the drug of choice because of sedation. This may be true for treatment in adults but not necessarily in children. Pediatricians, fearing potential liver toxicity with dantrolene and noting the *Physicians' Desk Reference*[10] statement that baclofen is not recommended for children under age 12, turn to diazepam because of its track record of safety in the treatment of seizures in children. In some settings it is the most commonly employed muscle relaxant drug for children. Yet, there are few well-designed studies on the use of diazepam for spasticity in children, and all are quite old. The first inkling of its possible clinical value as a relaxant came in 1962 from the work of Katz and associates,[27] who

Table 1 Summary of results of controlled, double-blind trials of dantrolene in patients with cerebral palsy

Number of Patients	Dosage Regimen	Duration of Therapy* (weeks)	Effect (No. of Patients)	Classification of Cerebral Palsy	Age of Patients (years)	Reference No.
Dantrolene versus placebo						
17	dantrolene 20–400 mg/day placebo	4	dantrolene>placebo (12) dantrolene = placebo (5)	dyskinetic	7–38	31
28	dantrolene 12 mg kg^{-1} d^{-1} placebo	3	dantrolene>placebo (5) dantrolene = placebo (23)	spastic	1.5–12	32
4	dantrolene 1–10 mg kg^{-1} d^{-1} placebo	1.5	dantrolene≈placebo	spastic	9–17	33
23	dantrolene 12 mg kg^{-1} d^{-1} placebo	1	dantrolene≥placebo	spastic	1.5–17	34
20	dantrolene 1–15 mg kg^{-1} d^{-1} placebo	6	dantrolene = placebo	spastic	4–15	35
Dantrolene versus Diazepam						
22	dantrolene ≤225 mg/day diazepam ≤12 mg/day	3	dantrolene>diazepam (9) dantrolene<diazepam (7) dantrolene = diazepam (4)	spastic	2–8	30

*On maximum dose only.
(Adapted with permission from Wuis.[26])

employed it in adult patients with muscle spasm and pain associated with deformity, limited movement, or paralysis.

Among the first to test this drug in children with cerebral palsy, Phelps[28] reported favorably on a group of 19 inpatients with predominantly athetoid cerebral palsy. Diazepam had as positive an effect on the emotional status of the children as on the hypertonia. Though there were only two patients with spasticity, he felt the response to diazepam was better in the athetoid type. Among a heterogeneous population of children with cerebral palsy, Keats and associates[29] also found the best response among those with athetosis. Nogen[30] reported that treatment with diazepam brought definite improvement in spasticity and activities of daily living in 20 to 22 patients in comparison to placebo. However, when diazepam was compared to dantrolene in the second part of his study, dantrolene was more effective in nine patients, and diazepam and dantrolene were equally effective in four. Side effects of lethargy and drowsiness were not bothersome after a short period of acclimation. Unfortunately, no actual data were presented in this article; nor were the outcome measures precisely described and quantified.

Dantrolene Many studies have been published on the use of dantrolene in spasticity. The heterogeneity of the patients treated, even within a study, and the lack of objective quantitative methods of measurement make the drawing of definite conclusions about its effectiveness for a specific type of spastic disorder a difficult task.[26] Table 1

Table 2 Summary of results of trials of baclofen in patients with cerebral palsy

Number of Patients	Dosage Regimen	Duration of Therapy* (weeks)	Effect	Classification of Cerebral Palsy (No. of Patients)	Age of Patients (years)	Reference No.
35	45 mg/day	2	baclofen>placebo	spastic	3–61	37
20	30–60 mg/day	2	baclofen>placebo	spastic (17) mixed (3)	2–16	38
18	2 mg·kg^{-1}·d^{-1}	1	baclofen = placebo	spastic (12) mixed (6)	7–16	39
36	30–70 mg/day	4	baclofen≥placebo	spastic (21) mixed (15)	2–17	40
20	10–60 mg/day	4	baclofen>placebo	spastic	2–16	41,42

*On maximum dose only
(Adapted with permission from Wuis.[26])

summarizes the results of controlled double-blind studies in children with cerebral palsy.

In most studies subtle benefits were found, but these seldom warranted continuation of the drug after the trial period. In cerebral palsy, dantrolene has not been compared with baclofen. These findings are difficult to interpret without controlling for likely changes in drug metabolism and/or excretion.

Hepatic injury is the most feared side effect of dantrolene. A recent review of all cases of hepatic adverse events associated with dantrolene therapy reported to the manufacturer through 1987 revealed that of 122 cases containing sufficient data to analyze, 38% had asymptomatic transaminase elevations, 10% had additional mild hyperbilirubinemia, 30% had jaundice, and 22% died.[36] Deaths were associated with administration for longer than 2 months, concomitant drug use, additional nonhepatic disease, and advanced age. There have been no deaths reported in children taking dantrolene. These experiences underscore the urgent need for controlled safety data for drugs administered to children.

Baclofen An overview of the use of baclofen in children with cerebral palsy is shown in Table 2. In most studies baclofen had some effect, mainly in patients with the spastic form of cerebral palsy. The present data do not help in the choice of either baclofen or dantrolene in a specific type of spastic disorder.

Intrathecal baclofen Although its use as an oral preparation spans almost two decades, administration of baclofen via the intrathecal route is relatively new. Penn and Kroin[43] first proposed the use of intrathecal baclofen in 1985 as an alternative to invasive neurosurgical techniques for the reduction of spasticity. Since then few studies have explored its use in the treatment of spasticity associated with cerebral palsy, especially among children. In a recent study by Albright and associates,[44] a 25 μg intrathecal dose given to 17 subjects, ages 5 to 27 years, was sufficient to produce a significant reduction in lower extremity tone in 13 children. Onset of action was apparent within 20 to 40 minutes following injection.

Because baclofen is believed to act at the level of the spinal cord by inhibiting the release of excitatory neurotransmitters presynaptically, intrathecal administration allows it to reach its site of action quickly. Furthermore, more than ten times greater drug concentrations have been achieved through intrathecal versus oral administration.[45,46] Low cerebrospinal fluid concentrations following oral dosing are explained by baclofen's low lipid solubility as well as its 30% binding to plasma proteins.[45,47] These attributes account for limited transport across the blood-brain barrier.

While the usual side effects of baclofen appear to be fewer with intrathecal administration, this technique is not without hazards. In addition to mechanical problems associated with continuous infusion pump failure, other complications include meningitis, localized infections, and catheter displacement.[48] The most serious complication encountered has been accidental overdose with respiratory depression and coma.[49] Obviously, the size of the pump is problematic for small children when continuous infusion is desired.

Intrathecal baclofen has been shown to be effective in reducing spasticity and increasing function in patients—primarily adults—suffering from multiple sclerosis, spinal cord injury, and cerebral palsy. Further study is needed to determine the efficacy, safety, and practicality of chronic intrathecal baclofen infusion in children.

Summary

Use of muscle relaxant drugs for treatment of spasticity in children with cerebral palsy has a rational physiologic basis. However, despite their widespread use, there has been very little study of the pharmacodynamics of these drugs, particularly in relation to the desired functional effects. Furthermore, little is known about optimal dosing, safety, and side effects of these compounds in young children. So little information about baclofen is available that the *Physicians' Desk Reference*[10] does not recommend its use for cerebral palsy or for children under 12. Intrathecal administration of baclofen offers promise, although there are considerable logistic and practical difficulties with this approach for small children.

Much work needs to be done to determine whether this often-used treatment modality for muscle tone reduction in children is effective, which drugs are most effective and at what doses, and what mode of administration achieves the best result with fewest unwanted side effects. At present, there are few guidelines for the clinician.

References

1. Blasco, PA: Cerebral palsy: Clinical diagnosis and natural history, in Park TS, Phillips LH II, Peacock WJ (eds): *Management of Spasticity in Cerebral Palsy and Spinal Cord Injury*. Philadelphia, Hanley & Belfus, 1989.
2. Healy A: Cerebral palsy, in Blackman JA (ed): *Medical Aspects of Developmental Disabilities in Children Birth to Three*, ed 2. Rockville, MD, Aspen Publications, 1990.

3. Blackman JA, Healy A: *The Early Needs of Children With Cerebral Palsy.* Iowa City, University of Iowa, 1983.

4. Blackman JA: Cerebral palsy, in Wolraich ML (ed): *The Practical Assessment & Management of Children With Disorders of Development and Learning.* Chicago, Year Book Medical Publishers, 1987.

5. Cruichshank WM: *Cerebral Palsy,* ed 3. Syracuse, NY, Syracuse University Press, 1976.

6. Lance JW: Symposium synopsis, in Feldman RG, Young RR, Koella WP (eds):): *Spasticity: Disordered Motor Control.* Chicago, Year Book Medical Publishers, 1980, p 485.

7. Nathan P: Some comments on spasticity and rigidity, in Desmedt JE (ed): *New Developments in Electromyography and Clinical Neurophysiology.* Basel, Switzerland, Karger, 1973, pp 13–14.

8. Young RR, Wiegner AW: Spasticity. *Clin Orthop* 1987;219:50–62.

9. Davidoff RA: Mode of action of antispasticity drugs. *Neurosurgery: State of the Art Reviews* 1989;4:315–324.

10. *Physicians' Desk Reference.* Oradell, NJ, Medical Economics Co, 1992.

11. Young RR, Delwaide PJ: Drug therapy: Spasticity. *N Engl J Med* 1981;304: 96–99.

12. Morselli PL, Principi N, Tognoni G, et al: Diazepam elimination in premature and full-term infants, and children. *J Perinat Med* 1973;1:133–141.

13. Agurell S, Berlin A, Ferngren H, et al: Plasma levels of diazepam after parenteral and rectal administration in children. *Epilepsia* 1975;16:277–283.

14. Meberg A, Langslet A, Bredsen JE, et al: Plasma concentration of diazepam and N-Desmethyldiazepam in children after a single rectal or intramuscular dose of diazepam. *Europ J Clin Pharmacol* 1978;14:273–276.

15. Greenblatt DJ, Divoll AM, Harmatz JS, et al: Diazepam disposition determinants. *Clin Pharmacol Ther* 1980;27:301–312.

16. Hainaut K, Desmedt JE: Effect of dantrolene sodium on calcium movements in single muscle fibers. *Nature* 1974;252:728–730.

17. Lietman PS, Haslam RHA, Walcher JR: Pharmacology of dantrolene sodium in children. *Arch Phys Med Rehabil* 1974;55:388–392.

18. Lerman J, McLeod ME, Strong HA: Pharmacokinetics of intravenous dantrolene in children. *Anesthesiology* 1989;70:625–629.

19. Inotsume N, Higashi A, Matsukane I, et al: Relationship between serum concentration and daily dose of dantrolene in cerebral palsy patients. *Ped Pharmacol* 1986;5:253–259.

20. Nogen AG: Effect of dantrolene sodium on the incidence of seizures in children with spasticity. *Childs Brain* 1979;5:420–425.

21. Rice GPA: Pharmacotherapy of spasticity: Some theoretical and practical considerations. *Can J Neurol Sci* 1987;14(suppl 3):510–512.

22. Kochak GM, Rakhit A, Wagner WE, et al: The pharmacokinetics of baclofen derived from intestinal infusion. *Clin Pharmacol Ther* 1985;38:251–257.

23. Gerkin R, Curry SC, Vance MV, et al: First order elimination kinetics following baclofen overdose. *Ann Emerg Med* 1986;15:843–846.

24. Milla PJ, Jackson AD: A controlled trial of baclofen in children with cerebral palsy. *J Int Med Res* 1977;5:398–404.

25. Lossius R, Dietrichson P, Lunde PKM: Effect of diazepam and desmethyldiazepam in spasticity and rigidity: A quantitative study of reflexes and plasma concentrations. *Acta Neurol Scand* 1980;61:378–383.

26. Wuis EW: Spasticity and drug therapy. *Pharm Weekbl (Sci)* 1987;9:249–260.

27. Katz RA, Aldes JH, Rector M: A new drug approach to muscle relaxation. *J Neuropsychiatry* 1962;3(suppl):S91-S95.

28. Phelps WM: Observations of a new drug in cerebral palsy athetoids. *Western Med* 1963;4(suppl):5.

29. Keats S, Morgese A, Nordland T: Role of diazepam in the comprehensive treatment of cerebral palsied children. *Western Med* 1963;4(suppl):22.

30. Nogen AG: Medical treatment for spasticity in children with cerebral palsy. *Childs Brain* 1976;2:304–308.

31. Chyatte SB, Birdsong JH, Roberson DL: Dantrolene sodium in athetoid cerebral palsy. *Arch Phys Med Rehabil* 1973;54:365–368.

32. Denhoff E, Feldman S, Smith MG, et al: Treatment of spastic cerebral-palsied children with sodium dantrolene. *Dev Med Child Neurol* 1975;17:736–742.

33. Ford F, Bleck EE, Aptekar RG, et al: Efficacy of dantrolene sodium in the treatment of spastic cerebral palsy. *Dev Med Child Neurol* 1976;18:770–783.

34. Haslam RHA, Walcher JR, Lietman PS, et al: Dantrolene sodium in children with spasticity. *Arch Phys Med Rehabil* 1974;55:384–388.

35. Joynt RL, Leonard JA Jr: Dantrolene sodium suspension in treatment of spastic cerebral palsy. *Dev Med Child Neurol* 1980;22:755–767.

36. Chan CH: Dantrolene sodium and hepatic injury. *Neurology* 1990;40:1427–1432.

37. VanHemert JCJ: A double-blind comparison of baclofen and placebo in patients with spasticity of cerebral origin, in Feldman RG, Young R, Koella WP (eds): *Spasticity: Disordered Motor Control*. Chicago, Year Book Medical Publishers, 1980, pp 41–49.

38. Jukes AM (ed): *Baclofen: Spasticity and Cerebral Pathology*. Northampton, Cambridge Medical Publications, 1978.

39. McKinlay I, Hyde E, Gordon N: Baclofen: A team approach to drug evaluation of spasticity in childhood. *Scot Med J* 1980;25(suppl):S26-S28.

40. Schwartzman JS, Tilbery CP, Kogler E, et al: Effects of Lioresal in cerebral palsy. *Folia Med* 1976;72:297–302.

41. Milla PJ, Jackson ADM: A controlled trial of baclofen in children with cerebral palsy. *J Int Med Res* 1977;5:398–404.

42. Calta RG, Sautomauro ET: The use of baclofen in children with cerebral palsy. *Folia Med* 1976;73:199.

43. Penn RD, Kroin JS: Continuous intrathecal baclofen for severe spasticity. *Lancet* 1985;2:125–127.

44. Albright AL, Cervi A, Singletary J: Intrathecal baclofen for spasticity in children with cerebral palsy. *JAMA* 1991;265:1418–1422.

45. Knutson E, Lindblom U, Martensson A: Plasma and cerebrospinal fluid levels of baclofen (Lioresal) at optimal therapeutic responses in spastic paresis. *J Neuro Sci* 1974;23:473–484.

46. Müller H, Zierski J, Dralle D, et al: Intrathecal baclofen in spasticity, in Müller H, Zierski J, Penn RD (eds): *Local Spinal Therapy of Spasticity*. Berlin, Springer Verlag, 1988, pp 155–214.

47. Gilman AG, Goodman LS, Gilman A: *Goodman and Gilman's The Pharmacological Basis of Therapeutics*, ed 8. New York, Macmillan Publishing, 1990.

48. Lazorthes Y, Sallerin-Caute B, Verdie JC, et al: Chronic intrathecal baclofen administration for control of severe spasticity. *J Neurosurgery* 1990;72:393–402.

49. Penn RD, Savoy SM, Corcos D, et al: Intrathecal baclofen for severe spinal spasticity. *N Eng J Med* 1989;320:1517–1521.

Chapter 19

Technology-Assisted Self-Care in the Treatment of Spastic Diplegia

Karen E. Pape, MD, FRCPC, FAAP
Susan E. Kirsch, MD, FRCPC, FAAP

Introduction

What is technology-assisted self-care? It is a new concept in rehabilitation management that consists of three important components.

Technology

Alvin Toffler in *The Third Wave* estimated that the pool of medical knowledge is doubling every five to ten years.[1] This rapid expansion of knowledge is matched by the development of new technologies in nearly every field. Initially, technology development is purpose driven but, once developed, new uses are often found for the product. Some of the best examples of this process are found in the NASA Technology Transfer Program where technologies initially developed for the space program are finding widespread use as consumer and medical devices.

In recent years there have been many developments in the area of peak performance athletics. The aim of The Magee Clinic is to identify these developments and technologies and transfer their use to the disabled population. Frequently this requires an adaptation of the technology to enable the disabled to perform at their peak. One such technology is electrical muscle stimulation.

Assisted

It is important to recognize that these technologies assist total management and do not replace or substitute for other modalities. The process of learning just how technology can be of assistance in the care of the physically disabled is in its infancy.

Self-Care

The last component of The Magee Clinic Program is self-care. It is obvious that health care is costly and resources are scarce both in money and, more importantly, in skilled time. We believe that by using professionally guided self-care we can improve the overall quality of care delivered to the individual with a physical handicap. It can also be extremely cost effective.

An important secondary benefit of a self-care home program is that the patient learns to take responsibility for his or her own treatment program. This produces an improvement in self-confidence and independence. These are important qualities for everyone but are not commonly available to the physically disabled.

Evolution of Disability

What causes the disability in cerebral palsy? One of the most common definitions of cerebral palsy is "a permanent, but not unchanging, disorder of movement and posture due to a non-progressive defect or lesion of the brain in early life."[2] While this definition has gained wide acceptance, it is no longer accurate.

In the past, much weight has been given to the description "permanent" with reference to the brain defect or lesion. This once vigorously defended position is now crumbling in response to advances in clinical and basic neuroscience that demonstrate evidence of neuroplasticity. There is a remarkable ability of the human brain, in contrast to a rat brain, to find a way to cope with neural loss. Clinically, the evidence is most obvious in individuals who have had a hemispherectomy in early life. These children, subjected to removal of one-half of the hemispheric component of the brain, have a near normal outcome with minimal physical or neuropsychological defects.[3] Equally, there is a growing body of evidence that preterm infants with massive brain lesions may develop normally.[4] Others, with apparently indistinguishable brain lesions, have severe cerebral palsy. The exact mechanism of why one infant is normal and one has severe hemiplegia as a result of a unilateral brain lesion is not immediately obvious. However, current knowledge indicates that some lesions do not lead to permanent sequelae.

The second part of the quotation, "but not unchanging disorder of movement and posture," expresses an interesting concept. The disorder of movement and posture in children with cerebral palsy changes in the developing child. First and foremost, it must be recognized that in some cases it goes away. Transient dystonia of prematurity was first described in 1972 by C. M. Drillien.[5] More recently, Nelson and Ellenberg[6] reported a high incidence of spontaneous recovery from motor defects in children who were diagnosed at 1 year of age. Taudorf and associates[7] reported that fewer children recovered if the primary diagnosis was made after 2 years of age.

These data are interesting but they beg the question of whether those cases who apparently recover had a "wrong diagnosis" or whether they represent neuroplasticity with spontaneous recovery. An equally possible hypothesis is that those children have recovered because they have had effective intervention.

Nonetheless, in persistent cases of cerebral palsy, the disorder itself changes in character over time. Spasticity evolves over the first years of life, producing secondary changes in bone and muscle growth.[8,9]

Imbalances commonly lead to altered biomechanics.[10,11] Shortened muscles are weak; elongated muscles even weaker.

How does this information fit with a ''disorder of movement and posture due to a non-progressive deficit or lesion of the brain in early life''? There is no argument that the deficit or lesion of the brain started the problem, initiating the abnormal growth and development. But the abnormal growth of muscle and bone are heavy contributors to the disorder of movement and posture. For example, the hemiplegic child who walks reasonably well at 2 to 3 years of age has a better pelvic orientation than the same child at 15 to 16 years of age when the effects of leg-length discrepancy produce unequal forces through the pelvis and back.

It seems clear that the traditional definition of cerebral palsy[2] lacks precision. It assumes a simple cause and effect relationship between brain deficit or lesion and the disorder of movement and posture. Adherence to this linear model has led to a prolonged search for ''the'' answer, ''the'' treatment, ''the'' procedure, or ''the'' surgical intervention. Not surprisingly, the quest is ongoing and the solution still distant.

It is now becoming clear that the problem of cerebral palsy is multifactorial, and all the numerous variables interact. While it is acceptable as a first principle that early brain deficit or lesion initiates the problem, it is impossible to predict the outcome of a particular brain lesion in the individual case. Evolution of signs and symptoms over time and in response to multiple interventions further complicates the picture. In other words, the child with cerebral palsy represents a complex self-organizing system. Within this system, physicians and therapists are unlikely to be able to tease out exactly which intervention is producing change. In fact, the search for a direct cause and effect relationship in the evaluation of new therapies may be limiting therapeutic possibilities.

In contrast to a simple linear model, chaos theory describes the behavior of systems characterized by complex interactions.[12] This scientific theory recognizes that a specific intervention may lead to widely varying outcomes in different subjects. The effect, named the ''butterfly phenomena,''[13] has been the topic of debate and discussion in many different fields of endeavor.[14] Over the past 10 to 15 years there has been a growing awareness that the insights derived from nonlinear dynamics and chaos theory may suggest a new approach to the study of biologic systems.[15-20] Rather than trying to identify and measure the changes in one variable that is part of a fluctuating system, it may be more fruitful to look for overriding principles and patterns of outcome that may be applied to a wide variety of cases.

One such overriding principle attributed to Hippocrates is ''that which is used grows and develops, that which is not used withers and atrophies away.'' Spastic muscle is weak and the nonspastic antagonist muscle is even weaker. In adult studies, several techniques have been used to strengthen muscles.[21-23] Electrical stimulation of muscle has been widely used in both injured athletes and adult disabled individuals.[24–27] In these cases, the investigators studied cooperative, adult subjects and targeted specific muscle groups for strengthening.

In children, the situation is very different; it can be described as an attempt to hit a moving target. Not only does the nature of the disability change with growth and development, but the child's cooperation, motivation, and ability to tolerate uncomfortable procedures varies with maturity and intelligence. For all these reasons, traditional electrical stimulation techniques cannot be easily used in young children. However, animal studies have shown a clear trophic effect of low intensity electrical fields.[28–32] In addition, growth hormone release occurs preferentially during sleep,[33,34] and, finally, children are most cooperative when asleep. Therefore, we developed a technique of low intensity nighttime electrical stimulation for the treatment of muscle weakness in cerebral palsy. We applied this technique to a broad range of children with spastic diplegia and have measured global functional change. We did not attempt to measure isolated muscle strength or to assess spasticity.

Outcome Trial

Patient Selection

During 1989, unselected children aged 2 to 10 years who had spastic diplegia were offered a treatment trial of nighttime transcutaneous electrical stimulation. The diagnosis of cerebral palsy was made by the staffs of unrelated treatment centers who referred patients to the clinic for evaluation. Patients with associated sensory disabilities and/or previous surgery were included. A broad range of cognitive ability was also accepted, although those with severe retardation, who were unable to tolerate nighttime application of the stimulation were excluded. We also excluded those children who were using antispasmotic drugs to control their seizures and those with uncontrolled seizure activity. These exclusion criteria applied, therefore, to the most severely involved, multihandicapped children.

The severity of neuromotor involvement was scored clinically. Mildly affected children had attained independent ambulation with or without bracing below the knee. Moderately affected children were able to walk only with an assistive device. Bracing was also frequently required for these patients. Severely affected children were either not ambulatory or were household ambulators with walking aids, who used wheelchairs outside of the house.

Protocol

Treatment was offered on a 12-month trial basis, using a single subject design with the patient acting as his or her own control.[35–37] Baseline and 6- and 12-month assessments were performed. No attempt was made to standardize physical therapy during the study. All continued their standard rehabilitation procedures as independently administered by community rehabilitation centers.

Electrical Stimulation

Low-level electrical stimulation was applied overnight through surface electrodes placed over the tibialis anterior and quadriceps femoris muscles on alternative legs on consecutive nights. Specific motor points were not used. Conductive silicone rubber electrodes were used that were $1'' \times 2''$ and were backed with a water-activated semisolid adhesive gum. After instruction, the childrens' parents applied the electrodes at home while the patients were awake to ensure correct electrode positioning. The stimulator was turned on either before or after the child fell asleep according to family preferences. Periods of sleep, duration of stimulation, functional changes, and any problems were recorded by the parents on diary sheets provided by the investigators. Electrode positioning was reviewed after 6 weeks and every 3 months thereafter.

A dual-channel, battery-operated electrical stimulator was used, which generated alternating coupled current pulses to balance for equal charge transport in both directions. Pulse width was 300 μsec; pulse frequency was between 35 and 45 Hz; peak intensity was <10 mA, with a 1:1 ON-OFF cycle. The stimulus intensity was just above sensory threshold so that the muscle showed no evidence of active contraction. A 2-second pulse envelope rise time avoided the induction of muscle cocontraction.

End Point Measurement

The end points of this trial were based on gross motor functional skills. Treatment was discontinued when the patient was within the normal range in testing. The Progressive Ambulation Scale (PAS) developed for this study consists of a ten-point descriptive ordinal scale as follows: (1) independent sitting (includes W-sitting, cross-legged sitting, and sitting with extended legs); (2) crawling (includes bunny hop and reciprocal crawling); (3) balancing in the tall kneeling position; (4) standing with support; (5) walker use; (6) crutch use; (7) cane use; (8) independent household ambulation; (9) use of a walking aid for distance only; and (10) independent walking.

Each child was scored at baseline, and the scoring was updated every six months. All changes to walking aids were prescribed by independent physicians and/or therapists who had no involvement with the study. Children scoring 1 to 5 on the PAS were in the severe category; scores of 5 to 9 represented moderate severity. By definition, all children scoring 10 on the PAS would be considered mildly affected. The mildly affected subjects were scored on the balance and locomotor subsections of the Peabody Developmental Motor Scales (PDMS).[38]

Data Analysis

The Progressive Ambulation Scale score was expressed as a mean ± standard deviation. The Wilcoxon Signed-Rank Test was used to compare baseline to 6- and 12-month results.

Table 1 Clinical trial patient characteristics

		Entry Characteristics				Study Patients	
	No.	**Sex**		**Age in Months***	**No. at 6 Mos**	**No. at 12 Mos**	**Age at Entry in Mos***
Severity		**Male**	**Female**				
Mild	19	11	8	63 ± 18	17	13	63 ± 20
Moderate	38	17	21	63 ± 20	34	28	65 ± 19
Severe	17	9	8	40 ± 9	14	11	39 ± 8
Total	74	37	37	57 ± 20	65	52	

*Mean ± 1 standard deviation

In the mildly affected group, the raw scores on the balance and/or locomotor subscales at entry into the study were compared with the 6- and 12-month scores. All data are shown as mean ± standard deviation. The paired Student's t Test was used to compare results within groups.

Results

During the calendar year 1989, 86 children with spastic diplegia were referred for treatment at The Magee Clinic. Seventy-four (86%) entered a clinical trial of nighttime electrical stimulation. Of the 12 children who did not start the trial following initial consultation, four were excluded for behavioral problems, two were too mild for treatment, two were too young (under 2 years of age), and four children, who were appropriate for the trial, elected not to start treatment.

Table 1 describes the clinical population. There was no clear sex predominance. The age at entry to the study was similar in the mild (63 ± 18 months) and moderate (63 ± 20 months) group, but younger in the severe (40 ± 9 months) group. Sixty-five children (88%) have completed six months of treatment and testing. Seven children were lost to follow-up and two treated children had missing data as they were uncooperative with baseline and follow-up testing. Fifty-two children (70%) have completed 12 months of treatment and testing. Data were incomplete in 13 children for the following reasons: Two of the children were lost to follow-up. Eight did not return at the appropriate time for repeat testing but are continuing in the ongoing trial. One child developed increased seizures after six months of electrical stimulation and stopped electrical stimulation for a prolonged period while anticonvulsants were adjusted. One child had a selective dorsal rhizotomy after nine months of electrical stimulation. One child stopped electrical stimulation for several months because of problems sleeping.

Group 1 Mild

Over the one year of electrical stimulation treatment, acquisition of new skills resulted in increased PDMS scores. The comparisons between 0 and 6 months, and 0 and 12 months in locomotor and balance scores were statistically significant ($p < 0.005$, Table 2).

These changes on serial testing were reflected in life skill changes.

Table 2 Raw scores of the Peabody Developmental Motor Scales for group I mild

	Baseline Raw Score	Six Months Raw Score	p	Twelve Months Raw Score	p
Balance subsection	32 ± 7	37 ± 11	0.0007	39 ± 10	0.0058
Locomotor subsection	50 ± 16	64 ± 19	0.0001	69 ± 21	0.0001

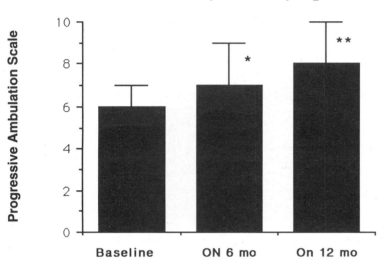

Fig. 1 *Progressive Ambulation Scale in moderately involved children. Change from baseline to 6 months (*) was significant at p = 0.0002 and to 12 months (**) at p = 0.0001.*

Parents reported decreased falling (four), increased endurance (two), transitions to standing independently (three), and the new skills of walking backwards or sideways, and jumping and balancing on one leg (eleven). Use of ankle-foot orthoses decreased to inserts (two), partial use during the day (three), or no braces (one).

Groups 2 & 3 Moderate & Severe

Functional changes were measured on the PAS. In the moderate group, mean scores changed from 6 ± 1 at baseline to 7 ± 2 at 6 months to 8 ± 2 at 12 months. These changes were significant at p = 0.0002 and p = 0.0001, respectively (Fig. 1). In the severe group, the baseline score on the PAS was 3 ± 2, which improved to 4 ± 1 at 6 months and 5 ± 1 at 12 months. These changes were also significant at p = 0.007 and p = 0.004 (Fig. 2).

In the moderately affected group, changes occurred in use of walking

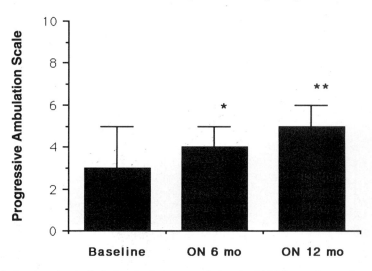

Fig. 2 *Progressive Ambulation Scale in severely involved children. Change from baseline to 6 months (*) was significant at p = 0.007 and to 12 months (**) at p = 0.004.*

aids. Walker use progressed to use of crutches (four), canes (three), use of walker in playground only (two), or independent walking (three). Crutch/cane use progressed to independent walking in three further patients. Two younger children who were taking steps with support but had not yet received an aid to walking, progressed to independent walking. Thus, 8 of 29 (28%) of the moderate group became independent ambulators, changing category from moderate to mild.

In the severely affected children, the following changes were reported: improved posture and balance for independent sitting (eight), controlled and faster four-point reciprocal crawl (six), and maintenance of tall kneel position (five). Eight of eleven (73%) were independently started on walker use by their community physiotherapists during this year. Improved sitting balance and reciprocal crawling were noted as leg spasticity decreased. None of these children changed in category from severe to moderate.

Discussion

How do we account for these motor changes during treatment with electrical stimulation? Previous investigators have used electrical stimulation to muscle groups to treat spasticity. Their approach differed from ours in that high levels of stimulation producing muscle contractions were used.[39-44] Although these approaches decreased spasticity, they did not produce a sustained effect.

Our use of low level nighttime electrical stimulation is a new technique. However, there is precedent animal work for this approach. In our subjects, applying electrical stimulation at night also takes advantage of a time window during sleep when spasticity is naturally reduced.

But the question remains as to whether we can be sure that the observed changes in function were caused by the electrical stimulation. The trial showed a positive effect across a broad range of subjects. The effect was maximal in the milder groups after 12 months of treatment. In the moderate and severe groups, sustained improvements were also seen. However, it is possible that all of the changes occurred as a result of ongoing growth and development. In growing children, it is impossible to separate the role of learning, motivation, and practice from the experimental intervention.

Our functional tests indirectly showed the effect of increased muscle strength and decreased spasticity but the most consistent change noted by the parents of the children participating in the trial was improved self-confidence, risk taking, and general levels of cooperation. We concluded that part of the effectiveness of nighttime electrical stimulation was the self-care component. By providing the technology in the home, we created a potent force to improve the child's and family's sense of confidence and control over the chronic disability of cerebral palsy. It is arguable whether the electrical stimulation or this positive self-care aspect of the program was more important in the development of functional improvements. In contrast to a more linear approach, chaos theory allows us to accept the interaction of multiple variables in the production of a beneficial effect.

Summary

One of the major challenges of the 1990s will be to integrate technology into the overall rehabilitation management of children. A clear recognition that the patient controls the rehabilitative process is also necessary. Because of the rapid pace of technologic developments, it is unlikely that any individual practitioner will be able to remain current with even selected areas of the field. Therefore, it is our responsibility to make the individual patients experts in their own disabilities so that they can actively seek out the new treatments and technologies that may help them achieve their peak performance.

Acknowledgments

This work was supported in part by grants from The Henry White Kinnear Foundation, The Ontario Easter Seal Research Institute, and The Loyal True Blue & Orange Research Institute.

References

1. Toffler A: *The Third Wave*. New York, William Morrow, 1980.
2. Christensen E, Melchor JC: *Cerebral Palsy: A Clinical and Neuropathological Study*, Clinics in Developmental Medicine. London, Spastics Society with Heinemann Medical, 1967, no 25, p 1.
3. Hoffman HJ, Hendrick EB, Dennis M, et al: Hemispherectomy for Sturge-Weber Syndrome. *Childs Brain* 1979;5:233–248.
4. Wigglesworth JS: Plasticity of the development brain, in Pape KE, Wigglesworth JS (eds): *Perinatal Brain Lesions*. Oxford, Blackwell Scientific Publications, 1989, pp 253–269.
5. Drillien CM: Abnormal neurologic signs in the first year of life in low-birthweight infants: Possible prognostic significance. *Dev Med Child Neurol* 1972;14:575–584.
6. Nelson KB, Ellenberg JH: Children who "outgrew" cerebral palsy. *Pediatrics* 1982;69:529–536.
7. Taudorf K, Hansen FJ, Melchior JC: Spontaneous remission of cerebral palsy. *Neuropediatrics* 1986;17:19–22.
8. Molnar GE: Cerebral palsy, in Basmajian JV (ed): *Pediatric Rehabilitation*. Baltimore, Williams & Wilkins, 1985, pp 420–467.
9. Castle ME, Reyman TA, Schneider ME: Pathology of spastic muscle in cerebral palsy. *Clin Orthop* 1979;142:223–232.
10. Sharrard WJ: Paralytic deformity in the lower limb. *J Bone Joint Surg* 1967; 49B:731–747.
11. O'Dwyer NJ, Neilson PD, Nash J: Mechanisms of muscle growth related to muscle contracture in cerebral palsy. *Dev Med Child Neurol* 1989;31:543–557.
12. Gleick J: *Chaos: Making A New Science*. New York, Penguin Books, 1987.
13. Lorens E: Predictability: Does the flap of a butterfly's wing in Brazil set off a tornado in Texas? Presented at the Annual Meeting of the American Association for the Advancement of Science, Washington, DC, Dec 29, 1979.
14. Pool R: Chaos theory: How big an advance? *Science* 1989;245:26–28.
15. Goldberger AL, Rigney DR, Mietus J, et al: Nonlinear dynamics in sudden cardiac death syndrome: Heart rate oscillations and bifurcations. *Experientia* 1988;44:983–987.
16. Denton TA, Diamond GA, Helfant RH, et al: Fascinating rhythm: A primer on chaos theory and its application to cardiology. *Am Heart J* 1990;120:1419–1440.
17. Goldberger AL, West BJ: Fractals in physiology and medicine. *Yale J Biol Med* 1987;60:421–435.
18. Wang LP, Pichler EE, Ross J: Oscillations and chaos in neural networks: An exactly solvable model. *Proc Natl Acad Sci USA* 1990;87:9467–9471.
19. Soong AC, Stuart CI: Evidence of chaotic dynamics underlying the human alpha-rhythm electroencephalogram. *Biol Cybern* 1989;62:55–62.
20. Hoppensteadt FC: Intermittent chaos, self-organization, and learning from synchronous synaptic activity in model neuron networks. *Proc Natl Acad Sci USA* 1989;86:2991–2995.
21. Milner-Brown HS, Miller RG: Muscle strengthening through high-resistance weight training in patients with neuromuscular disorders. *Arch Phys Med Rehabil* 1988;69:14–19.
22. Grimby G: Physical activity and muscle training in the elderly. *Acta Med Scand Suppl* 1986;711:233–237.
23. Palmer SS, Mortimer JA, Webster DD, et al: Exercise therapy for Parkinson's Disease. *Arch Phys Med Rehabil* 1986;67:741–745.
24. Leiber RL: Skeletal muscle adaptability III: Muscle properties following chronic electrical stimulation. *Dev Med Child Neurol* 1986;28:662–670.

25. Milner-Brown HS, Miller RG: Muscle strengthening through electrical stimulation combined with low-resistance weights in patients with neuromuscular disorders. *Arch Phys Med Rehabil* 1986;67:530–535.

26. Boutille D, Smith B, Malone T: A strength study utilizing the Electro-Stim 180. *J Orthop Sports Phys Ther* 1985;7:50–53.

27. Eriksson E, Haggmark T: Comparison of isometric muscle training and electrical stimulation supplementing isometric muscle training in the recovery after major knee ligament surgery. *Am J Sport Med* 1979;7:169–171.

28. Pette D, Vrbová G: Invited Review: Neural control of phenotypic expression in mammalian muscle fibers. *Muscle Nerve* 1985;8:676–689.

29. Cabric HS, Appell Resic A: Effects of electrical stimulation of different frequencies on the myonuclei and fibre size in human muscle. *Int J Sports Med* 1987;8:323–326.

30. Gibson JNA, Rennie MJ, Smith K: Prevention of disuse muscle atrophy by means of electrical stimulation: Maintenance of protein synthesis. *Lancet* 1988; 11:767–769.

31. Dodd L, Gray SD, Hudlicka O, et al: Evaluation of capillary density in relation to fibre types in electrically stimulated rabbit fast muscles. *J Physiol (Lond)* 1980;301:11P-12P.

32. Myrhage R, Hudlicka O: Capillary growth in chronically stimulated adult skeletal muscle as studied by intravital microscopy and histological methods in rabbits and rats. *Microvasc Res* 1978;16:73–90.

33. Weitzman ED, Boyar RM, Kaplan S, et al: The relationship of sleep stages to neuroendocrine secretion and biological rhythms in man, in *Recent Progress in Hormone Research*. New York, Academic Press, 1975, pp 399–446.

34. Rose SR, Municchi G, Barnes FM, et al: Spontaneous growth hormone secretion increases during puberty in normal girls and boys. *J Clin Endocrinol Metab* 1991;73:428–435.

35. Barlow DH, Hersen M: *Single Case Experimental Design Strategies for Studying Behaviour Changes*, ed 2. New York, Pergamon Press, 1984.

36. Martin JE, Epstein LH: Evaluating treatment effectiveness in cerebral palsy. *Phys Ther* 1976;56:285–294.

37. Ottenbacher KJ: *Evaluating Clinical Change. Strategies for Occupational and Physical Therapists*. Baltimore, Williams & Wilkins, 1986.

38. Folio MR, Fewell RR: *Peabody Developmental Motor Scales and Activity Cards* (manual). Allen, TX, DLM Teaching Resources, 1983.

39. Glenn MB, Whyte J: *The Practical Management of Spasticity in Children and Adults*. Philadelphia, Lea & Febiger, 1990.

40. Alfiori V: Electrical treatment of spasticity. *Scand J Rehabil Med* 1982;14: 177–182.

41. Levine MG, Knott M, Kabat M: Relaxation of spasticity by electrical stimulation of antagonist muscles. *Arch Phys Med Rehabil* 1952;33:668–673.

42. Solomonov M, Ambrosia R, King AD, et al: Studies toward spasticity suppression with high frequency electrical stimulation. *Orthopedics* 1984;7: 1284–1288.

43. Chan EWY: Some techniques for the relief of spasticity and their physiological basis. *Physiother Canada* 1986;38:85–89.

44. Dubowitz L, Finnie N, Hyde SA, et al: Improvement of muscle performance by chronic electrical stimulation in children with cerebral palsy. *Lancet* 1988; 1:587–588.

Consensus

Nonsurgical intervention techniques used to treat children with spastic diplegia include physical therapy, muscle relaxant drugs, electrical stimulation and biofeedback, and orthotics (particularly ankle-foot orthoses). Although many of these intervention techniques are widely used throughout North America, there currently is little evidence of efficacy in improving function, nor have they been the subject of scientifically designed studies.

Physical Therapy

Virtually all children with spastic diplegia eventually see a physical therapist, either for evaluation or for treatment. Although evidence suggests that physical therapy may improve postural adaptations, to date no study evaluating its effect in spastic diplegia has demonstrated unequivocal efficacy. Physicians expect the primary effects of physical therapy on the disability in spastic diplegia to be increased independence through the use of assistive and mobility devices and improved parental ability to manage a child with a disability. Technical aspects are well taught, but the current curriculum has not provided the physical therapist with much formal training in how to be a primary source of parental support.

The effect of physical therapy on the function of the child with spastic diplegia should be evaluated in three primary areas: (1) following orthopaedic surgery or rhizotomy; (2) during growth spurts in the two- to four-year-old age group as well as the prepubertal period; and (3) in a preventive approach before weightbearing. Controlled studies of ambulatory patients with spastic diplegia who were undergoing specific types of orthopaedic surgical procedures would be ideal. These studies should be problem specific and may address a number of different operative procedures on the lower extremities in spastic diplegia.

In most of North America, physical therapy for children with spastic diplegia requires a referral and signature of a physician. There must be increased responsibility on the part of the physician as well as the physical therapist in prescribing physical therapy. Before signing the referral, the physician must insist that goals be set for the physical therapy. If the treatment plan includes an attempt to improve walking ability and to strengthen the lower extremities, physical therapy should be provided at least three times a week over the prescribed period. Reevaluation at the end of a specified time period is required to determine whether or not the goals have been met. If goals have not been met, the intensity or type of physical therapy should be modified or physical therapy should be stopped for a specified period during which monitoring of function continues.

Other areas that require an objective evaluation include: (1) the use of physical therapy in the neonatal intensive care unit; (2) the use of flexibility exercises and the age at which they may be most appropriate; and (3) the use of inhibitive casting. This discussion group agrees that it is ethical to use an untreated control group in evaluating treatments for spastic diplegia.

Improvement is needed in education of physical therapists in the area of treatment of spastic diplegia. Adding this information to the physical therapy curriculum would be helpful, but because pediatrics is such a small part of the entry-level curriculum, pediatric orthopaedists need to organize either local or regional teaching conferences to provide the pediatric physical therapist with information on treating spastic diplegia from the orthopaedists' viewpoint. At the present time, many of the conferences that physical therapists attend that deal with this area are organized by special interest groups with focus on either a specific technique, such as neurodevelopmental treatment, or are commercially sponsored. Pediatric orthopaedists dealing with neuromuscular disease must become more involved in the education of physical therapists who assess and treat children with spastic diplegia.

Muscle Relaxant Drugs

The muscle relaxant drugs used to treat spastic diplegia are principally diazepam, dantrolene, and baclofen. These medications are used less often in spastic diplegia than in spastic quadriplegia. These medications are currently used on an empirical basis, and some orthopaedists use them, especially diazepam, after orthopaedic surgical procedures. However, the pharmacokinetics have not been described for the use of these drugs in children with spastic diplegia.

Nakom, which is a medication that includes L-dopa, has been used with reported improvement in the Soviet Union to treat children who have spastic diplegia with extrapyramidal features. This treatment has been effective primarily for patients with akinesia, bradykinesia, and slow hyperkinesis associated with elevation of serum cortisol levels.

More specific evaluation of the pharmacokinetics of muscle relaxants is needed, as are clinical trials to determine efficacy for use in treatment of children who have spastic diplegia. Goals of treatment should be established before initiation of muscle relaxant medication, and the effect of the medication should be reevaluated in a specific time period after initiation of the drug treatment. If the medications, particularly intrathecal baclofen, effectively reduce spasticity, they

may provide some indication of the potential effect of rhizotomy.

Biofeedback

Recently, emphasis has been placed on the weakness that exists in spastic diplegia after orthopaedic surgical procedures or rhizotomy. In spite of previous concerns regarding the presumption that muscle strengthening would increase muscle tone and decrease joint mobility, new interest has arisen in strengthening the muscles of children with spastic diplegia. To date there is no reported evidence in the North American literature of a controlled study on the effect of biofeedback on spastic diplegia, although this technique has been used to improve function and activities of daily living in other neurologically impaired patients of various ages.

Professionals involved with evaluation of spastic diplegia must be aware of the associated muscle weakness in the lower extremities. Also, methods are needed for measuring strength in these children, and controlled studies must be undertaken to determine the effect of treatments such as functional electrical stimulation, exercise programs, and the like.

Orthotics

The use of orthotics for children with spastic diplegia is widespread and costly. Although the use of ankle-foot orthoses (AFO) improves some parameters of gait as assessed by computer based gait analysis, more controlled studies are needed to demonstrate functional gains.

Those who deal with children with spastic diplegia realize that there is a wide variation in how AFOs are fabricated. Reports of studies in which AFOs are used should include specific information on each AFO used. This should include the material (polyethylene versus polypropylene), foot plate design, length of calf portion, and cutouts and other design features that may have an impact on the child's function.

It is important to define the goal for the orthotic before initiating its use. The principal reasons for use of an AFO are to control the joint for improvement in postural control and gait and/or to decrease the amount of overflow of spasticity to other areas of the lower extremities. The orthotic should be used for a prespecified length of time, after which functional gains associated with its use should be evaluated. If use of the orthotic has not met the goals specified, consideration needs to be given to discontinuing the use of orthotics.

Large annual expenditures are made for the use of nonsurgical intervention techniques in the care of children with spastic diplegia. With increasing budgetary constraints, controlled studies are needed of all the nonsurgical interventions described above as well as many surgical interventions, not only to guide us in the best treatment for our patients, but also to provide data for appropriate allocation of resources.

Section Six
Surgical Interventions

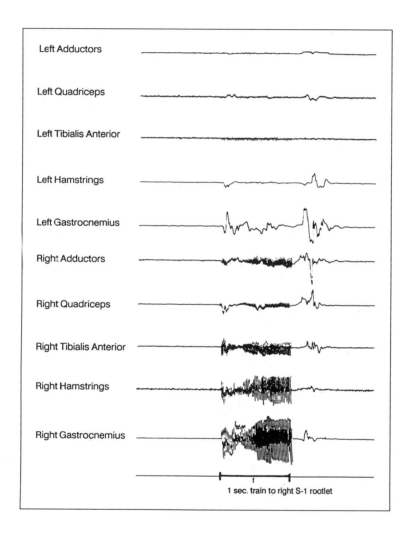

Left Adductors

Left Quadriceps

Left Tibialis Anterior

Left Hamstrings

Left Gastrocnemius

Right Adductors

Right Quadriceps

Right Tibialis Anterior

Right Hamstrings

Right Gastrocnemius

1 sec. train to right S-1 rootlet

Chapter 20

Physiologic Effects of Soft-Tissue Surgery

Colin F. Moseley, MD

Introduction

Most of the orthopaedic surgical procedures performed for patients with cerebral palsy include the release, lengthening, or transfer of muscles or their tendons. To understand the short- and long-term effects of such surgery, it is necessary to understand the mechanics and biology of muscle and, in particular, the responses of muscle to these types of procedures.

Mechanics of Muscle

The basic contractile unit of muscle is the sarcomere, which is composed of variable numbers of interdigitating strands of the proteins actin and myosin. Much work has been done by Huxley[1] and others to define the microstructural basis of muscle contraction, but that subject is outside the scope of this chapter. A number of sarcomeres attached to each other in series, end to end, constitute a myofibril, and a number of myofibrils in parallel, lying side to side, constitute a muscle fiber, the basic anatomic unit of muscle. Although the number of fibers in a given muscle does not change significantly throughout life, the number of fibrils in a fiber may increase and decrease, and the number of actin-myosin contractile units in a given sarcomere may also vary.[2] It is these variations that occur with atrophy and hypertrophy.

The strength of a muscle is related to the number of contractile units in parallel and, therefore, to both the number of sarcomeres in parallel and the cross-sectional areas of those sarcomeres. Actually, the cross-sectional area of the sarcomeres is relatively constant because, in the process of hypertrophy, the addition of new actin-myosin units will bring the size of the sarcomere to the point where it splits in two.

It is a reasonable first approximation, therefore, to say that the strength of a muscle is related to its cross-sectional area, and that the strengths of different muscles are proportional to their relative cross-sectional areas. This approximation, however, ignores the effect of muscle architecture, and it is possible that two muscles of the same

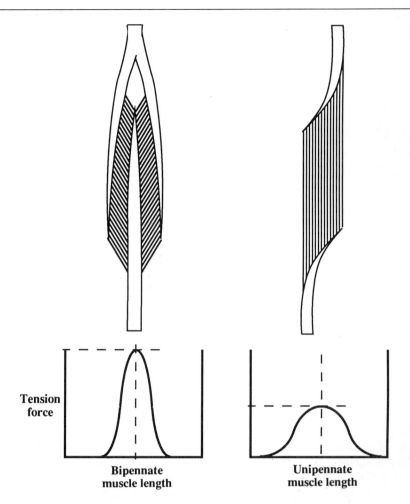

Fig. 1 *Two muscles of the same cross-sectional area can have different strengths because of their differences in architecture. The muscle with a large number of short fibers is very strong through a short excursion, and the muscle with a smaller number of long fibers is not as strong but has a greater excursion, and therefore maintains its strength over a greater range of lengths.*

shape and bulk will have very different strengths (Fig. 1). The bipennate muscle, which has relatively short muscle fibers that pass obliquely to the anatomic axis of the muscle, is much stronger than the unipennate muscle, which is the same size but has a smaller number of fibers. The length of the fibers in the unipennate muscle, however, is greater than that of the fibers in the bipennate muscle and, therefore, the excursion of the muscle is greater.

Silver and associates[3] assessed the relative strengths and fiber lengths of the muscles of the leg in a fashion similar to that used by Brand,[4] who studied upper limb muscles. Like Brand, they found that the fibers

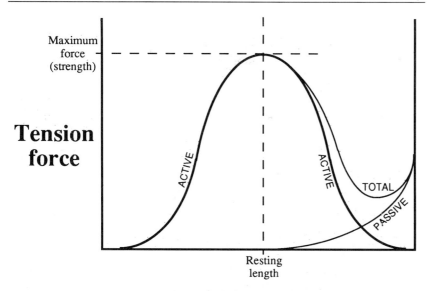

Fig. 2 *The Blix curve represents the maximum tension force exerted by a muscle as a function of length. The active component is that force generated by the contraction of the muscle, and the passive component is the elastic tension that results from stretching the muscle beyond its resting length. The muscle is able to generate the greatest tension at its resting length.*

of a given muscle were of consistent length and were not directly related to the length of the muscle itself. They found that the soleus muscle is more than 50% stronger than the gastrocnemius, and that the total strength of the plantar flexors is approximately six times that of the dorsiflexors. This latter finding is in keeping with the clinical finding that the strength of the plantar flexors cannot be reestablished by posterior transfer of extensor muscles.[3]

It has long been recognized that the maximum tension force that a given muscle can develop is related to its starting length, and is maximum at the resting length of the muscle. The classic experiment in physiology is to affix the two ends of an excised muscle to two posts, to provide the muscle with maximum electrical (tetanic) stimulation, and to measure the tension force that is developed. The test can then be repeated by altering the distance between the posts to generate a curve relating muscle length to maximum force. Such an experiment shows that the active force is a function of length in the shape of a bell curve, and that there is also a passive component of tension that increases as the muscle is lengthened beyond its resting length (Fig. 2). This curve, known as the Blix curve, has been reproduced numerous times by numerous investigators.[5,6]

The Blix curve reflects the anatomy of the muscle. Strong muscles with short excursions show a narrow curve with a high peak, whereas weaker muscles with longer excursions show a wide bell shape with a lower peak. The sensitivity of muscle strength to deviations from the resting length of the fibers suggests that all fibers in one muscle must be approximately the same length, and this has been confirmed by anatomic dissection.

It is important to remember that the Blix curve reflects only the particular parameters of the experiment, specifically one muscle at one moment in time provided a maximum stimulus. The curve reflects the maximum force that the muscle can generate, which usually is defined as muscle strength. It does not represent the long-term effect of shortening or lengthening.

It is also important to remember that while muscles are the only active motors in the musculoskeletal system, they are only that. They are not autonomous, and they operate under the direction of the brain, which, when it is sending signals to muscles to contract, is receiving and interpreting feedback not on the strength of the muscle but on the effects of its messages. This consideration is doubly important in the context of cerebral palsy.

It is also worth noting that there are other mechanical factors besides its strength involved in how well a muscle performs its function. These factors include the muscle's lever arm about the joint under consideration and the number and positions of the other joints that the muscle may cross.

Biology of Muscle

In humans, unlike some animals, the number of muscle fibers present at birth in one individual remains fairly constant throughout life, although the number of fibers differs significantly from one individual to another.[7] However, the number of fibrils in a fiber and the number of actin-myosin units in a sarcomere are variable, and this variability is expressed anatomically and functionally as atrophy and hypertrophy.

Increasing the load on a muscle (active tension force, perhaps integrated over time) stimulates that muscle's sarcomeres to add myosin-actin units. When the addition of such units brings the cross-sectional area of the sarcomere to a critical point, perhaps related to nutrition, the fibril, with its sarcomeres, splits in two, with the result that the cross-sectional areas of the fibrils in a given muscle remain more or less constant.[8]

The mechanisms of muscle growth and the controlling factors have been extensively studied, particularly by Goldspink.[8-11] It is obvious that muscles grow in length as an infant grows to become an adult, but, in contrast to bones, there is no obvious anatomic or histologic growth plate. It appears that muscles, again unlike bones, do not have any independent, congenitally-controlled growth pattern, but appear to elongate only in response to their circumstances. It appears that there is some mechanism within muscle that tends to maintain sarcomeres at a constant length, and this may have something to do with the length of the actin and myosin proteins and their degree of overlap. In any case, if a muscle is maintained at a length longer than its usual resting length, for example, by casting a joint in a fixed position away from its resting position, then the muscle will accommodate in the immediate phase by stretching with elongation of its sarcomeres. In the longer term it enters an anabolic phase with the addition of sarcomeres in series so that the number of sarcomeres in the length of a fibril increases to the point where the sarcomeres recover their normal length.[10,11] Conversely, if a tendon of a muscle is transected so that the muscle can no longer recognize the growth of its adjacent bone, then no sarcomeres will be added to the muscle and the muscle will not grow. Sarcomeres will, in fact, be lost and muscle fibers will shorten.[10]

The stimulus for muscle growth is often said to be tension, but, if that were the case, spastic muscles would be expected to grow faster than their normal counterparts. It is much more likely that the stimulus is, in fact, the elongation of the muscle and the stretching of its sarcomeres, although the issue is more complex than that. Immobilization in an elongated position causes induction of the genes responsible for the production of muscle proteins in rats, but different muscles show different patterns of response.[12] In the normal person, therefore, muscle growth occurs in response to the bone growth and elongation of the limb to which it is attached. This would also suggest that if immobilization of a joint in an extreme position causes stretching of a muscle, then that muscle can be expected to grow longer more rapidly than normal by the addition of new sarcomeres to its fibrils.

While certain animals can add sarcomeres at any point in their muscle fibrils,[13] in humans new sarcomeres tend to be added only at the ends of fibrils.[14] It appears, in rabbits, that the relative rates of growth of a muscle and its tendon depend on the excursion of the muscle.[13,15] Studies suggest that tendons grow interstitially throughout their lengths, but perhaps maximally at the tendon-bone and musculotendinous junctions.[15,16] Ziv and associates[17] concluded that the growth of spastic muscles is similar to that of normal muscles, and they coined the term ''muscle growth plate'' to refer to the areas of growth at the musculotendinous junctions.

This hypothesis of muscle growth leads to an understanding of the mechanism for the development of contractures in spastic patients. Spastic muscles tend to hold the joint about which they function in an abnormal position that allows that muscle to be shorter than normal for most of the time. The excursion of that muscle, and thereby the stimulus for muscle growth are reduced. As a result, the muscle does not grow as rapidly as its adjacent bone, and a relative contracture develops. The word relative is important here, because the muscle is not actually getting shorter, but is only failing to grow appropriately. This is at least a partial explanation for the observed clinical fact that the progression of contractures in cerebral palsy tends to stop after maturity.

Understanding that muscle is a reactionary tissue that grows or even shortens in response to its circumstances puts surgeons in a position to consider the effects of the surgery that they perform on muscles or their tendons.

Muscle and Tendon Surgery

Orthopaedists perform three types of surgery on muscles and their tendons: release, lengthening, and transfer. Following a release, either the muscle will reattach itself to surrounding soft tissues and begin to function as it did prior to the release, or it will not reattach itself, and will, therefore, remain functionless. If the muscle does reattach itself and begin to function once again, the effect of the surgery on the muscle and the result in the patient will be identical to a lengthening procedure. Because complete loss of muscle function by release does not have important physiologic effects, and because muscle transfers will be covered extensively elsewhere in this text, this chapter will concentrate on lengthening procedures.

Tendon lengthening is performed either to correct deformity or to weaken the muscle. The heel cord may be lengthened, for example, because of a gastrocnemius contracture that prevents the ankle from being dorsiflexed to the neutral position or because of a functional deficit in a child who is a persistent toe walker even in the absence of a severe fixed contracture. In the first case, the goal of the surgery is to allow the joint to resume a more normal range of motion without actually affecting the length of the muscle. If that is the case, then there will be no physiologic effects of the surgery on the muscle and its Blix curve can be expected to be unchanged. The muscle will have the same strength and excursion as it did preoperatively, which was less than normal.

Somewhat more complex is the situation in which a tendon is lengthened to the extent that the muscle actually becomes shorter than it was preoperatively. This is probably the situation with most adductor releases, and perhaps, inadvertently, with some formal tendon lengthenings as well.

The immediate effect on the muscle is that it becomes shorter by virtue of its sarcomeres decreasing their lengths. Because there is a natural tendency for sarcomeres to regain their normal length, sarcomeres will disappear from the muscle, probably at its ends, so that the reduced muscle length will be exactly compensated for by the reduction in the number of sarcomeres.

The immediate effect of the surgery is exactly analogous to the experimental conditions that gave rise to the Blix curve. The muscle is acutely shortened and postoperatively will be asked to perform at a length somewhat shorter than preoperatively. The Blix curve for that muscle will not be changed, but the muscle will function on the downslope of the curve instead of at its peak so that its strength will be reduced.

In the long term, once the muscle has adjusted its sarcomere length, the entire Blix curve will have shifted to the left so that the muscle, in its new range of excursion, will once again be functioning at the peak of the curve. Because the muscle is shorter, however, the bell shape will be somewhat narrower, and, for a given deviation from its resting length, the strength of the muscle will drop off faster than it did preoperatively.

Orthopaedists should remind themselves of what this means. To say that a muscle is weakened by 50% does not mean that it will perform all of its functions half as well. Those functions that used to require more than 50% muscle strength will be impossible to perform with this reduction, and those functions that required less than 50% will be able to be performed more or less normally, although perhaps with increased fatigue. Suppose, for example, that it requires 70% of gastrocnemius strength to stand on the toes of one leg, that it takes 30% of gastrocnemius strength to provide useful push-off in gait, and that a given patient has had an operation that has reduced the strength of that muscle by 50%. This patient will no longer be able to stand on his toes, but will be able to develop useful push-off in gait.[18]

It is again interesting to consider the effect of muscle architecture on the result of tendon lengthening. Consider, for example, two muscles that are identical in cross-sectional area, bulk, and shape: one unipennate with a relatively small number of long fibers and one bipennate with a relatively large number of short fibers. If the tendons of these muscles are lengthened by equal amounts, the effect on the bipennate muscle will be more profound, because that lengthening will represent a greater portion of the excursion of its fibers.

Among the treatment options available for significant contractures are surgical lengthening of the tendon or repeated application of corrective casts (Fig. 3). Among the pros and cons that the orthopaedist must consider in determining treatment strategy are the long-term outcomes of the two procedures. The patient whose contracture has been completely corrected by repeated courses of serial casting will have a musculotendinous unit of normal length in which both the muscle and tendon will be of normal length and, presumably, the muscle will have normal strength and normal excursion. The patient whose contracture has been completely corrected by tendon lengthening, however, will be left with a musculotendinous unit that is normal in length, but whose muscle is shorter than normal and whose tendon is longer than normal. The muscle will have normal strength, but, because it is shorter, will have decreased excursion. This will be reflected by a narrowing of the Blix curve and a more rapid than normal fall-off in strength in positions away from the neutral position (Fig. 4). This is an example in principle only and should not be construed as a recommendation for casting over tendon lengthening.

The Motor Unit

This discussion has dealt with muscles as autonomous motor units and has neglected what is perhaps the most important aspect of muscle

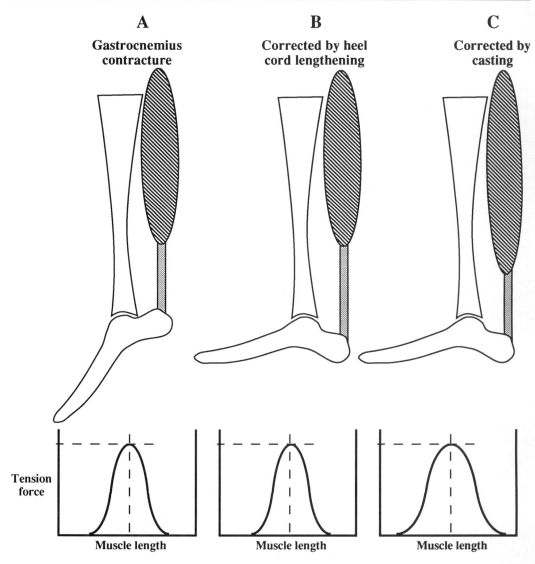

A
Gastrocnemius contracture

B
Corrected by heel cord lengthening

C
Corrected by casting

Tension force

Muscle length   Muscle length   Muscle length

Fig. 3 *The long-term mechanical results of correcting a gastrocnemius contracture (**left**). The correction by heel-cord lengthening (**center**) changes neither the configuration nor the mechanical characteristics of the muscle, leaving it in its preoperative, abnormally short state. The correction by gradual elongation by serial casting (**right**) increases the length of the muscle and brings its mechanical characteristics back to normal.*

function in cerebral palsy. The muscle exists as the last item in a chain of command that begins with the brain. Muscle activity begins in the brain as a high-level command, ''stand on tip toes to reach the top shelf;'' is broken down into mid-level commands, ''plantarflex the ankle;'' and finally to low-level commands, ''stimulate the gastrocne-

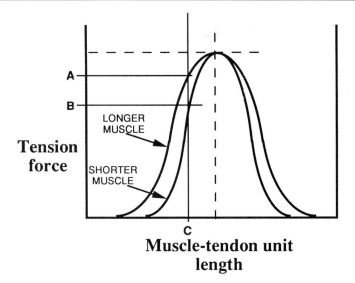

Fig. 4 *The long-term mechanical effect of shortening of the muscle component of a musculotendinous unit. The peak strength of the muscle at its resting length is not affected, but, because of the shortened excursion and narrowed Blix curve, the maximum strength of the shorter muscle (B) is less than that of the longer muscle (A) at all other lengths (C).*

mius and, to counteract its inversion effect, also stimulate the peroneals.'' These low-level commands are then translated into neural activity that ends in muscle stimulation. If any one of these steps is not handled appropriately, the stimulus to the muscle will be inappropriate.

It is important, particularly in the context of cerebral palsy, to understand how the brain decides how much stimulation to apply to the muscle. There is a tendency to think that the brain somehow analyzes the situation, determines how much stimulation the muscle needs, sends out that amount, and that's it. The system does not work that way. The brain is a part of a servomechanism in which its activities are dependent on its perceived results of those activities in a feedback loop. In such a mechanism, the brain does not send out a calculated amount of stimulation, but monitors the degree of ankle plantarflexion and sends out whatever amount of stimulation is required to produce the desired effect, the degree of ankle plantarflexion and standing on toes that allows reaching the top shelf. The relationship between brain and muscle is not like that between a rifle and its bullet, but like that between a thermostat and its furnace.

Such servo systems imply the presence of a feedback loop, and it is extremely important in cerebral palsy to recognize that the function of a given muscle begins with perception, not only proprioception but perception of the horizon, the floor, and the vertical. The brain is, therefore, involved in converting the sensations from the extremities into the perceptions that can be useful in the servomechanism, and then in suitably integrating all of that information into muscle stimulation. In cerebral palsy, the muscle may be the only part of this complicated system that is functioning normally. The acceptance of sensory information, its processing into perceptions, the utilization of perceptions to construct an appropriate motor strategy, and the breakdown of that motor strategy into low-level commands and suitable muscle stimulation may all be impaired in ways that are not understood. To complicate matters further, it is likely that surgery to change the length of muscles and tendons also has profound effects on this feedback system, effects that are unpredictable and can produce unexpected effects following surgery.

One problem with analysis of patients who have cerebral palsy is determination of the level of the demand that is causing abnormal function. If the patient with a crouched gait is crouching because of a contracture of the hip flexors and does not have significant abnormalities in the servo system, then it is reasonable to expect that a simple release or lengthening of the flexors would improve his/her gait. If, on the other hand, the patient is crouching because his/her servo system works best with all joints flexed, then releasing the patient's flexors may not have the desired effect, and the crouching may continue postoperatively for the same high-level reasons that were causing it preoperatively.

Conclusions

Cerebral palsy is a complex and challenging disease, and muscle function is perhaps the best understood and least important component of the system. The surgeon treating cerebral palsy must constantly be aware that although muscles move joints, it is the brain that moves muscles.

References

1. Huxley HE: Molecular basis of contraction in cross-straited muscles, in Bourne GH (ed): *The Structure and Function of Muscle.* Atlanta, Academic Press, 1972, pp 301–387.
2. Jones DA, Round JM: Growth, development and ageing of muscle, in *Skeletal Muscle in Health and Disease.* New York, Manchester University Press, 1990, pp 78–97.
3. Silver R, de la Garza J, Rang M: The myth of muscle balance. *J Bone Joint Surg* 1985;67B:432–437.
4. Brand PW, Beach RB, Thompson DE: Relative tension and potential excursion of muscles in the forearm and hand. *J Hand Surg* 1981;6:209–219.
5. Jones DA, Round DA: The mechanism of force generation, in *Skeletal Muscle in Health and Disease.* New York, Manchester University Press, 1990, pp 18–40.
6. Monod H: How muscles are used in the body, in Bourne GH (ed): *The Structure and Function of Muscle.* Atlanta, Academic Press, 1972, pp 23–74.
7. Penney RK, Prentis PF, Marsall PA, et al: Differentiation of muscle and the determination of ultimate tissue size. *Cell Tissue Res* 1983;228:375–388.
8. Goldspink G: Malleability of the motor system: A comparative approach. *J Exp Biol* 1985;115:375–391.

9. Goldspink G: Postembryonic growth and differentiation of striated muscle, in Bourne GH (ed): *The Structure and Function of Muscle*. Atlanta, Academic Press, 1972, pp 179–236.

10. Goldspink G: The adaptation of muscle to a new functional length, in *Mastication: Proceedings of a Symposium on the Clinical and Physiological Aspects of Mastication*. University of Bristol, John Wright & Sons, 1976, pp 90–99.

11. Goldspink DF: A comparative study of the effects of denervation, immobilization, and denervation with immobilization on the protein turnover of the rat soleus muscle. *J Physiology* 1978;280:64p–65p.

12. Loughna PT, Izumo S, Goldspink G, et al: Disuse and passive stretch cause rapid alterations in expression of developmental and adult contractile protein genes in skeletal muscle. *Development* 1990;109:217–223.

13. Crawford GNC: An experimental study of muscle growth in the rabbit. *J Bone Joint Surg* 1954;36B:294–303.

14. Carlson DS, Ellis E III, Dechow PC: Adaptation of the suprahyoid muscle complex to mandibular advancement surgery. *Am J Orthod Dentofac Orthop* 1987;92:134–143.

15. Crawford GNC: An experimental study of tendon growth in the rabbit. *J Bone Joint Surg* 1950;32B:234–243.

16. Wessels WE, Dahners LE: Growth of the rabbit deltoid ligament. *Clin Orthop* 1988;234:303–305.

17. Ziv I, Blackburn N, Rang M, et al: Muscle growth in normal and spastic mice. *Dev Med Child Neurol* 1984;26:94–99.

18. Lockhart RD: Anatomy of muscles and their relation to movement and posture, in Bourne GH (ed): *The Structure and Function of Muscle*. Atlanta, Academic Press, 1972, pp 1–21.

Chapter 21

The Rationale for Rhizotomy

William L. Oppenheim, MD
Loretta A. Staudt, MS, PT
Warwick J. Peacock, MD

Selective posterior rhizotomy (SPR) is a neurosurgical procedure designed to reduce spasticity by dividing posterior spinal nerve rootlets. Rootlets are selectively cut on the basis of intraoperative electromyographic responses to their electrical stimulation. Until recently, neurosurgical treatment for cerebral palsy was limited to attempts to facilitate inhibition with cerebellar stimulators[1-2] or to the use of stereotactic procedures to reduce abnormal tone and involuntary movements.[3-5] As early as 1889, Abbe[6] reported the use of rhizotomy for neuralgic pain relief, in which entire posterior roots were divided. He credited the first use of the procedure as well as the term rhizotomy to Dr. C. L. Dana, who used a one-cell dry pocket battery to stimulate a root in order to establish the neurologic level at which he was working. The use of posterior rhizotomy for the treatment of spasticity was proposed in 1908 by Förster,[7] who divided the L2-L4 posterior nerve roots. In 1913, Förster[8] reported a series of 159 patients in whom he avoided dividing three contiguous levels by skipping level L4, and adding S1. He emphasized the identification of "real" spasticity, he excluded cases associated with athetosis or paralysis, and he obtained improved results in patients whose involvement was primarily in the lower extremities. These remain important considerations today.

Rhizotomy was not further explored until the mid 1960s, when Gros and associates[9] revised the procedure, preventing the loss of sensation by sectioning only a fraction of the rootlets constituting the posterior root. Gros[10] further refined the technique, using electrical stimulation to map out rootlets related to useful muscles such as the gluteus maximus, quadriceps, gastrocnemius, and abdominal muscles, which were spared, and those rootlets deemed to be related to handicapping muscles such as the hip flexors and adductors, which were sacrificed. Other neurosurgical procedures for reduction of spasticity, such as anterior rhizotomy and myelotomy, have been described;[11-13] however, anterior procedures led to flaccid paralysis and attempting to divide sensory fibers within the substance of the cord risks pyramidal tract and bladder denervation. Cervical rhizotomy was performed in the early 1970s[14-17] with some reported success but with cortical, respiratory, and urinary complications. Cervical spine instability may result from multilevel laminectomies performed in this region.[18]

In 1976, Fasano and associates,[19,20] introduced a method of posterior rhizotomy in which electrical evaluation of the sensitivity of the posterior rootlets was used as the basis for selective ablation. This approach was suggested by an animal model that demonstrated that recurrent electrical stimulation of the afferent fibers of a monosynaptic pathway decreased the amplitude of the reflex response.[21] In Fasano's initial series of 62 patients, 25% to 50% of the rootlets were divided in the majority of patients.[20] The procedure was reviewed by Ouaknine,[22] and Laitinen and associates,[23] and it was recently popularized in North America by Peacock and associates.[24–28] Peacock modified the procedure by moving the site of the laminectomy from the level of the conus to the cauda equina (L2 to S1) to facilitate identification of levels to prevent potential bowel and bladder complications.

Physiologic Rationale

Voluntary motion in the presence of normal muscle tone is achieved by balancing suprasegmental facilitatory and inhibitory impulses at the segmental spinal cord level. Local spinal cord circuits are also important. The physiology of the central and peripheral nervous systems and the connections between them are still being elucidated. Thus, any attempt to fully explain the efficacy of selective posterior rhizotomy on the basis of what is known can be challenged at a more basic level. In spite of this, it is useful to review the basic neuroanatomy and neurophysiology in order to lay out a rational framework for discussion and potential future research.

Spasticity has been defined as a motor disorder characterized by a velocity-dependent increase in resistance to passive stretch associated with hyperactive tendon reflexes.[29] It is one feature of the upper motoneuron lesion that may occur at the level of the brain or spinal cord. Spasticity is characterized by: (1) hypertonia of the clasp-knife type in which resistance to passive stretch gives way with continued force, as opposed to rigidity where resistance is felt throughout the range of motion; and (2) exaggerated tendon reflexes with or without clonus. Associated features of the upper motoneuron lesion may include: (1) a loss of isolated muscle control and fine voluntary movements; (2) weakness; (3) lack of normal postural reactions; (4) presence of abnormal associated movements; (5) depression of superficial reflexes; and (6) presence of specific abnormal reflexes (for example, Babinski, Oppenheim).[30]

Skeletal muscle is composed of large extrafusal force-generating fibers that make up the main contractile mass. The muscle spindles are specialized sensory organs that lie scattered throughout the muscle belly and contain small intrafusal muscle fibers.[31] Extrafusal fibers are innervated by type I-alpha (Ia) efferent neurons of the ventral horn. When the fibers are active, the entire muscle shortens and the muscle spindle is relatively relaxed. Conversely, when the extrafusal muscle fibers are passively stretched, the muscle spindle is also stretched resulting in an increase in the firing frequency of the associated afferent neurons (especially type Ia from the annulospiral structures). These afferent impulses are transmitted via the posterior spinal nerve root to the spinal cord. They cause the alpha motoneuron of the stretched muscle to effect contraction, restoring the spindle to its prestretched state. This is the classic monosynaptic stretch reflex. The intrafusal fibers of the spindle are also under the control of gamma efferent motoneurons, which adjust spindle sensitivity.

As a result of collateral connections within the spinal cord, afferent fibers associated with the reflex arc can affect adjacent or even remote segments of the cord. Sherrington[32] showed that while some muscles are contracting, others are reciprocally and automatically relaxing (reciprocal innervation). Thus, the same afferent neurons that trigger extensor muscle contraction at one level may inhibit flexor muscles at another. An example is the triceps reflex in which the extensor muscles are activated and the biceps are momentarily inhibited. Similarly, under normal circumstances, reciprocal excitation occurs. In pathologic conditions, including cerebral palsy, reciprocal excitation may occur to an abnormal degree, causing inappropriate cocontraction of muscle groups.[33,34] Dietz[35] found that children with cerebral palsy, as well as very young normal children, exhibited abnormally increased cocontraction during the stance phase of gait. There was reduced amplitude of electromyograph (EMG) recordings in spastic muscles. These children also exhibited the absence of normal polysynaptic reflexes and the presence of type Ia neuron-mediated monosynaptic stretch reflexes during movement.

While the final common pathway of both activating and inhibiting activity is the anterior horn cell and its axon, other factors are also important in regulating tone. The spindle itself is modulated and adjusted by the gamma efferent motoneuron, but there is little experimental support suggesting that the gamma system is primarily involved in development of spasticity.[36] Afferent impulses from the Golgi tendon organ are carried in type Ib fibers through the posterior root to the dorsal horn, and then through internuncial fibers to inhibit the alpha motoneurons of the originating muscle. The Golgi tendon organ was initially thought to be important as a protective mechanism responding to muscle stretch, but is now viewed as a possible feedback loop when a muscle is contracting against a significant load.[36,37] Renshaw cells in the ventral horn are innervated by recurrent collaterals of the alpha motoneuron and act to provide inhibitory feedback to the same alpha motoneuron. They are also under the influence of supraspinal centers. Disruption of recurrent inhibition could conceivably result in a net gain in the spinal reflex arc, but there is no direct proof of this, and there are arguments to the contrary.[38] Finally, presynaptic inhibition reduces the transmission of impulses in the type Ia fiber through an interneuron that depolarizes the terminal before its synapse with the alpha motoneuron. These interneurons are controlled by both supraspinal and peripheral inputs, and loss of presynaptic inhibition has been hypothesized as a possible mechanism for spastic hyperreflexia.[36]

In summary, muscle activity is activated primarily by muscle spindle afferent neurons and inhibited through the combined influences of descending tracts and peripheral mechanisms. Integration of these competing influences takes place at the level of the spinal cord through complex circuitry, much of which is known but continues to require further elucidation. The proper balance between these influences results in optimal tone and posture.[24]

In cerebral palsy, inhibition from descending tracts is decreased, tilting the balance in favor of facilitation by the spindle afferent neurons through the posterior root. In addition to this disinhibition, it has been suggested that sprouting of type Ia afferent neurons can occur in response to loss of descending motor tracts increasing the hyperexcitability of the motoneuron pools.[39] Selective posterior rhizotomy (SPR) attempts to lessen the facilitatory influence of these afferent fibers in order to balance the loss of inhibition, or augmentation, of the reflex arc by whatever mechanism is responsible. This is based on the belief that the reflex arc itself is normal and that the influences on it are distorted and can be rebalanced by resection of rootlets containing muscle spindle afferent neurons.

While this scheme is convenient in explaining the efficacy of SPR, it must be borne in mind that there is a difference between voluntary control of muscles and the control of resting muscle tone in a patient with an upper motoneuron lesion. Simply reducing tone is unlikely to restore voluntary motor control. For example, Lee and associates[40] found that stretch reflex enhancement was not responsible for stiffness of voluntarily activated elbow muscles of adult spastic hemiplegic patients. Sahrmann and Norton[41] concluded that impairment of movement in adult hemiplegics was primarily related to poor agonist control, rather than to limitation of movement due to antagonistic stretch reflexes. Burke[36] believed that mechanical changes in the muscle contribute to the clinical picture of hypertonia, rather than neuronal changes alone. In normal patients, tone must be related to compliance of soft tissues because background motor unit activity disappears with complete relaxation. He argued that if normal tone is a function of the mechanical nature of muscle, factors other than hyperreflexia should be considered as contributors to stiffness in the spastic patient.[36] Although children with lower extremity spasticity are not equivalent to adults with hemiplegia, spasticity alone is not the only cause of motor dysfunction in patients with upper motoneuron lesions. Exaggerated cocontraction, inappropriate timing of muscle activity, and weakness can play a major role.

The success of surgical reduction of spasticity is dependent on the degree to which spasticity interferes with function as well as underlying factors such as strength, selective muscle control, and balance. If contractures, subluxation of the hips, scoliosis, and other orthopaedic problems are present, they will continue to influence function even when spasticity is eliminated. Patients with underlying weakness, who rely on spasticity for antigravity support, may lose function if that spasticity is eliminated. The reduction of spasticity as an aim in itself is discouraged in favor of a comprehensive program of goal-oriented management based on a complete understanding of each patient.

Relation to Traditional Orthopaedic Surgery

Although the indications for orthopaedic surgery and SPR may initially appear similar, the procedures are not equivalent. The goal of releasing muscles and tendons is to eliminate contractures. The goal of severing dorsal rootlets is to eliminate spasticity. Individuals with extensive fixed contractures requiring multiple tendon lengthening should be referred for orthopaedic surgery rather than rhizotomy. Because the procedures are complimentary, rather than competing, traditional treatment plans may need to be revised. For example, if spasticity is controlled, casting, as opposed to surgical release, may suffice for correcting residual deformity. Or, perhaps, with the patient under anesthesia and undergoing rhizotomy, the orthopaedist can address any severe residual contractures by performing the tendon lengthening under the same anesthesia.

It is difficult to imagine how hip dysplasia or scoliosis, once established, can benefit from rhizotomy, and the effect of rhizotomy in preventing such problems will have to be elucidated. Children who have undergone orthopaedic procedures and who have a full active and passive range of motion are unlikely to require further surgery. If spastic postures have recurred after previous orthopaedic surgery, rhizotomy may be considered provided that strength is good. Most children have some combination of spasticity and soft-tissue tightness. If rhizotomy is advised, parents are reminded that rhizotomy addresses only the spasticity, and additional orthopaedic surgery may be required at some point. If scoliosis fusion is contemplated, consideration is first given to rhizotomy, though SPR is rarely performed in the presence of severe spinal deformity. This is an important consideration in children with spastic quadriplegia or total body involvement. When it is not clear whether the more appropriate approach is neurosurgical or orthopaedic, it is wise to commence with an orthopaedic program if the focus is relatively limited (for example, simple hamstring release versus a combined release of hip, knee, and ankle musculature). Hip subluxation or bony deformity should not be expected to respond to rhizotomy, and, in fact, there is some suggestion that if an underlying weakness is unmasked, hip subluxation may be accelerated following SPR in individuals with spastic quadriplegia, which is a relatively rare indication.[42] Overall, two thirds to three quarters of patients who have undergone SPR will still require some type of orthopaedic surgery.

Patient Selection

No surgical procedure can succeed unless it is directed toward specific goals and limited to those patients who have the actual potential to reach those goals. The goal of SPR is to reduce spasticity. Clearly then, the best candidates for SPR are purely spastic children who had a low birth weight and were born prematurely. Such children are usually identified by the age of one year. They normally display an initial hypotonic stage that progresses to frank spasticity, with persistence of primitive reflexes and other features of the upper motoneuron lesion as enumerated above. Full-term children are more likely to have dystonia or athetosis along with the spasticity and are less responsive to SPR. The ideal patient is an intelligent, motivated child with spastic diplegia and no severe fixed contractures, who is already walking independently and is attempting to improve his/her gait pattern and endurance. SPR does not create the potential for ambulation, which is the primary goal of many families. However, SPR can improve the gait of a child who is walking or developing that skill. Bleck's[43] criteria for ambulation prognosis are useful as guidelines. Other candidates for SPR are severely involved quadriplegic patients whose spasticity interferes with comfort, sitting, dressing, perineal care, or various classroom activities, and other activities. Improvement in upper extremity function and speech are not primary goals of the procedure but may accompany an overall reduction in tone. Moderately-affected children with spastic cerebral palsy should be very carefully evaluated because many factors other than spasticity interfere with function in these patients.

Because cerebral palsy is a multifaceted disorder, assessment for patient selection should emphasize the identification of features of cerebral palsy that will persist following surgical reduction of spasticity. First, the evaluation team determines that spasticity is present and interfering with function. Other forms of abnormal tone and movement should be identified so that patients with rigidity, dystonia, athetosis, ataxia, and truncal hypotonia can be eliminated as candidates. Rigidity is characterized by a "lead-pipe" type of resistance to passive motion. Dystonia involves fluctuating tone, and often is associated with persistent primitive reflexes. Athetosis is punctuated by involuntary movement around a joint axis, orofacial movement, and finger fanning. Ataxia is recognized by the findings of dysequilibrium, intention tremors, and past pointing. In those with mixed lesions, the results will be mixed. Patients with pure spasticity are the best candidates.

Next, the range of motion is evaluated and the presence of any apparent contractures and bony deformities recorded. Individuals with extensive fixed contractures are referred for orthopaedic surgery. Most children have some combination of spasticity and soft-tissue tightness. If fixed contractures are obviously present but rhizotomy is otherwise desirable, a tentative plan may be developed to reduce contractures through serial casting or surgery between 6 months and 1 year following the rhizotomy to allow time for surgical recovery and maximal rehabilitation.

The preoperative determination of underlying strength and motor control is a difficult but critical area in the evaluation of patients for the rhizotomy procedure, because weakness is often a major problem after surgery. Some children depend on spasticity for antigravity sup-

Outline 1 Selection criteria for rhizotomy candidates

Positive selection criteria
    Prematurity
    Pure spasticity
    Good trunk control
    Good strength and motor control
    Minimal fixed contractures
    Keen motivation and intelligence
    Availability of therapy
Negative selection criteria
    Weakness of antigravity musculature
        Neurectomy and overlengthening
        Truncal weakness and hypotonia
        Lower extremity weakness
        Unilateral weakness: hemiplegia
    Rigidity, dystonia, athetosis, ataxia
    Marked fixed contractures
    Fixed spinal deformity/prior spinal fusion

port. Reducing spasticity in these situations can be detrimental and may interfere with goals of standing, or walking. Evaluation of trunk musculature, hip abductors and extensors, quadriceps, and calf muscles is particularly important. In sitting, the control of head and trunk is noted, followed by application of slow and fast challenges in all directions to determine the presence of righting, protective, and equilibrium responses. The Rancho Los Amigos Hospital test of upright motor control is useful in estimating antigravity control in the presence of synergistic movement patterns.[44] Antigravity control of the lower extremities is assessed in the upright position to determine if the child can activate hip, knee, and ankle flexors for clearance in swing and to observe hip, knee, and ankle control for stability in unilateral stance. Asking the child to perform activities such as squatting-to-standing and heel raises in a slow controlled manner can help to distinguish the use of reflexes, such as the positive supporting reaction, from voluntary motor control. Children should be observed in a variety of developmental postures and during transitional movements and gait to estimate their strength and functional skill levels. Finally, selective motor control, for example, the ability to isolate movement such as ankle dorsiflexion with the knee extended, is evaluated to determine if there is some freedom from the synergistic patterns of movement that tend to persist following surgery.[45]

Outline 1 provides a summary of both positive and negative selection criteria in the assessment of patients as candidates for rhizotomy.

The Surgical Procedure

The procedure is performed under endotracheal anesthesia without the use of long acting muscle relaxants. The patient is positioned prone, and the EMG team (neurologist and physical therapist) is allowed access to the lower extremities as necessary while sterility is maintained on the operative field. In order to safely identify specific nerve roots, a narrow midline laminectomy or laminotomy is performed from L2 to L5, taking care to leave the facet joints intact. In addition, some of the dorsum of S1 is reflected to allow identification of nerve roots from L2 to S2.

After the dura is opened, the posterior root is separated from the anterior root and then subdivided with a blunt microprobe into 4 to 10 rootlets, depending on the spinal level and size of the root. Each rootlet is electrically stimulated, and the response is analyzed using electromyography as described below. Levels are identified using bony landmarks and regional anatomy, with confirmation through electrical stimulation of the anterior nerve roots. In marking out the incision, the iliac crest is used as a reference to the level of the L4 spine or the L4-L5 interspace. This may be confirmed using a cross-table radiograph. During surgery, the L5 spine usually is identified as the last mobile spinous process. After the dura is opened, the largest nerve root should be identified as that of S1.

Stimulation of the anterior nerve root of S1 should result in knee flexion and ankle plantarflexion, while stimulation of the anterior nerve root of S2 should elicit ankle plantarflexion with toe flexion. The anterior nerve root is differentiated from the posterior nerve root by noting its position, color, vascularity, shape, and threshold of electrical stimulation. The posterior nerve root is broader, flatter, and lighter in color than the anterior nerve root and enters the back of the spinal cord. The threshold for motor response from electrical stimulation is much lower for the anterior root than for the posterior root.

For the usual bilateral case, 50 to 70 posterior rootlets are tested and approximately one fourth to one half are subsequently divided. Some dysesthesias may be felt transiently (2 days to 3 weeks) following surgery, but significant sensory loss has not been observed even when a whole posterior nerve root was divided. Several contiguous complete posterior root sections are necessary to result in anesthesia over a central dermatome.

Electrical Analysis

The selectivity of the procedure derives its name from the implied ability of the surgeon to differentiate between nerve rootlets believed to be associated with an abnormal spinal cord reflex arc and those judged to be normal. Only rootlets associated with abnormal intraoperative electromyograms (EMGs) are sacrificed. Two insulated microprobe electrodes are used to electrically stimulate each nerve rootlet, and needle electrodes placed in lower extremity muscles are used to make EMG recordings. Simultaneous bilateral EMGs from multiple muscle groups are most effective. An initial stimulus of a 0.1 millisecond burst is applied to the whole posterior nerve root at increasing voltages until the threshold for stimulation is found. This may range from approximately 10 to 50 V. The surgeon then isolates the first rootlet, and this stimulation procedure is repeated. After the threshold

Decremental Response   **Incremental Response with Proximal Spread**

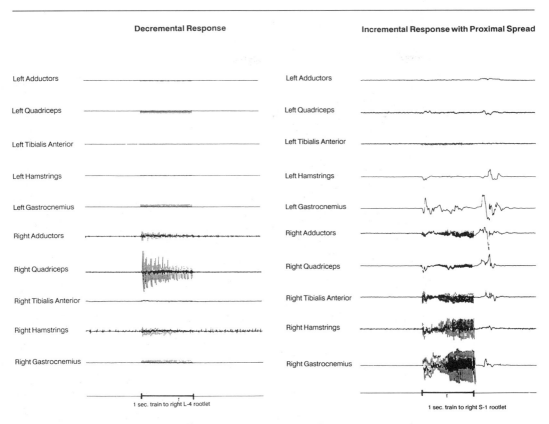

1 sec. train to right L-4 rootlet   1 sec. train to right S-1 rootlet

Fig. 1 *Left*, *Demonstrated is a normal ideal decremental response seen when the L4 rootlet is stimulated.* **Right**, *Here an S'1 rootlet is stimulated and an abnormal incremental response is seen along with spread to muscles not associated with the S'1 rootlet. This would be considered an abnormal response. (Reproduced with permission from Oppenheim W: Selective posterior rhizotomy for cerebral palsy.* Clin Orthop *1990;253:20–29.)*

to a single stimulus is identified, the process is repeated using trains of electrical stimuli that are applied at a frequency of 50 Hz for 1 second. The EMG response to these trains of stimuli is analyzed. In the normal response, there is a decreasing magnitude seen in the serial muscle action potentials. In the abnormal case, the amplitude of the potentials may actually increase and at times persist after the 1-second stimulus application has ceased. Other abnormal patterns include clonic responses and spread of activity to muscle groups not normally innervated by the rootlet being tested (Figs. 1 and 2).

In summary, an electrical response is generated at threshold voltage for each rootlet, and the quality of the response is evaluated. Rootlets associated with abnormal responses generally are divided, and those with more normal responses are spared. In all cases, the EMG information is used along with clinical information based on careful pre-

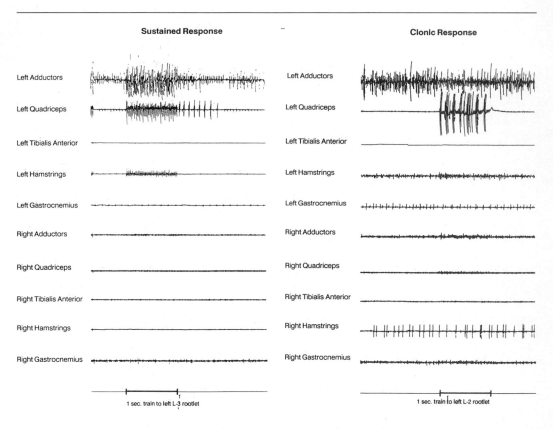

Fig. 2 *Left, This is a typical sustained response in which the response continues after the stimulus has ceased. It is abnormal. **Right**, In this patient, in addition to a sustained response a crossover quadriceps clonic response is seen as well. In practice it is sometimes difficult to tell an abnormal from a normal response so that clinical correlation is always warranted and therefore the electrophysiologist and the surgeon must both be familiar with the patient preoperatively. (Reproduced with permission from Oppenheim W: Selective posterior rhizotomy for cerebral palsy.* Clin Orthop *1990;253:20–29.)*

operative assessment. Clinical judgment is an integral part of the intraoperative decision as to how many and which rootlets should be sacrificed. In addition to the surgeon, at least one member of the EMG team should be very familiar with the child's clinical picture. The degree and location of spastic muscles, areas of weakness, functional abilities, and goals of the procedure are important factors to consider along with EMG evaluation. In the more severely involved child, in whom a huge percentage of the rootlets are associated with an abnormal response, care should be taken to avoid excessive deafferentation.

Postoperative Considerations

Weakness is a feature of the early (6 months) postoperative period. Ankle-foot orthoses, a walker, proper preparation, and a knowledgeable therapist are helpful in restoring function during this time. Physical and occupational therapy considerations have been described by several authors.[46–48] Typical problems encountered by the therapist are described below.

Hypersensitivity of the Feet and Legs This occurs in the early postoperative period and usually resolves spontaneously within 7 to 10 days. Firm pressure, footwear modifications, and early weightbearing may be helpful.

Flexor Spasms These may be seen in the early days to weeks following surgery and tend to resolve with time. They occur more frequently in children with moderate to severe involvement. Pressure on the flexor surfaces should be avoided.

Crouched Posture This frequently results from calf weakness and poor tibial control. Orthotic support and strengthening exercises are recommended. A hinged orthosis may be used if initially locked and gradually unlocked with time. An elastic strap can assist the calf muscle in intermediate stages. If crouch is severe or persistent, an ''anticrouch'' design of orthosis should be considered.

Excessive Pronation of Foot and Ankle This is frequently seen preoperatively and may appear exaggerated postoperatively. Children use this motion as a substitute for dorsiflexion when range is limited or cannot be obtained rapidly. Alignment may be improved through orthotic design once adequate dorsiflexion range is available.

Weakness of Hip Girdle and/or Quadriceps Muscle Weakness of the hip girdle and/or quadriceps muscle may occur. Active exercise and provision of external support during walking help to bolster hip musculature. Climbing activities, side stepping, bridging exercises, sit-to-stand activities, and cycling can help promote strength and endurance. Isokinetic exercises can be used if selective control is good.

Trunk Weakness or Imbalance Trunk weakness or imbalance may occur. Proper trunk alignment over the pelvis should be encouraged in positioning and during activities, and the ability to weight shift in all directions should be addressed. Forward weight shifting is important for transition from sitting to standing and for transfers. Some activities that provide exercise for the trunk are self-pumping on a swing, push/pull activities, prone extension, supine flexion, and the use of therapy balls.

Therapy Burnout This may be exhibited by the child, family, and/or therapist. Realistic goals and consideration of the family's lifestyle and the child's interests are important to assess preoperatively. Introduction of recreational activities such as swimming, cycling, horseback riding, and dance exercises are often helpful in promoting balance, strength, and endurance, as well as motivation.

Results

When patients are properly selected, reduction of spasticity allows increased function and facilitates the activities of daily living. To date, most evaluation of progress after rhizotomy has been based on subjective clinical assessment. Muscle tone has been rated on such clinical scales as those proposed by Ashworth and modified by Bohannon.[49] Additional objective assessments of muscle tone and patient function are being performed.[27,28,45]

Perhaps the longest series to date is that of Peacock and associates.[24,25] They noted the best results in patients who were purely spastic, who had more involvement in the lower extremities than the upper extremities, who had no prior orthopaedic surgery, and who could side sit independently. Tone was reduced to normal in 35 children who were rated as having a high or very high level preoperatively. Of 40 patients with spastic diplegia, 18 experienced postoperative hypotonia that returned to a more normal level with time and physical therapy. Weakness was commonly observed in these patients, and it is presumed that this weakness was present preoperatively and became unmasked following reduction of spasticity. In terms of gait, improvement was seen in most patients, either in degree of smoothness, velocity, or stride length. Some patients advanced from one level of support to a lesser level of support.

More involved patients (those with spastic quadriplegia) also benefitted, but in terms of ease of care, positioning, sitting ability, and range of motion, rather than in individual functional activities of daily living. Long-term follow-up for up to 7 years revealed that reduction of spasticity and functional improvement were maintained in these patients.[50] Berman and associates[51] studied 29 of these children before and after SPR and reported a decrease in muscle tone and joint stiffness, and an increase in functional movement patterns. Kinematic studies of gait were performed in 16 of these patients, confirming improvements in joint motion, stride length, and walking speed. Gait studies were repeated 3 years after surgery, revealing further improvement in the arc of motion used during walking.[28] A recent study of 25 individuals undergoing SPR revealed decreased tone, increased range of motion, and functional gains including improvement in gait parameters.[27] Baseline studies performed preoperatively to help control for the effects of maturation and therapy showed no significant changes in the same parameters.

Other authors have noted improvements in patients following SPR. Sutherland[52] described a gait study that revealed increased range of motion at the hip, knee, and ankle of a child with spastic diplegia who had undergone rhizotomy. Tippets and associates[53] stated that 80% of spastic patients undergoing rhizotomy attained a goal of improved quality of function, and that the best candidates were those with only mild or moderate restriction of motion. Gage (Symposium on Rhizotomy, American Academy of Cerebral Palsy and Developmental Medicine, San Francisco, 1989) used three-dimensional gait analysis to confirm the efficacy of rhizotomy in selected patients. He reported an increase in range of motion of the hips and knees, velocity, and stride length. Cahan and associates[45] and Perry and associates[54] reported similar gait analysis findings following rhizotomy. They also demonstrated reduced clonic activity in spastic muscles on EMG and improved foot-floor contact patterns during gait.

Summary

SPR appears to be effective in reducing spasticity in highly-selected children with cerebral palsy. The current explanation for this effectiveness focuses on the spinal reflex arc and its modulation at the level of the anterior horn cell by supraspinal and segmental influences. Selective division of posterior spinal nerve rootlets is believed to balance the decrease of normal inhibitory influences on the motoneurons. Diminished inhibition of motoneurons is not the only effect of the upper motoneuron lesion in cerebral palsy, and the multifaceted nature of the disorder must be realized to achieve the desired surgical outcome. Factors such as weakness, retention of primitive movement patterns, poor balance reactions, and impaired selective motor control will remain after surgical reduction of spasticity and will continue to affect motor function. Secondary problems such as joint contractures and bony deformities will require further orthopaedic management. A team approach to this complex disorder is necessary, and the success of the intervention will depend on the team's ability to predict the effects of diminished spasticity on the function of each patient.

References

1. Ivan LP, Ventureyra EC: Chronic cerebellar stimulation in cerebral palsy. *Childs Brain* 1982;9:121–125.
2. Miyasaka K, Hoffman HE, Froese AB: The influence of chronic cerebellar stimulation on respiratory muscle coordination in a patient with cerebral palsy. *Neurosurg* 1978;2:262–265.
3. Speelman JD, van Manen J: Cerebral palsy and stereotactic neurosurgery: Long term results. *J Neurol Neurosurg Psychiatry* 1989;52:23–30.
4. Laitinen L, Singounas E: Longitudinal myelotomy in the treatment of spasticity of the legs. *J Neurosurg* 1971;35:536–540.
5. Nashold BS Jr, Slaughter DG: Effects of stimulating or destroying the deed cerebellar regions in man. *J Neurosurg* 1969;31:172–186.
6. Abbe R: Resection of the posterior roots of spinal nerves to relieve pain, pain reflex, athetosis and spastic paralysis-Dana's operation. *Med Record (NY)* 1911;79:377–381.
7. Förster O: Uber eine neue operative Methode der Behandlung spastischer Lähmungen mittels Resektion hinterer Rückenmarkswurzeln. *Z Orthop Chir* 1908;22:203–223.
8. Förster O: On the indications and the results of the excision of posterior spinal nerve roots in men. *Surg Gynecol Obstet* 1913;16:463–474.
9. Gros C, Ouaknine G, Vlahovitch B , et al: La radicotomie sélective postérieure dans le traitement neuro-chirurgical de l'hypertonie pymidale. *Neurochirurgie* 1967;13:505–518.

10. Gros C: Spasticity: Clinical classification and surgical treatment. *Adv Techn Stand Neurosurg* 1979;6:55–97.

11. Bischof W: Die longitudinale myelotomie. *Zentralblat Neurochir* 1951;11:79–88.

12. MacCarty CS, Kiefer EJ: Thoracic, lumbar and sacral spinal cordectomy: Preliminary report. *Mayo Clin Proc* 1949;24:108–115.

13. Munro D: The rehabilitation of patients totally paralyzed below the waist: With special reference to making them ambulatory and capable of earning their living. I. Anterior rhizotomy for spastic paraplegia. *N Engl J Med* 1945;233: 453–461.

14. Benedetti A, Carbonin C, Columbo F: Extended posterior cervical rhizotomy for severe spastic syndromes with dyskinesias. *Appl Neurophysiol* 1977/1978; 40:41–47.

15. Frailoli B, Nucci F, Baldassarre L: Bilateral cervical posterior rhizotomy: Effects on dystonia and athetosis, on respiration and other autonomic functions. *Appl Neurophysiol* 1977/1978;40:26–40.

16. Heimburger RF, Slominski A, Griswold P: Cervical posterior rhizotomy for reducing spasticity in cerebral palsy. *J Neurosurg* 1973;39:30–34.

17. Kottke FJ: Modification of athetosis by denervation of the tonic neck reflexes, abstract. *Dev Med Child Neurol* 1970;12:236–237.

18. Yasuoka S, Peterson HA, MacCarty CS: Incidence of spinal column deformity after multilevel laminectomy in children and adults. *J Neurosurg* 1982;57:441.

19. Fasano VA, Barolat-Romana G, Ivaldi A, et al: La radicotomie postérieure fonctionnelle dans le traitement de la spasticité cérébrale. Premieres observations sur la stimulation electrique peroperatoire des racines postérieures, et leur utilisation dans le choix des racines ā sectionner. *Neurochirurgie* 1976;22:23–34.

20. Fasano VA, Broggi G, Barolat-Romana G, et al: Surgical treatment of spasticity in cerebral palsy. *Childs Brain* 1978;4:289–305.

21. Decandia M, Provini L, Taborikova H: Mechanisms of the reflex discharge depression in the spinal motor neuron during repetitive orthodromic stimulation. *Brain Res* 1967;4:284–291.

22. Ouaknine GE: Le traitement chirurgical de la spasticite. *Union Med Can* 1980; 109:1424–1444.

23. Laitinen LV, Nilsson S, Fugl-Meyer AR: Selective posterior rhizotomy for treatment of spasticity. *J Neurosurg* 1983;58:895–899.

24. Peacock WJ, Arens LJ: Selective posterior rhizotomy for the relief of spasticity in cerebral palsy. *S Afr Med J* 1982;62:119–124.

25. Peacock WJ, Arens LJ, Berman B: Cerebral palsy spasticity: Selective posterior rhizotomy. *Pediatr Neurosci* 1987;13:61–66.

26. Peacock WJ, Staudt LA: Spasticity in cerebral palsy and the selective posterior rhizotomy procedure. *J Child Neurol* 1990;5:179–185.

27. Peacock WJ, Staudt LA: Functional outcomes following selective posterior rhizotomy in children with cerebral palsy. *J Neurosurg* 1991;74:380–385.

28. Vaughan CL, Berman B, Peacock WJ: Cerebral palsy and rhizotomy. A three year follow-up evaluation with gait analysis. *J Neurosurg* 1991;74:178–184.

29. Lance JW: Symposium synopsis, in Feldman RG, Young RR, Koella WP (eds): *Spasticity-Disordered Motor Control*. Chicago, Year Book Medical Publishers, 1980, p 45.

30. Samilson RL (ed): *Orthopedic Aspects of Cerebral Palsy*. Philadelphia, JB Lippincott, 1975, p 8.

31. Boyd IA: The isolated mammalian muscle spindle. *Trends Neurol Sci* 1980;3: 258–265.

32. Sherrington CS: On reciprocal innervation of antagonistic muscles. *Proc R Soc* 1896;60:414–417.

33. Myklebust BM, Gottlieb GL, Penn RD, et al: Reciprocal excitation of antagonistic muscles as a differentiating feature in spasticity. *Ann Neurol* 1982; 12:367–374.
34. Myklebust BM, Gottlieb GL, Agarwal GC: Stretch reflexes of the normal infant. *Dev Med Child Neurol* 1986;28:440–449.
35. Dietz V: Role of peripheral afferents and spinal reflexes in normal and impaired human locomotion. *Rev Neurol (Paris)* 1987;143:241–254.
36. Burke D: Spasticity as an adaptation to pyramidal tract injury. *Adv Neurol* 1988;47:401–423.
37. Burke D, Lance JW: Studies of the reflex effects of primary and secondary spindle endings in spasticity, in Desmedt JE (ed): *New Developments in Electromyography and Clinical Neurophysiology.* Basel, Switzerland, Karger, 1973, pp 475–495.
38. Katz R, Pierrot-Deseilligny E: Recurrent inhibition of alpha-motoneurons in patients with upper motor neuron lesions. *Brain* 1982;105:103–124.
39. McCouch GP, Austin GM, Liu CN, et al: Sprouting as a cause of spasticity. *J Neurophysiol* 1958;21:205–216.
40. Lee WA, Boughton A, Rymer WZ: Absence of stretch reflex gain enhancement in voluntarily activated spastic muscle. *Exp Neurol* 1987;98:317–335.
41. Sahrmann SA, Norton BJ: The relationship of voluntary movement to spasticity in the upper motor neuron syndrome. *Ann Neurol* 1977;2:460–465.
42. Green W, Dietz F: Rapid progressive hip subluxation in cerebral palsy after selective posterior rhizotomy. *J Pediatr Orthop* 1991;11:494–497.
43. Bleck EE: Locomotor prognosis in cerebral palsy. *Dev Med Child Neurol* 1975;17:18–25.
44. Montgomery J, Gillis MK, Winstein C, et al: *Physical Therapy Management of Patients With Hemiplegia Secondary to Cerebrovascular Accident.* Downey, CA, Professional Staff Association of Rancho Los Amigos Hospital, 1983.
45. Cahan L, Adams J, Perry J, et al: Instrumented gait analysis following selective posterior rhizotomy, abstract. *Phys Ther* 1989;69:386.
46. Elk B: Preoperative assessment and postsurgical occupational therapy for children who have undergone a selective posterior rhizotomy. *SA J Occup Ther* 1984;14:45–50.
47. Irwin-Carruthers SH, Davids LM, Van Rensburg CK, et al: Early physiotherapy in selective posterior rhizotomy. *Fisioterapie* 1985;41:45–49.
48. Staudt LA, Peacock WJ: Selective posterior rhizotomy for treatment of spastic cerebral palsy. *Pediatr Phys Ther* 1989;1:3–9.
49. Bohannon RW, Smith MB: Interrater reliability of a modified Ashworth scale. *Phys Ther* 1987;67:206.
50. Arens LJ, Peacock WJ, Peter J: Selective posterior rhizotomy: A long-term follow-up study. *Childs Nerv Syst* 1989;5:148–152.
51. Berman B, Peacock W, Vaughan CL, et al: Assessment of patients with spastic cerebral palsy before and after rhizotomy. *Dev Med Child Neurol* 1987;29:24.
52. Sutherland DH: Utilization of gait analysis for clinical decision making in cerebral palsy II. Presented at the Workshop of the American Academy of Cerebral Palsy and Developmental Medicine, Boston, MA, October 1987, p 20.
53. Tippets RH, Walker ML, Liddell KL: Long-term follow-up of selective dorsal rhizotomy for relief of spasticity in cerebral-palsied children, abstract. *Dev Med Neurol* 1989;31(suppl 59):19.
54. Perry J, Adams J, Cahan LD: Foot-floor contact patterns following selective dorsal rhizotomy, abstract. *Dev Med Neurol* 1989;31(suppl 59):19.

Chapter 22
Selective Posterior Rhizotomy

Luciano S. Dias, MD
Gerard R. Marty, MD

Introduction

Cerebral palsy is the most common of all pediatric neuromuscular disorders in the United States with a prevalence of approximately two cases per 1,000 births. In 1987, Bleck[1] reviewed 423 patients with cerebral palsy and found that 66% fit into the class of spastic diplegia. Of those with spastic diplegia, 79% were independent ambulators, 19% walked with external assistance, and 2% were nonambulators.

Hypertonicity and joint contractures, which are typical in patients with spastic diplegia, limit the development of functional independent gait. Orthopaedic surgery has traditionally been used to alleviate this problem by releasing fixed joint contractures, reducing the effect of spasticity on a muscle group, and balancing agonist-antagonist muscle interaction.[2-16]

In 1984, selective posterior rhizotomy (SPR) was introduced in the United States by Peacock[17-20] as a means of improving the gait pattern of children with spastic diplegia by reducing the underlying spasticity in the lower extremity. This procedure was introduced at the Chicago Children's Memorial Hospital in 1987, and since that time more than 150 children with spastic cerebral palsy have been carefully selected to undergo this procedure. In this chapter, we will retrospectively review the results of the first 50 patients to undergo rhizotomy, and compare them with the results of 42 patients who underwent soft-tissue procedures.

Literature Review

Between 1908 and 1913, Förster[21-23] reported on a series of 159 patients who had undergone rhizotomy to reduce spasticity. Fasano,[24,25] in the late 1970s, reported on 109 patients with a three-year follow-up. Peacock,[17-20] in 1987, reported on three- to seven-year follow-up of his first 60 cases done through an L1-L5 laminectomy. Fifty-one cerebral palsy patients were classified as being mainly spastic. Thirty-four of the patients were ambulatory after the surgery, compared with 16 before

Table 1 Summary of soft-tissue procedures (group II)

Procedure	No. Performed*
Tendon Achilles lengthening	70
Vulpius	38
Sliding	32
Hamstrings lengthening	28
Medial hamstrings	19
Medial and lateral hamstrings	9
Adductor release	46
Iliopsoas release	36
Peroneal tendon lengthening	4
Posterior tibial tendon lengthening	4

*There were 42 patients in the soft-tissue procedures group.

surgery; 24% of the 51 patients were treated with standard orthopaedic procedures after their rhizotomy. Vaughan and associates[26] prospectively reported on 14 of Peacock's cerebral palsy patients who had undergone gait analysis before and after rhizotomy. They reported statistically significant improvements in stride length, gait velocity, and range of motion during gait at both the hip and knee levels.

There have been no studies comparing the results of this procedure with the results of tendon lengthening and transfer procedures used in the orthopaedic surgery community.

Purpose

Currently, SPR is being performed at more than 18 medical centers around the country, although there are limited hard data describing its specific indications or comparing its benefits with those of the standard orthopaedic procedures. Complicating this issue is lack of specific SPR outcome measurements for the spastic diplegic patient who has had no previous surgery or for the patient who has had the standard orthopaedic surgery. This study retrospectively examines preoperative and postoperative range of motion and videotape gait analysis, as well as postoperative computerized gait analysis, to compare the outcomes of one group of patients treated with SPR and another treated with soft-tissue procedures.

Materials and Methods

Ninety-two patients were studied. Group I consists of 50 consecutive spastic diplegic cerebral palsy patients who underwent SPR to reduce the spasticity. There were 28 boys and 22 girls, ranging in age at the time of surgery from 2.5 to 12.6 years (mean: 5.7 years).

Group II consists of 42 consecutive spastic diplegic cerebral palsy patients who underwent soft-tissue procedures including adductor myotomy, iliopsoas release/lengthening, hamstring lengthening, and/or Achilles tendon lengthening by Dr. Luciano Dias (Table 1). At the time these surgeries were performed, the distal rectus femoris transfer[27] was not yet an available procedure. There were 23 boys and 19 girls, ranging in age from 1.1 to 12.8 years (mean: 5.2 years) at the time of the surgery.

Patients undergoing rhizotomy were evaluated preoperatively by a team consisting of the neurosurgeon, the orthopaedic surgeon, the pediatric rehabilitation physician, and the physical therapist. The criteria for inclusion in this study were that the patient be classified as spastic diplegic, have near-normal intelligence, ambulatory potential, no history of previous bony surgery, and no joint dislocation. Patients in the SPR group underwent surgery between 1987 and 1989, with an average follow-up of 1.5 years. Patients in the soft-tissue group underwent surgery between 1983 and 1989, with an average follow-up of two years. Twenty-three of the 92 patients had additional orthopaedic surgery during the postoperative period that we are reviewing. In these cases, the postoperative data were obtained from the last office visit before the additional surgery, and the follow-up period was limited to that time. No data from these patients were collected after the additional surgery.

Range of motion data were collected from each patient's preoperative and postoperative evaluations. Included in these data were hip abduction with the hips in flexion, hip flexion contracture using the Thomas test, popliteal angle measurement, and ankle dorsiflexion with the knee in extension. Hip rotation and tibial torsion data were not collected.

The second part of our study involves the evaluation of preoperative and postoperative videotapes of 33 patients in the SPR group and 26 patients in the soft-tissue group. Using a rating system which we developed (Table 2), we compared the preoperative and postoperative gait of the two groups.

For the final part of this study, we reviewed the computerized gait analysis studies of 16 spastic diplegic patients who had undergone SPR. We also reviewed studies of 18 spastic diplegic patients who had undergone soft-tissue procedures prior to the availability of the rectus transfer. We compared their stride length, cadence, gait velocity, single limb stance times, and joint range of motion measurements during the gait cycle.

Postoperative Management

Patients in the selective posterior rhizotomy group underwent a four- to six-week intensive inpatient physical therapy program in the Rehabilitation Institute of Chicago. Patients in the soft-tissue group were casted for approximately two to three weeks postoperatively. Almost all of them underwent an intensive inpatient physical therapy program for about four weeks.

Results

In the rhizotomy group, average preoperative hip abduction was 47 degrees; hip flexion contracture, 7.5 degrees; popliteal angle, 41

Table 2 Rating scale to quantitatively assess overall function and quality of gait

Observation	Points
Patient's ability to walk:	
No abnormal gait pattern seen on clinical examination	30
Patient walks alone with good balance	25
Patient walks alone but has poor balance	20
Patient walks with minimal assistance (eg, holding someone's hand lightly for balance)	15
Patient walks with moderate assistance (eg, external device such as a walker needed to ambulate)	10
Patient is able to walk a few steps, but only with pelvic support	5
Patient is not able to take a step, even with maximum assistance	0
Maximum points possible	30
Quality of gait:	
Each hip	
No abnormal adduction during gait	10
Increased adductor thrust during stance	8
Adduction brings knee to midline of body	6
Adduction brings knee past midline	4
Adduction causes crossing of feet	2
Maximum for two hips	20
Each knee	
No significant crouching, normal flexion during swing	10
No significant crouching, decreased flexion in swing	8
Crouching between 10–20 degrees (late stance)	6
Crouching between 20–45 degrees (late stance)	4
Crouching between 45–90 degrees (late stance)	2
Crouching greater than 90 degrees	0
Maximum for two knees	20
Each ankle (initial foot contact)	
Normal heel toe gait pattern	10
Plantigrade	8
Toes first, heel off ground less than 1 inch	6
Toes first, heel off ground between 1 and 2 inches	4
Toes first, heel off ground greater than 2 inches	2
Maximum for two ankles	20
Foot progression (for each foot)	
Intoeing or outtoeing less than 45 degrees	5
Intoeing or outtoeing greater than 45 degrees	0
Maximum for two feet	10
Maximum points possible	70
Combined scales	
Maximum possible points	100

degrees; and ankle dorsiflexion, minus 4 degrees. Postoperatively, these patients demonstrated an average hip abduction of 60 degrees, hip flexion contracture of 2.5 degrees, popliteal angle of 34 degrees, and ankle dorsiflexion of 4 degrees. In the soft-tissue group, the average preoperative hip abduction was 50 degrees; hip flexion contracture, 10 degrees; popliteal angle, 35 degrees; and ankle dorsiflexion, minus 9 degrees. Postoperatively, the average hip abduction was 62 degrees;

Table 3 Patients in selected posterior rhizotomy group requiring additional surgery

Procedure	No.*
Hamstring lengthening	13
Iliopsoas lengthening	3
Achilles tendon lengthening	12
Adductor myotomy	5
Peroneus lengthening	3
Rectus transfer	4
Rectus release	1
Posterior tibial lengthening	1

*Twenty-two patients in this group required soft-tissue surgery.

hip flexion contracture, 1 degree; popliteal angle, 27 degrees; and ankle dorsiflexion, 8.6 degrees.

There are no statistically significant differences in preoperative and postoperative range of motion at the 0.05 confidence level. It appears that equinus contractures of the ankle and tightness of the hamstrings are least affected by SPR. This correlates well with the need for additional orthopaedic surgery in the rhizotomy group (Table 3). All three of the 50 SPR patients reviewed who were over the age of nine years required soft-tissue procedures after the rhizotomy. Nine other patients showed progressive decrease in range of motion after the rhizotomy. The other 13 patients who required soft-tissue procedures showed no improvements in the contractures after the rhizotomy.

We also reviewed the need for additional surgery in the soft-tissue group. Ten of the 42 patients in this group had a stiff knee gait pattern, requiring rectus transfer procedures, which were not available at the time of their original soft-tissue procedures. Three other patients had further soft-tissue release procedures during the follow-up period.

Videotape Analysis

Preoperative and postoperative videotapes were taken of 33 patients in the SPR group. The average time of the postoperative videotape was 18 months after surgery. Preoperative and postoperative videotapes were also taken of 26 patients in the soft-tissue group, with an average postoperative videotape time of 25 months. A rating scale was devised (Table 2). The videotapes were randomly reviewed for scoring purposes. Patients in the SPR group improved from an average of 47.6 to 56.8 on the gait scale. In the soft-tissue group, the improvement was from an average of 48.0 to 57.6 on a 70-point scale. On the 30-point functional scale, patients in the SPR group improved from an average of 15.3 to 17.1, while patients in the soft-tissue group improved from an average of 15.6 to 20.2.

In addition to comparing overall scores, we compared the number of patients in each group who were independent ambulators preoperatively and postoperatively as well as the number of patients in each group

Table 4 Comparison of gait analyses following rhizotomy and soft-tissue release

Parameter	Rhizotomy	Soft-Tissue Release
Stride length (% of age-matched nl value)	73.5%	52.5%
Gait velocity (%of age-matched nl value)	63.5%	52.3%
Hip range of motion	47.7 degrees	32.9 degrees
Knee range of motion	49.18 degrees	26.17 degrees

with improved function versus those whose functional capacity remained the same or became worse. In the SPR group, 16 patients remained in the same functional category, 16 improved, and one patient deteriorated. In the soft-tissue group, 11 patients remained in the same category and 15 improved.

Before surgery, 19 patients in the rhizotomy group required external support (walker, crutches, or cane) for walking, and 14 were independent ambulators. Postoperatively, 14 required external support and 19 were independent. Therefore, only five of the 19 patients who required external support were able to ambulate without support after the rhizotomy. In the soft-tissue group, 13 patients required external support before surgery. At follow-up, only five required external support, and 21 patients were able to walk without support.

Although the differences between the two groups are not statistically significant, these data give the impression that in the early postoperative period (one to two years), patients in the soft-tissue release group function better than those in the SPR group.

Computerized Gait Analysis

We compared the stride length, cadence, and gait velocity of those patients on whom we had done computerized gait analysis, and studied the joint range of motion of the hip, knee, and ankle during gait. We found that patients in the SPR group had a longer stride length and greater gait velocity than patients in the soft-tissue release group. We also found that the hip and knee range of motion was closer to normal in the SPR group than in the soft-tissue group. In summary, the rhizotomy groups showed a lower incidence of stiff-legged gait (Table 4).

Discussion

There is a great deal of concern in the orthopaedic community that SPR is now being performed too frequently without any demonstration of its long-term effectiveness. In addition, concern has been raised over whether neurosurgeons with limited experience dealing with cerebral palsy should be managing this problem. In this study, we have tried to examine some of the early results of SPR in the spastic diplegic child and compare them with the results of more traditional orthopaedic soft-tissue release procedures.

Preliminary data obtained from short-term follow-up visits (one and one-half years) seem to indicate that, in the selected cases, patients undergoing rhizotomy do as well as those who have soft-tissue release procedures. However, it seems that in spite of the rhizotomy, 40% to 50% of the patients will require soft-tissue procedures. What is still unknown is the long-term outcome of patients who underwent rhizotomy followed by soft-tissue procedures.

Careful selection of patients remains the key to obtaining a successful result.[28] The results of this study point to the need for a carefully designed, randomized prospective study using preoperative and post-operative gait analysis.

As described by Rang,[29] the pathogenesis of deformity in cerebral palsy has three known stages. In stage I, the deformity begins with muscles that are not fully lengthened; this is the spastic stage. In stage II, there are fixed shortening contractures, and in stage III, the muscles are shortened and joints are dislocated. It seems appropriate to believe that the prime indication for SPR is at stage I of the disease, usually when the patient is between the ages of 3 and 6.

Conclusion

Based on this retrospective study, we believe that SPR has a role in the management of the child with spastic diplegia; however, when compared with the usual soft-tissue procedures, the end result is quite similar as far as improvement in the passive range of motion. The functional gains are also quite similar but the soft-tissue group showed a better outcome in the area of unsupported walking. The postoperative computerized gait analysis showed slightly better gait parameters in the SPR group.

It is important to emphasize that the SPR is only part of the overall management of spastic diplegia; at least 40% to 50% of the patients will require further orthopaedic procedures. It is also important to remember that, in spite of constant review of our cases and improvement in our selection criteria, we still see children after rhizotomy with an unpredictable outcome (for example, progressive hip subluxation). Such problems are not encountered in the soft-tissue cases.

Further studies with longer follow-up are needed before we can really evaluate the results of this new surgery. The need for a well trained SPR team cannot be overemphasized.

References

1. Bleck EE: Spastic diplegia, in Bleck EE (ed): *Orthopaedic Management in Cerebral Palsy,* Clinics in Developmental Medicine. Philadelphia, JB Lippincott, 1987, no 99, p 282.
2. Baker LD: A rational approach to the surgical needs of the cerebral palsy patient. *J Bone Joint Surg* 1956;38A:313–323.
3. Banks HH: The knee and cerebral palsy. *Orthop Clin North Am* 1972;3:113–129.
4. Banks HH: Management of spastic deformities of the foot and ankle. *Clin Orthop* 1977;122:70–76.

5. Banks HH, Green WT: The correction of equinus deformity in cerebral palsy. *J Bone Joint Surg* 1958;40A:1359–1379.

6. Banks HH, Green WT: Adductor myotomy and obturator neurectomy for the correction of adduction contracture of the hip in cerebral palsy. *J Bone Joint Surg* 1960;42A:111–126.

7. Bleck EE: Hip deformities in cerebral palsy, in American Academy of Orthopaedic Surgeons *Instructional Course Lectures, XX*. St. Louis, CV Mosby, 1971, chap 3, pp 54–82.

8. Conrad JA, Frost HM: Evaluation of subcutaneous heel-cord lengthening. *Clin Orthop* 1969;64:121–127.

9. Drummond DS, Rogala E, Templeton J, et al: Proximal hamstring release for knee flexion and crouched posture in cerebral palsy. *J Bone Joint Surg*, 1974; 56A:1598–1602.

10. Gaines RW: A systematic approach to the amount of Achilles tendon lengthening in cerebral palsy. *J Pediatr* 1985;4:448.

11. Graham HK, Fixsen JA: Lengthening of the calcaneal tendon in spastic hemiplegia by the White slide technique: A long term review. *J Bone Joint Surg* 1988;70A:472–475.

12. Grant AD, Feldman R, Lehman WB: Equinus deformity in cerebral palsy: A retrospective analysis of treatment and function in 39 cases. *J Pediatr Orthop* 1985;5:678–681.

13. Green WT, McDermott LJ: Operative treatment of cerebral palsy of spastic type. *JAMA* 1942;118:434–440.

14. Griffin PP, Wheelhouse WW, Shiavi R: Adductor transfer for adductor spasticity: Clinical and electromyographic gait analysis. *Dev Med Child Neurol* 1979;19:783–789.

15. Beals RK: Spastic paraplegia and diplegia: An evaluation of nonsurgical and surgical factors influencing the prognosis for ambulation. *J Bone Joint Surg* 1966;48A:827–846.

16. Thometz J, Simon S, Rosenthal R: The effect on gait of lengthening of the medial hamstrings in cerebral palsy. *J Bone Joint Surg* 1989;71A:345–353.

17. Peacock WJ, Arens LJ, Berman B: Cerebral palsy spasticity: Selective posterior rhizotomy. *Pediatr Neurosci* 1987;13:61–66.

18. Peacock WJ, Arens LJ, Berman B: An assessment of selective posterior rhizotomy as a procedure for relieving spasticity in cerebral palsy. *Dev Med Child Neurol* 1987;29(suppl 55):22.

19. Peacock WJ, Eastman RW: The neurosurgical management of spasticity. *S Afr Med J* 1981;60:849–850.

20. Peacock WJ, Arens LJ: Selective posterior rhizotomy for the relief of spasticity in cerebral palsy. *S Afr Med J* 1982;62:119–124.

21. Förster O: Ueber eine neue operative Methode der Behandlung spastischer Lahmungen mittels Resektion hinterer Ruckenmarks-swurzhenn. *Z Orthop Chir* 1908;22:203–223.

22. Förster O: Resection of the posterior nerve roots of spinal cord. *Lancet* 1911;2: 76–79.

23. Förster O: On the indications and results of the excision of posterior spinal nerve roots in men. *Surg Gynecol Obstet* 1913;16:463–474.

24. Fasano VA, Urciuoli R, Broggi G, et al: New aspects in the surgical treatment of cerebral palsy. *Acta Neurochir Suppl* 1977;24:53–57.

25. Fasano VA, Broggi G, Barolat-Romana G, et al: Surgical treatment of spasticity in cerebral palsy. *Childs Brain* 1978;4:289–305.

26. Vaughan CL, Berman B, Peacock WJ: Gait analysis of spastic children before and after selective lumbar rhizotomy. *Pediatr Neurosci* 1988;14:297–300.

27. Gage JR: Surgical treatment of knee dysfunction in cerebral palsy. *Clin Orthop* 1990;253:45–54.

28. Oppenheim WL: Selective posterior rhizotomy for spastic cerebral palsy: A review. *Clin Orthop* 1990;253:20–29.

29. Rang M: Cerebral palsy, in Morrissy RT (ed): *Lovell and Winter's Pediatric Orthopaedics*, ed 3. Philadelphia, JB Lippincott, 1990, vol 1, pp 465–506.

Consensus

One of the important goals of treatment of children with cerebral palsy is the improvement of function. Thus, the desired outcome of selective dorsal rhizotomy is similar to that of orthopaedic surgery, to improve function. However, the mechanism by which selective dorsal rhizotomy attempts to improve function (the reduction of spasticity by decreasing neural stimulation) is different from the mechanisms by which orthopaedic surgery does so (release of contractures, rerouting muscles, and realignment of the skeleton).

Selective dorsal rhizotomy can be expected to reduce spasticity. Rhizotomy may also improve function in some patients. However, the duration of post-rhizotomy benefits is not known.

A team approach should be used in choosing candidates for selective dorsal rhizotomy. A neurosurgeon skilled in the techniques of selective dorsal rhizotomy must be a member of the team. Other team members should include, but are not limited to, an orthopaedic surgeon, a pediatrician, and a physical therapist. All team members should have experience and expertise in the care of children with cerebral palsy and other childhood disabilities. The team should establish the diagnosis, set goals for the patient, and be prepared to discuss all treatment options. In addition, the team should agree that the patient would benefit from a reduction in spasticity, and there should be agreement among the team members whenever selective dorsal rhizotomy is recommended.

Intelligent, ambulatory patients with spastic diplegia are candidates for selective dorsal rhizotomy, and choreoathetosis is a contraindication to the procedure. More information and results of surgery are needed for decisions about patients with the various other patterns of cerebral palsy. It is not known whether selective dorsal rhizotomy should be used in patients with quadriplegia, hemiplegia, poor balance, dystonia, scoliosis, or mental retardation or seizures. It also is not known whether rhizotomy should be used in very young patients or adolescent patients, or in patients who have had prior orthopaedic procedures. Although these findings may be considered relative contraindications, and their presence certainly should be considered before undertaking surgery, data concerning benefits and adverse outcomes are not available at this time. Unrealistic parental expectations constitute a serious contraindication.

New ways should be developed to improve selection of patients for rhizotomy. Specific techniques to unmask a patient's spasticity while accurately assessing that patient's underlying strength should be evaluated. These investigations should include, for example, the use of pharmacologic agents such as baclofen or midazolam.

Criteria for selecting rootlets for section or for preservation currently seem to vary from one institution to another. The electrophysiologic criteria as well as the role of clinical judgment during the surgery itself must be refined and delineated.

Physical therapy is needed following selective dorsal rhizotomy. The intensity, the duration, and the optimal location (inpatient or outpatient) for administering physical therapy are not known. As with other major surgical procedures, selective dorsal rhizotomy has the potential for serious complications. Moreover, it does not eliminate the need for subsequent orthopaedic surgery.

Because long-term follow-up is lacking, and both the preoperative selection criteria and the intraoperative techniques need to be defined, centers offering selective dorsal rhizotomy are obliged to develop formalized protocols and collect follow-up data. Selective dorsal rhizotomy studies are, for the most part, case series without control. There are some reports of nonrandomized concurrent, cohort comparisons between contemporaneous patients who did and did not receive treatment.

The process of critical scrutiny of indications, technique, and outcomes should not be focused on selective dorsal rhizotomy alone but should apply to all treatment techniques.

Section Seven
Crouched Gait

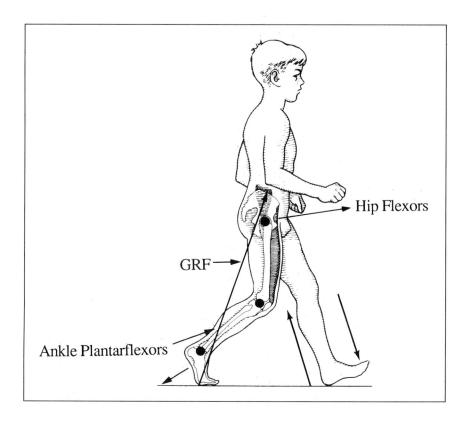

Chapter 23

Function of the Hamstrings in Cerebral Palsy

Jacquelin Perry, MD
Craig Newsam, MPT

Overactivity of the hamstrings has long been recognized as a cause of excessive knee flexion in the gait of cerebral palsy patients. The potential surgical answers are lengthening, release, or transfer of the offending muscles. None of these procedures has proved totally satisfying. One difficulty is the biarticular nature of the hamstring muscles. Lengthening or release of the muscles reduces their effectiveness as hip extensors. All too often, the result is excessive anterior tilt of the pelvis, which may lead to a painful lordosis. Conversely, transfer of the hamstrings to the femur may cause genu recurvatum by removing all posterior restraint at the knee. Compromises include mixing the techniques or surgically modifying only some of the hamstrings.

Unanswered is the question of which muscle or muscles should be modified. Three long hamstrings cross both the knee and hip. Medially there are the semimembranosus and semitendinosus. On the lateral side is the biceps femoris. An electromyograph (EMG) in a normal subject shows that the three long hamstrings have a similar pattern of action (Fig. 1). Peak action occurs in terminal swing to decelerate hip flexion. Secondary knee hyperextension also is prevented. Activity continues for a brief time at the onset of stance (loading response). Then the muscles relax for the rest of the stride.

Two muscles share the biceps tendon. The biceps femoris long head is biarticular while the biceps femoris short head crosses only the knee. Very different timing is displayed on an EMG by the short head of the biceps (Fig. 2). It is active only in initial swing to assist knee flexion for toe clearance. Hence, the two biceps, which share a common tendon, have very distinct actions.

If the long hamstring muscles normally work in synergy, is this true for their pathologic state as well? Clinical testing for spasticity and contracture suggests an affirmative answer, but differences sometimes are noted. To clarify hamstring muscle action as a guide for performing more definitive surgery, gait EMG was done as a presurgical test. These data have been reviewed to see if some common rules can be formulated.

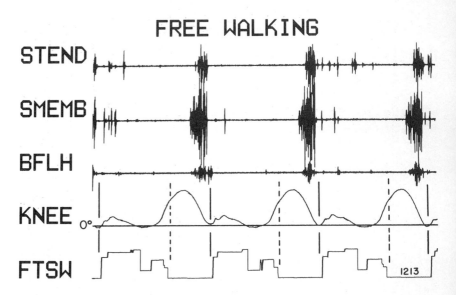

Fig. 1 *Normal EMG function of the long hamstrings: semitendinosus, semimembranosus, and biceps femoris long head. Solid vertical line denotes initial contact; dashed vertical lines denotes the beginning of swing (toe-off).*

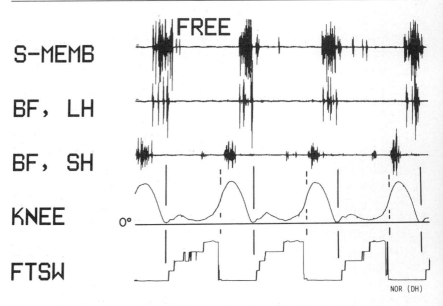

Fig. 2 *Normal EMG showing difference in function of two heads of the biceps femoris.*

Method

The material for this chapter represents a retrospective review of the dynamic EMG records of the children with cerebral palsy most recently tested in the Rancho Los Amigos Medical Center pathokinesiology laboratory. Thirty records with adequate data were selected. All patients had a diagnosis of a crouch gait secondary to spastic cerebral palsy, and the purpose of the test was presurgical planning.

Timing of muscle action during walking was recorded with paired fine wire electrodes inserted in the muscles of interest. Accuracy of placement was determined by mild electrical stimulation through the electrode and palpation of muscle action. Following manual testing of strength, spasticity, and passive range, muscle action during walking was recorded. Gait data were gathered as the subjects traversed a 10 m long walkway, the middle 6 m of which were delineated by photoelectric cells as the steady-state data collection segment.

The total testing protocol included eight muscles. For this study, records that included the semimembranosus and the two heads of the biceps femoris were selected. The EMG records were processed with the EMG analyzer to display quantitatively the timing and amplitude profile of each muscle. These data were compiled according to the timing pattern of the EMGs. Timing profiles that exceeded the normal on or off times by more than one standard deviation were classified as excessive. The EMG records showing normal or less duration were grouped as mild.

The motion data for the hip, knee, and ankle, were used to identify the peak values for terminal stance and terminal swing, the phases where knee extension is normally maximal. These values were related to the different EMG patterns per muscle and per muscle group to determine the functional significance of the abnormal modes of muscle action.

Results

Excessive muscle activity was the most frequent EMG pattern found for both of the long hamstrings in this group of patients with cerebral palsy. The incidence was 100% for the biceps femoris long head, and 80% for the semimembranosus. In contrast, the short head of the biceps femoris displayed excessive activity in only 31% of the records.

Three major forms of excessive EMG activity were identified; continuous, prolonged, and premature combined with prolonged (premature/prolonged). Prolonged action was the most common pattern within the excessive group (44%). This was followed by the continuous EMG pattern (26%) and premature/prolonged (26%). For the biceps femoris long head, prolonged action was the most frequent gait abnormality. This was followed by premature/prolonged, while continuous action was less frequent. The semimembranosus had an equal incidence of continuous and prolonged, with premature/prolonged action being

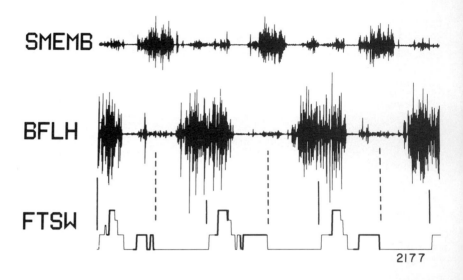

Fig. 3 *Reverse phasing of semimembranosus combined with premature onset and prolonged cessation of biceps femoris long head in a cerebral palsy patient.*

much less frequent. Reversed phasing, also considered a form of excessive action, was an infrequent occurrence (4%) (Fig. 3).

The muscle patterns falling within the mild category included normal, premature/curtailed, and absent action. Six of the semimembranosus records (20%) showed some form of mild action. This was not seen in any of the biceps femoris long head recordings. Hence, among the two long hamstrings studied, the semimembranosus showed the greater variability. In contrast to the long hamstrings, a majority (73%) of the biceps femoris short head EMG patterns fell into the mild category. These were almost equally divided between normal and premature/curtailed.

When the timing of the semimembranosus and long head of the biceps were compared within subjects, nine pairs (30%) showed the same pattern of excessive activity (Fig. 4), both continuous in three, both prolonged in five, and premature/prolonged in one. Eleven pairs of muscles (36%) showed different mixtures of excessive activity: Continuous with prolonged (Fig. 5), continuous with premature/prolonged, and the mixture of prolonged action in one muscle and premature/prolonged in the other. The other combinations (10) showed a pattern of mixed excessive and mild (Fig. 6).

The timing of activity by the short head of the biceps generally was distinctly different from that of the long head of the biceps, although both share the same tendon (Fig. 7). EMG activity of the biceps femoris short head was available in 26 of the 30 patient records studied. In four

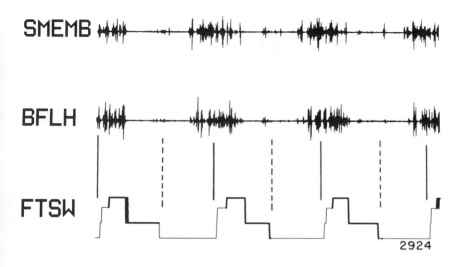

Fig. 4 *A patient showing premature onset as well as prolongation of activity in both the semimembranosus and biceps femoris long head.*

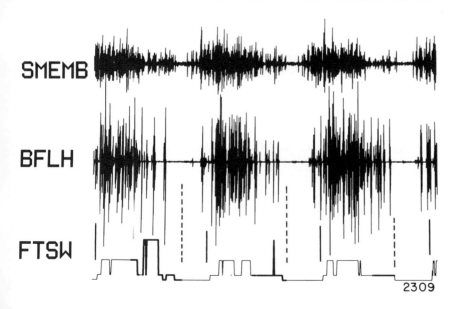

Fig. 5 *Cerebral palsy patient showing continuous EMG activity of the semimembranosus along with prolonged EMG of the biceps femoris long head. Both muscles show forms of excessive phasing.*

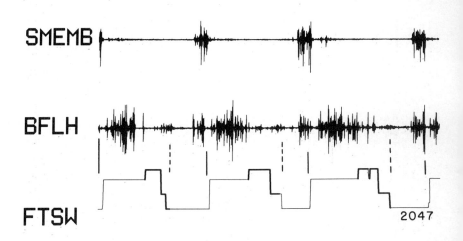

Fig. 6 *Mixture of mild and excessive EMG within one subject. Semimembranosus shows normal phasing (mild) while the biceps femoris long head is prolonged (excessive).*

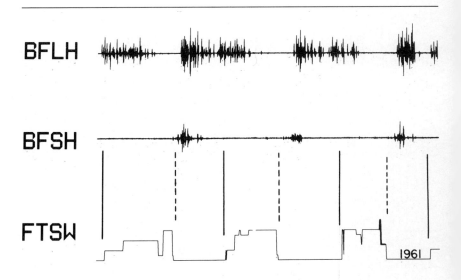

Fig. 7 *Example of difference in phasing of the two heads of the biceps femoris in a cerebral palsy patient. Biceps femoris short head is active in initial swing only (normal); biceps femoris long head is active throughout swing and into midstance (premature/prolonged).*

cases, the EMG testing protocol was modified to study another muscle in lieu of the biceps femoris short head. Normal swing phase timing occurred in 10 of the 26 muscles studied (38%). Abnormal swing action (premature/curtailed) was the dominant timing for another nine subjects (33%). Stance phase action was displayed by just seven patients (26%). A direct comparison of the two heads of the biceps (long and short) found only two pairs with the same timing (continuous action for both). In 18, or 69%, action of the short head of the biceps related to swing while the long head of biceps displayed prolonged stance phase action.

Residual hip flexion in terminal stance was seen with each type of excessive biceps femoris long head action (24 degrees) but was associated only with continuous semimembranosus activity (10 degrees). Terminal swing hip flexion was not significantly different from normal in any patient. The relative knee flexion occurring in terminal stance (40 versus 21 degrees) and terminal swing (50 versus 35 degrees) was notably greater when there was premature muscle action in addition to the prolonged EMG. With only five samples in each of the four groups, this greater knee flexion has to be considered a strong trend that only approached statistical significance. There also was notably less terminal stance knee flexion when the EMG of the semimembranosus was in the mild category (10 degrees for the mild group versus 31 degrees for the severe group). A similar difference was not seen in terminal swing. At the ankle, continuous action of either muscle—semimembranosus or biceps femoris long head—is associated with an increase in the maximum stance phase dorsiflexion (14 degrees). This contrasted with the mean 4-degree dorsiflexion and 5-degree plantarflexion occurring with the other pathologic EMG patterns.

Discussion

The clinical assumption that overactivity of the hamstring muscles is a basic finding in the cerebral palsy crouch gait was substantiated. It occurred in every child tested. The second common assumption that the medial (semimembranosus) and lateral (biceps femoris) hamstrings act the same is less valid. Twenty percent of the semimembranosus muscles showed normal or less than normal activity while this was the case in only 3% of the biceps femoris long head muscles studied. A second dissimilarity was in the type of overactivity recorded. Both the occurrence and severity of excessive knee flexion varied with the different types of hamstring activity.

In cerebral palsy patients with prolonged hamstring activity, rather than following the normal pattern of reaching peak intensity in terminal swing and then rapidly decreasing in loading response to avoid excessive knee flexion, the hamstring muscles fire at maximum intensity from terminal swing through the entire stance phase. This prolonged hamstring activity thereby accentuates the normal loading response knee flexion and leads to maintenance of a flexed position in mid and terminal stance as was demonstrated in this study. In order to counterbalance the overactive hamstrings, greater quadriceps activity is required to preserve weightbearing stability.

The addition, in some patients, of premature hamstring activation (premature/prolonged) was found to cause even greater knee flexion (50 versus 35 degrees) in terminal swing, which carried through into terminal stance (40 versus 21 degrees). This early mid swing activation adds dynamic knee flexion at a time when the knee is expected to passively extend. This effect is continued through terminal swing if the muscle intensity remains at the same level, a characteristic of the all-or-none mode of primitive locomotor control. The greater knee flexion present at initial foot contact tends to be maintained by the prolonged hamstring activity, leading to greater terminal stance flexion as well. Those patients who demonstrate continuous hamstring muscle action are likely to possess even more severely deranged pathomechanics as a result of the unrelenting abnormal flexor effect. Unfortunately, because there were only three patients with continuous activity in both hamstrings, little can be said at present.

In those instances where only the biceps femoris long head registered excessive action, persistent knee flexion in terminal stance was notably less (10 degrees). However, terminal swing knee flexion in this group (25 degrees) was similar to that found in patients with prolonged action in both hamstrings.

EMG analysis may allow a more selective approach in the lengthening of the hamstrings, in the hope of preserving pelvic control. With such a plan, the preferred muscle to be lengthened should be the one showing continuous or premature activity. When both muscles, semimembranosus and biceps femoris long head, show prolonged activity, only the most persistent one would be lengthened. To make such discriminating decisions, however, it is necessary to record the medial and lateral hamstrings separately. Whether surface electrodes can make this differentiation needs to be determined, particularly for the medial hamstrings where the activity in the adductors may be picked up by a surface electrode (cross-talk).

A second significant finding with surgical implications is the phasic difference in the actions of the short and long head of the biceps among the cerebral palsy patients. While swing phase knee flexion is normally initiated passively by rolling over the forefoot during the preswing phase of stance, cerebral palsy patients seldom have this degree of mobility. Thus, they must directly flex the limb with a deliberate flexor pattern. Having the short head of the biceps to assist knee flexion is an important asset that should be preserved. Only five of the cerebral palsy patients failed to have some useful swing phase biceps femoris short head muscle action. Hence, surgical lengthening of the biceps femoris long head should not violate the tendon of the short head if optimum initiation of knee flexion in swing is to be preserved.

The conclusion from this study of hamstring muscle function during gait is that, although 80% of the patients displayed excessive activity in both the semimembranosus and biceps femoris long head, there is considerable variability in the pathology contributing to the cerebral palsy crouch gait. Despite this excessive hamstring activity, hip flexion patterns were not significantly altered. In contrast, knee flexion at terminal stance was significantly increased to 32 degrees flexion and terminal swing flexion to 40 degrees. Current surgical practice of lengthening the semimembranosus aponeurosis and not altering the biceps femoris long head is supported both by the EMG data in this study and by the fact that the semimembranosus produces more of a deforming force owing to its greater cross-sectional area.[1] Biceps femoris short head and long head activity often differ significantly and must be differentiated surgically. Use of dynamic EMG should allow for more selective surgery, which may lead to better preservation of useful function following hamstring surgery.

Reference

1. Weber EF: *Ueber die Langenverhaltnisse der Fleischfasern der Muskeln im Allgemeinen.* Ber verh K Sachs Ges Wissensch, Math-Phys Cl, 1851.

Chapter 24

Distal Hamstring Surgery in Cerebral Palsy

Leon Root, MD

Introduction

Indications for surgery in cerebral palsy are never limited to a single muscle or body region. All parts are related to the whole. Therefore, it is the effect on the whole of each part and the effect on each individual part of every other part that make surgical decision making extraordinarily challenging. This is especially true of muscles that affect two joints. The hamstring muscles exemplify this complexity: They flex the knee and extend the hip, performing two different functions separately or simultaneously. The hamstrings also can adduct the hip, internally rotate the thigh, and externally rotate the leg. In spastic cerebral palsy patients, clinicians have observed every aspect of their function and, because of the underlying spasticity and muscle imbalance, have seen every possible deformity caused by this activity. Clinicians' deductions, based on observation and examination, have been confirmed objectively by gait analysis. Rather than dwelling upon the normal and abnormal function of the hamstrings, which has been described by Gage[1] and Sutherland and associates[2,3] this chapter focuses on: (1) the functional deformities caused by spastic hamstring muscles; (2) the goals of corrective surgery; (3) the complications or disadvantages of hamstring lengthenings; and (4) the effectiveness of distal hamstring surgery.

Functional Deformity

The hamstrings, in conjunction with related muscles and antagonists, may cause or be a significant factor in crouched gait pattern, limit stride length, contribute to an internal rotation gait pattern, and potentiate ankle equinus. When associated with abnormal function of the rectus femoris, the hamstrings contribute to a stiff knee gait pattern. By preventing normal lumbar lordosis, tight hamstrings can interfere with good sitting posture and prohibit long sitting. Contracted hamstrings can also be a factor in the development of hip subluxation and dislocation.

Goals of Surgical Treatment

The goals of treatment derive from the deformities to be corrected: eliminate or diminish the inefficient crouched gait pattern, improve stride length, decrease compensatory ankle equinus and hip flexion, minimize internal rotation gait, improve sitting balance and posture, and decrease the abnormal muscle pull that can cause hip dislocation.

Undesirable Effects of Hamstring Lengthenings

Awareness of what happens at the hip and ankle and in the front of the knee will help the surgeon avoid the problems that can result from hamstring lengthening. For example, lordosis will be increased after hamstring lengthening if hip flexors are tight or contracted. Spastic quadriceps may become tighter, leading to a stiff knee gait pattern. Excessive lengthening may result in loss of knee flexion and subsequent genu recurvatum. In addition, as the child grows, the muscles might contract again, requiring repeat surgery.

Distal Hamstring Surgery: A Clinical Review

Methods

The basic approach that I have used for hamstring surgery at The Hospital for Special Surgery for the past 25 years has been to perform a distal tenotomy of the semitendinosus and gracilis, aponeurectomy of the semimembranosus, and, when indicated, an aponeurectomy of the distal biceps femoris tendon. The surgery is generally done in the supine position so that straight leg raising and popliteal angles can be clinically evaluated. I always lengthen the medial hamstrings first, and if I am unable to achieve straight leg raising of 70 degrees or achieve a popliteal angle of 20 degrees, I then do an aponeurectomy of the biceps femoris. Simon[4] has stated that he can lengthen the hamstrings in the prone position and still obtain sufficient straight leg raising postoperatively.

Over the years I have changed my postoperative management. My mentor, Dr. William Cooper, casted the knee in extension for six weeks. I reduced cast immobilization to three weeks and, for the past five years, in patients that do not require casting at the hip, I have used a removable knee immobilizer and started active motion in five days. A study of 242 knees in 126 cerebral palsy patients has just been completed at The Hospital for Special Surgery. Minimum follow-up was 3 years (range 3 to 14 years), with an average of 5.9 years.[5] The age at operation ranged from 27 months to 20 years with a mean of 7.3 years. Forty-five patients were community ambulators, 19 were household ambulators, and 62 were essentially nonambulators. Preoperative straight leg raising varied from 30 to 70 degrees with a mean of 52 degrees. The popliteal angle ranged from 90 to 30 degrees with a mean of 66 degrees.

The mean preoperative flexion contracture of 36 knees in ten patients was 20 degrees (range 5 to 45 degrees). Fifty-two patients had a mean hip flexion contracture of 19 degrees, and 53 patients had an equinus deformity averaging − 3 degrees.

Of these patients, 87 had only distal medial hamstring surgery, 39 had both medial and lateral hamstring surgery, and 116 had bilateral procedures. Simultaneous hip and/or foot surgery was done in 107 patients (85%).

Results

Results of the hamstring lengthenings on ambulation are influenced by the fact that 85% of the patients had simultaneous surgery in other areas of the lower extremity that would influence their walking ability. After surgery, the number of community ambulators improved from 45 to 73; household ambulators decreased from 19 to 15; and nonambulators decreased from 62 to 38. No patient regressed in ambulation level. Of the 15 patients with typical crouched gait, only five cases persisted postoperatively.

Straight leg raising was improved from a presurgery mean of 52 degrees to a mean of 70 degrees one year after surgery, but decreased to a mean of 67 degrees by three years. The mean preoperative popliteal angle improved from 66 degrees to 20 degrees at one year and regressed to 39 degrees at three years. Of the 30 knees with preoperative knee flexion contracture, which averaged 20 degrees, only 15 had postoperative knee flexion contractures, with a mean of 9 degrees.

Recurrence, defined as regression to the preoperative straight leg raising value, occurred in 82 knees (33%) in 46 patients. Of these, only 22 patients (42 knees or 17%) required additional hamstring lengthenings. Three patients required a third hamstring lengthening, one of which was done proximally. Twenty-two patients subsequently had a distal rectus femoris transfer or release.

Multiple variables were analyzed for their effect upon recurrence: age at operation, disease severity, pattern of involvement, severity of straight leg raising limitation, duration of immobilization, medial versus medial and lateral releases, and concomitant operations (Table 1). Recurrence rate was lower in patients with a straight leg raising restriction of 45 degrees or less preoperatively than in those who had a mild or moderate restriction of 45 to 70 degrees (p = 0.001).

Genu recurvatum occurred in 18 knees in 10 patients postoperatively, an incidence of 7.9%. The range of recurvatum was from 3 to 10 degrees with a mean of 5 degrees. Age at surgery, length of postoperative immobilization, level of ambulation, severity of straight leg raising limitation, release of both medial and lateral hamstrings, and concomitant surgery had no statistically significant effect upon the rate of recurvatum.

Discussion

The decision as to which surgical procedure to use for lengthening the hamstring muscles depends on: (1) the effectiveness of the proce-

Table 1 Concomitant surgical procedures

Procedure	No. of Patients
Varus rotation osteotomy—proximal femur	10
Hip plate removal	12
Adductor tenotomy	11
Adductor transfer	48
Iliopsoas release	5
Salter osteotomy	3
Proximal rectus femoris release	6
Tendon Achilles lengthening	55
Posterior tibial tendon transfer or recession	13
Peroneus brevis transfer/lengthening	6
Peroneus longus lengthening	5
Supramalleolar osteotomy of tibia	3
Triple arthrodesis	1
Elbow flexor release and flexor carpiulnaris transfer	1
Mitchell procedure—great toe	1

dure in achieving the desired goals; (2) the incidence of complications and undesirable results; (3) the rate of recurrence and recurvatum; and (4) the technical simplicity and consistency of the procedure.

Complex transfers of the hamstrings have been largely abandoned. These include Silverskiöld's[6] proximal transfer of the origin of the hamstrings to the proximal femur, Eggers'[7] transfer of the distal hamstrings to the distal femur, and Evans' modification of the Eggers procedure.[8] Occasionally, medial hamstring transfers to the lateral femoral condyle are performed to improve external rotation of the thigh.[2,9]

Reimers[10] has compared the results of the modified Eggers procedure, distal hamstring lengthenings, and proximal release. The modified Eggers procedure consists of Z lengthening of the biceps femoris, tenotomy of the gracilis, and transposition of the semitendinosus and semimembranosus to the posterior femoral condyles with no shortening of the patellar ligament or division of the patellar retinaculum. One of the patients who had a modified Eggers procedure developed hip hyperextension bilaterally, and three patients who had distal hamstring lengthenings developed a recurrence three months postoperatively. Reimers recommends the proximal release of hamstrings in patients who do not have knee flexion contractures greater than 5 degrees.

Baumann and associates[11] prefer distal hamstring lengthenings. They caution that postoperative hyperlordosis and genu recurvatum are usually caused by excessive lengthenings and by impairment of the function of the semimembranosus and biceps femoris muscles.

Hsu and Li[12] reported on 49 distal hamstring elongations, 36 of which involved both medial and lateral hamstrings lengthenings. They employed a Z-plasty lengthening for the semitendinosus and an aponeurectomy of the semimembranosus and biceps tendons. Ten of their patients developed a stiff knee gait pattern, eight had increased lordosis, and one patient had excessive lumbar lordosis.

Campos da Paz and associates[13] reported a 40% incidence of recurrence in patients who had distal hamstring lengthenings and a 40% rate of recurvatum in hamstring transfers. They found no correlation between age at surgery and rate of recurrence. Proximal hamstring releases have been described in the literature by other authors.[10,14–16]

The complexity of the operation and the need to perform other surgeries simultaneously must be considered in selecting the most successful method of hamstring elongation with the smallest incidence of undesirable effects. In my opinion the direct, posterior approach for visualization of the distal hamstrings is simple and safe. The semitendinosus and gracilis require only tenotomies. The semimembranosus can be fractionally lengthened by an aponeurectomy, thereby partially preserving its function in extending the hip and flexing the knee. If it is necessary for achievement of an adequate straight leg raising of 70 degrees, the biceps femoris can be approached through a separate small lateral incision and an aponeurectomy performed. The lateral popliteal or common peroneal nerve in this area is easily identified and protected.

Operating on the hamstrings with the patient in the supine position allows measurement of straight leg raising and popliteal angles. These measurements enable the surgeon to determine how much the semimembranosus must be lengthened and whether or not the biceps femoris requires elongation as well. Although no postoperative nerve palsies were encountered with the distal lengthenings, two patients had painful paresthesias in their feet for as long as 6 months after surgery. These patients had medial and lateral hamstring lengthenings for preoperative straight leg raising of 45 and 50 degrees and popliteal angles of 90 and 80 degrees. Final straight leg raising after surgery was 70 and 75 degrees. I believe that the paresthesias resulted from the lateral popliteal nerve being stretched when testing for straight leg raising range. Both patients recovered completely. A compartment type syndrome for the peroneal nerve has been described and may contribute to this complication.[17–20]

Because this study of distal hamstring lengthenings is retrospective, gait analysis is not included in the evaluation of the results. However, Thometz and associates,[21] in describing the effect upon gait of lengthening of the medial hamstrings, reported no change in velocity, stride length, or cadence. They did report marked improvement in extension of the knee during the stance phase of gait, but noted that the arc of motion remained unchanged, with an increase of knee extension accompanied by a decrease of knee flexion. An average 5-degree increase in anterior pelvic tilt was observed but not found to be significant. Their study demonstrated only two statistically significant correlations: (1) improvement in straight leg raising correlated strongly with improvement in maximum extension of the knee (0.45); and (2) final straight leg raising and final maximum knee extension had the strongest correlation (0.65). Another important point in their paper was that patients whose preoperative knee flexion was normal by midstance were at highest risk for recurvatum. The results and conclusions derived from the clinical study at The Hospital for Special Surgery correlate well with this gait analysis study.

Conclusions

A retrospective study of 242 knees in 125 cerebral palsy patients, with a minimum three-year follow-up, indicated that distal tenotomy of the semitendinosus and gracilis and aponeurectomy of the semimembranosus are a safe and effective method of improving straight leg raising and the popliteal angle. An aponeurectomy of the biceps femoris was added in 39 patients. The incidence of recurvatum was 7.9% (18 knees in 10 patients), and the range was from 3 to 10 degrees. Although regression to the preoperative straight leg raising value occurred in 33% (82 knees in 46 patients), only 17% (42 knees in 22 patients) required additional hamstring lengthenings. None of the many variables studied correlated with the occurrence of genu recurvatum, and the only significant correlation with the recurrence of hamstring tightness was the degree of severity preoperatively, ie, those knees with 45 degrees or less of straight leg raising had a statistically smaller incidence of recurrence than those with straight leg raising of greater than 45 degrees (p = 0.001). Concomitant surgery on the hip, foot, or ankle was performed on 85% of the population (107 patients). There was no correlation with either recurrence rate or recurvatum. When all these factors are considered, I recommend that distal hamstring lengthenings, as described in this chapter, be performed for those patients who have limited straight leg raising and exhibit either a crouched pattern of walking or show interference with sitting due to hamstring tightness.

References

1. Gage JR: Surgical treatment of the knee dysfunction in cerebral palsy. *Clin Orthop* 1990;253:45–54.
2. Sutherland DH, Cooper L: The pathomechanics of progressive crouch gait in spastic diplegia. *Orthop Clin North Am* 1978;9:143–154.
3. Sutherland DH, Schottstaedt ER, Larsen LJ, et al: Clinical and electromyographic study of seven spastic children with internal rotation gait. *J Bone Joint Surg* 1969;51A:1070–1082.
4. Simon SR: Symposium: Management of cerebral palsy in the lower extremities. *Contemp Orthop* 1988;16:79–110.
5. Dhawlikar SH, Root L, Mann RL: Long-term retrospective analysis of distal hamstrings lengthening in cerebral palsy. *J Bone Joint Surg*, in press.
6. Silverskiöld N: Reduction of the uncrossed two-joint muscles of the leg to one-joint muscles in spastic conditions. *Acta Chir Scand* 1923;56:315–330.
7. Eggers GWN: Transplantation of hamstring tendons to femoral condyles in order to improve hip extension and to decrease knee flexion in cerebral spastic paralysis. *J Bone Joint Surg* 1952;34A:827–830.
8. Evans EB, Julian JD: Modification of the hamstring transfer. *Dev Med Child Neurol* 1966;8:539–551.
9. Ray RL, Ehrlich MG: Lateral hamstring transfer and gait improvement in the cerebral palsy patient. *J Bone Joint Surg* 1979;61A:719–723.
10. Reimers J: Contracture of the hamstrings in spastic cerebral palsy. A study of three methods of operative correction. *J Bone Joint Surg* 1974;56B:102–109.
11. Baumann JU, Ruetsch H, Schurmann K: Distal hamstring lengthening in cerebral palsy: An evaluation by gait analysis. *J Int Orthop* 1980;3:305–309.
12. Hsu LCS, Li HSY: Distal hamstring elongation in the management of spastic cerebral palsy. *J Pediatr Orthop* 1990;10:378–381.

13. Campos da Paz A, Nomura AN, Braga LW, et al: Speculations on cerebral palsy. *J Bone Joint Surg* 1984;66B:283.

14. Drummond DS, Rogala E, Templeton J, et al: Proximal hamstring release for knee flexion and crouched posture in cerebral palsy. *J Bone Joint Surg* 1974; 56A:1598–1602.

15. Seymour N, Sharrard WJW: Bilateral proximal release of the hamstrings in cerebral palsy. *J Bone Joint Surg* 1968;50B:274–277.

16. Sharps CH, Clancy M, Steel HH: Long term retrospective study of proximal hamstring release for hamstring contracture in cerebral palsy. *J Pediatr Orthop* 1984;4:443–447.

17. Adkison DP, Bosse MJ, Gaccione DR, et al: Anatomical variations in the course of the superficial peroneal nerve. *J Bone Joint Surg* 1991;73A:112–114.

18. Kernohan J, Levack B, Wilson JN: Entrapment of the superficial peroneal nerve. Three case reports. *J Bone Joint Surg* 1985;67B:60–61.

19. Mubarak SJ, Owen CA: Double-incision fasciotomy of the leg for decompression in compartment syndromes. *J Bone Joint Surg* 1977;59A:184–187.

20. Styf J: Entrapment of the superficial peroneal nerve. Diagnosis and results of decompression. *J Bone Joint Surg* 1989;71B:131–135.

21. Thometz J, Simon S, Rosenthal R: The effect on gait of lengthening of the medial hamstrings in cerebral palsy. *J Bone Joint Surg* 1989;71A:345–353.

Chapter 25

Distal Hamstring Lengthening/Release and Rectus Femoris Transfer

James R. Gage, MD

Normal Function

Before discussing the pathology of the knee in cerebral palsy, it is necessary to understand its function in normal gait.

Knee Function in Stance

During stance, the knee has three principal functions: (1) Because the foot is fixed on the floor and the upper segments are rotating, the knee allows the necessary transverse rotation between the shank and the thigh. (2) The knee provides one of the two principal sources for shock absorption during initial contact and loading response through a gradual flexion of about 15 degrees in early stance. (3) Knee flexion during initial contact and progressive extension during midstance and terminal stance allow energy conservation by reducing the vertical excursion of the body's center of mass.

Knee Function in Swing

During the swing phase of walking, the primary function of the knee is to provide clearance for the foot. This is necessary in normal gait because the pelvis drops about 5 degrees on the swing side, which prevents excessive vertical excursion of the center of gravity. Therefore, to obtain foot clearance, the limb must be shortened on the swing side via knee flexion. Furthermore, the foot is still in relative equinus during initial swing, necessitating an even greater amount of knee flexion. As a result, about 62 degrees of knee flexion is required to clear the swinging foot during swing phase.

Knee Kinematics and Kinetics

Kinematics: Stance and Swing

The normal kinematics of the knee in the sagittal plane are seen in Figure 1. There are two periods of flexion. The initial flexion wave

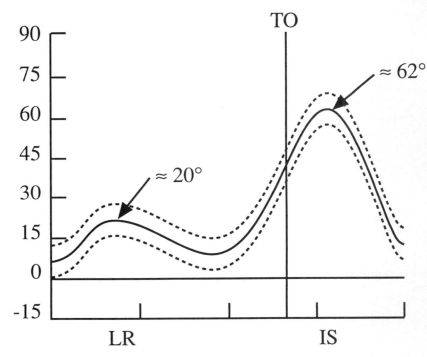

Fig. 1 *Knee kinematics. Gait cycle is on the axis and degrees of motion is on the abscissa. The vertical line represents toe-off. The sold line represents the mean, and the dotted lines one standard deviation. There are two periods of flexion; the first, during loading response, is for shock absorption, and the second, which peaks during initial swing, is to provide foot clearance. (Reproduced with permission from Gage JR: Gait Analysis in Cerebral Palsy. London, MacKeith Press with Blackwell Scientific Publications, 1991, p 86.)*

begins from a position of nearly full extension at initial contact and reaches a maximum of 15 degrees during loading response, a condition that helps decelerate the inertia forces of the body. Then, progressive extension continues until the end of terminal stance. With the onset of double support (preswing), the knee shows rapid flexion to a position of about 40 degrees by toe-off. Flexion continues to a peak of just over 60 degrees to allow toe clearance in initial swing. Then the knee continues to extend during midswing and terminal swing so that it is once again in a position of nearly full extension by the beginning of the next gait cycle.

Kinetics: Stance

The kinetics of the knee during a normal gait cycle are fairly complex. At initial contact the ground-reaction force (GRF) passes at or close to the center of the knee joint. Both hamstrings and quadriceps are active at this time for two reasons: (1) The GRF is roughly neutral

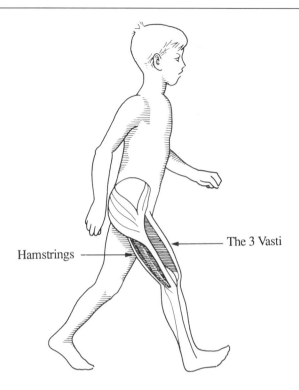

Hamstrings

The 3 Vasti

Fig. 2 *Hamstrings as hip extensors. During loading, response weight is accepted via knee flexion. Thus, the GRF falls behind the knee joint. Because this moment must be balanced or the knee would collapse into flexion, the quadriceps must be active to provide the needed extension moment at the knee. The hamstrings are also active at this time. It would appear that with the quadriceps (particularly the three vasti) preventing collapse of the knee, the hamstrings can act at the hip to assist the gluteus maximus in exerting the extension moment, which is necessary during this portion of the gait cycle both to stabilize the hip from the flexion moment created by the GRF and to provide the acceleration necessary for forward propulsion of the trunk.*

with respect to flexion and extension. If it moves anteriorly or posteriorly only a few millimeters, muscle action will be necessary to stabilize the knee. Thus, both muscle groups must be ready to exert control. (2) If the hamstrings are to act as accelerators of the hip joint, they must function as monoarticular muscles, ie, they must actively extend the hip but cannot flex the knee, or stance phase stability will be lost. This can be accomplished if the three vasti, the vastus intermedius, the vastus lateralis, and the vastus medialis, fire concurrently with the hamstrings (Fig. 2).

During midstance, the GRF is maintained anterior to the knee joint and posterior to the hip joint, making both joints inherently stable via their ligamentous structures, ie, the knee is prevented from hyperextension by the posterior capsule and cruciate ligaments and the hip is

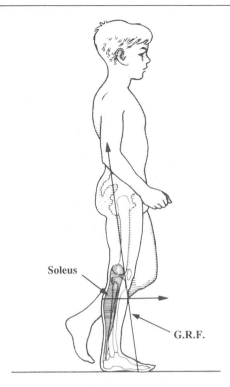

Fig. 3 *The function of the soleus. If the GRF is maintained posterior to the hip and anterior to the knee, both joints are stable in the sagittal plane via the iliofemoral ligament and the posterior knee capsule, respectively. Therefore, the soleus can stabilize all three major joints of the lower extremity (ankle, hip, and knee) by eccentrically retarding the forward progress of the tibia in midstance so that no other muscle action is necessary to stabilize the hip and/or knee.*

prevented from hyperextension by the iliofemoral ligament. Thus, all three major joints of the lower extremity (ankle, hip, and knee) can be stabilized by eccentric action of the triceps surae, and no sagittal plane muscle action is necessary at the hip or knee (Fig. 3). In terminal stance, gastrocnemius and soleus muscles, acting together, reverse the eccentric contraction at the ankle that was present in midstance, and concentric contraction (acceleration) begins. The knee is still stable because both GRF and inertial forces are maintaining it in extension. Preswing begins with the onset of double support (initial contact of the opposite limb) (Fig. 4). The hip flexors now begin concentric contraction, which accelerates the thigh into flexion. The body has also moved forward sufficiently so that the GRF now passes posterior to the knee, producing a strong flexion moment. As weight is unloaded onto the other side, the combination of thigh flexion and the posterior GRF drives the knee into flexion. At the time of toe-off, the knee is flexed approximately 40 degrees and stance phase is over.

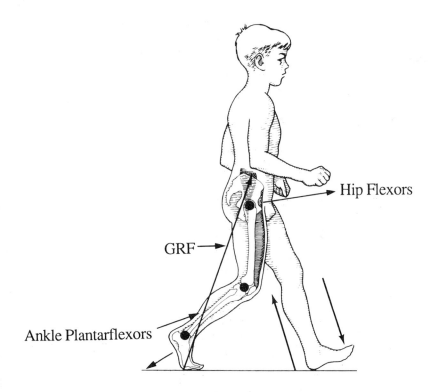

Fig. 4 *Knee flexion in preswing. Because the gastrocnemius originates in the posterior femur, it acts as a powerful knee flexor once the body's mass starts to be transferred to the forward limb. In addition, the hip flexors now begin concentric contraction that accelerates the thigh into flexion. Finally, the body has moved forward sufficiently that the GRF now passes well posterior to the knee, producing a strong flexion moment. As weight is unloaded onto the other side, these three factors combine to drive the knee into flexion. By the time of toe-off, the knee is flexed approximately 40 degrees and stance phase is over.*

Kinetics: Swing

At normal walking cadence, flexion and extension of the knee during swing are completely passive, and the leg acts as a simple pendulum with its point of fixation at the knee. If no muscles crossed the knee, the period of the pendulum would be dependent only on gravity and the mass moment of inertia of the leg.[1] In that situation, cadence could not be altered except perhaps by changing the mass of the leg by adding or subtracting a heavy shoe. However, cadence can be altered by muscle action. Because knee flexion is passive, walking speed can be increased

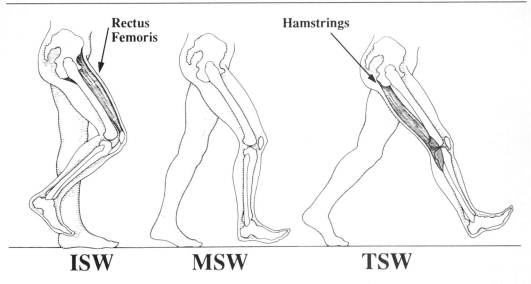

Fig. 5 *The swing phase of gait consists of three periods known as initial swing (ISW), midswing (MSW), and terminal swing (TSW). Midswing is a switching period when no muscles are active. During running or fast walking, the rectus femoris accelerates the shank in initial swing, and the hamstrings decelerate it in terminal swing. (Reproduced with permission from Gage JR:* Gait Analysis in Cerebral Palsy. *London, MacKeith Press with Blackwell Scientific Publications, 1991, p 74.)*

by putting more energy into the hip flexors and triceps surae. If this were done, however, the knee would flex excessively, just as in the prosthetic knee joint of an above-knee amputee when there is too little friction built into the joint.

The rectus femoris originates in the anteroinferior spine of the pelvis and inserts into the patella. Thus, if it were contracting concentrically at both ends, it would be a flexor of the hip and an extensor of the knee. During rapid gait, however, the rectus femoris contracts concentrically at the hip to assist with acceleration and eccentrically at the knee as a decelerator; at the knee it works like a door spring to prevent excessive flexion. The muscle, therefore, is working relatively isometrically as a spring and acts to transfer energy from the shank to the hip. Its major period of activity is during preswing and initial swing. Midswing is a switching period between the rectus femoris and the hamstring, hence, there is no muscle activity across the knee during this period. With the onset of terminal swing, eccentric hamstring activity begins to decelerate both the hip and knee (Fig. 5). In the opposite scenario, when the cadence is slower than normal, passive knee flexion is inadequate during initial swing and must be augmented by the gracilis, sartorius, and short head of the biceps; at the end of swing, knee extension must be augmented by the quadriceps. Because the period of required rectus femoris activity occupies approximately 20% of the gait cycle, at a cadence of 120 steps per minute the muscle would be active for only

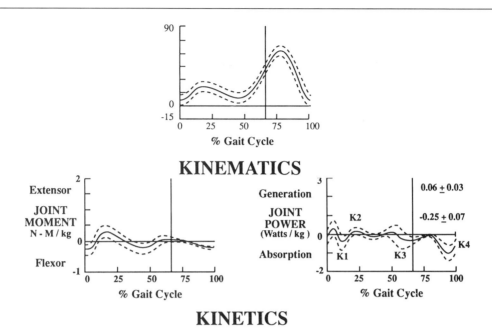

KINEMATICS

KINETICS

Fig. 6 *An illustration of normal knee kinematics and kinetics. The solid line represents the mean, and the dotted line one standard deviation. Throughout the period of knee flexion that occurs in loading response, there is an extensor moment indicating that the flexion is under quadriceps control. At the end of loading response until toe-off, a flexor moment begins, which indicates that throughout the remainder of stance, the quadriceps are inactive. During this latter portion of stance, knee stability is provided by the triceps surae via a plantarflexion/knee-extension couple. The joint power graph indicates that very little power is generated by the knee during normal walking, rather power is being transferred through the knee to the segment above or below. (Reproduced with permission from Gage JR:* Gait Analysis in Cerebral Palsy. *London, MacKeith Press with Blackwell Scientific Publications, 1991, p 86.)*

one tenth of a second and the period of hamstring activity would be similar. Therefore, in order to achieve normal gait, the control and timing of these muscles must be very precise. The normal kinematic and kinetic graphs of the knee are shown in Figure 6, and a schematic illustration of the timing and type of muscle action required for normal function is shown in Figure 7.

Pathologic Gait

Characteristics of cerebral palsy include abnormal tone, muscle imbalance between agonists and antagonists across joints, loss of selective muscle control, and dependence on primitive reflexes for ambulation. Because of these abnormalities, cospasticity of agonists and antagonists occurs during gait. In the tug-of-war created between the hamstrings and the quadriceps, normal sleeping and sitting positions

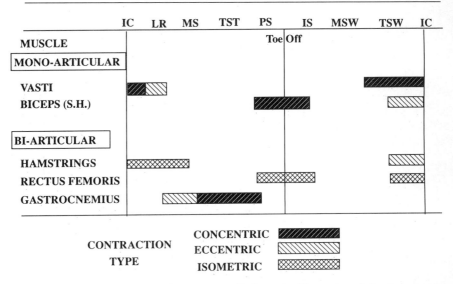

Fig. 7 *Muscle control of the knee in sagittal plane. An illustration of the timing and type of action of the muscles that control knee flexion-extension during one gait cycle. Initial contact (IC), toe-off (TO), and the subphases of stance and swing are labeled across the top. Notice that quadriceps activity ends with the end of loading response (LR) and that knee extension is maintained by the restraining action of the triceps surae throughout the remainder of stance (midstance (MS) and terminal stance (TST). The short head of the biceps and rectus femoris act during preswing (PS) and initial swing (ISW). The former acts to augment knee flexion during slow walking, whereas the latter acts to restrain excessive knee flexion during rapid gait. (Reproduced with permission from Gage JR:* Gait Analysis in Cerebral Palsy. *London, MacKeith Press with Blackwell Scientific Publications, 1991, p 87.)*

favor knee flexion (hamstrings). Gravitational forces also favor knee flexion; hence, hamstring contracture with knee flexion in stance is common in cerebral palsy. The high tone setting of both agonists and antagonists and their cospasticity produce an effect similar to that obtained by greatly increasing the friction setting in the knee of an amputee. The result is a restricted arc of swing and limited flexion-extension motion. This, in turn, results in difficulty in foot clearance during swing. The level of control necessary for normal function of muscles that cross more than one joint is significantly greater than the level of control necessary to manage a muscle that crosses only one joint. The hamstrings, gastrocnemius, and rectus femoris are all two-joint muscles that cross the knee, and must work in a coordinated fashion to provide the control required for normal function of this joint in gait. Given the pathology outlined, optimal treatment would need to be directed toward reducing the knee flexion forces during stance and augmenting sagittal plane motion during swing.

Crouch Gait

Knee flexion during stance can arise from several causes: (1) contracted hamstrings with resultant knee flexion contracture; (2) contrac-

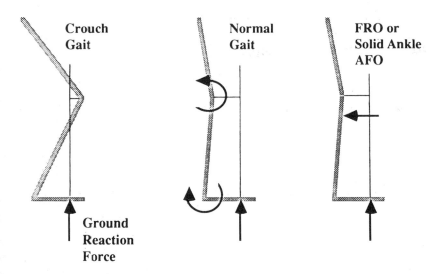

Crouch Gait

Normal Gait

FRO or Solid Ankle AFO

Ground Reaction Force

Fig. 8 *Excessive knee flexion in stance. In normal gait the knee is rendered stable in midstance and terminal stance via a plantarflexion/knee extension couple. If there is excessive knee flexion in midstance, the GRF moves behind the knee and generates a flexion moment that must be resisted by an internal (muscle) moment. The quadriceps are the principal muscles employed, but hip extensors can assist to some degree. AFO is ankle-foot orthosis, and FRO is floor reaction orthosis. (Reproduced with permission from Gage JR: Gait Analysis in Cerebral Palsy. London, MacKeith Press with Blackwell Scientific Publications, 1991, p 105.)*

ture of the hip flexors, which draws the upper end of the femur into flexion that must be balanced by an equal amount of flexion at the knee to keep the upper body centralized over the base of support; (3) inadequate strength of the triceps surae to decelerate the advancement of the tibia against the relatively stronger hamstrings and hip flexors; and (4) difficulties with balance and/or control.

In the past there has been a tendency to lengthen only one major muscle group at a time and then assess the result before doing more surgery. Because these children frequently walk on tiptoe, the most frequent operation has been Achilles tendon lengthening. However, if the triceps surae is lengthened in the presence of a static or dynamic contracture of either the hip flexors or the hamstrings, even more imbalance will be created at the knee, and with time and growth, the triceps surae will be unable to resist the contractures that develop at the joints above. In orthopaedic terms, overlengthened heel cords is a misnomer, as the triceps surae may well have been appropriately lengthened. However, if contractures or even excessive spasticity are left at the joints above, imbalance between agonists and antagonists will be increased, and therefore the magnitude of the flexion moment created by the GRF at the knee will be increased (Fig. 8). This results in increased tension forces on the triceps surae in midstance. Because muscles grow in response to tension,[2] (see chapter 20) the weakened triceps surae rapidly

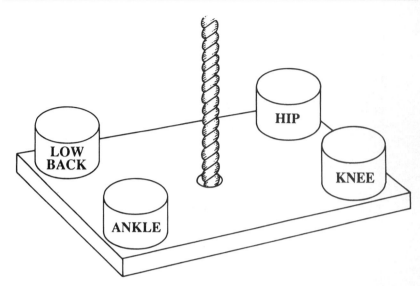

Fig. 9 *Balance between joints. A board suspended from a rope with a weight at each corner illustrates the concept of balance between the lower extremity joints and lumbar spine. For example, if surgery, such as Achilles tendon lengthening, is done in isolation it will upset the balance between the ankle below and the knee and hip above. The usual result is a reduction in the plantarflexion/knee extension couple such that the hip and knee flexors become dominant and contractures develop at those joints. The triceps surae is no longer strong enough to restrain the tibia in the face of the contractures above and the knee passes through the plane of the GRF so that it now generates an external flexion moment. The result is a crouch gait that is progressive over time. (Reproduced with permission from Gage JR: Gait Analysis in Cerebral Palsy.* London, MacKeith Press with Blackwell Scientific Publications, 1991, p 121.)

elongates further, and a vicious cycle is created, leading to progressive crouch.

The importance of balance in the surgical treatment of cerebral palsy is extremely important.[3,4] For example, isolated lengthening of the triceps surae will almost invariably lead to crouch, whereas isolated lengthening of hamstrings will lead to a stiff-limbed gait with increased lumbar lordosis and/or a forward trunk lean such that the patient requires crutches for balance.[5] In the sagittal plane, it is good to think of the low back, hip, knee, and ankle as four weights on the corners of a suspended board. If weight is removed from any corner in isolation, the board will tip. The only way to keep the board balanced is to add or subtract weight evenly at all four corners (Fig. 9). In general, the hip flexors, hamstrings, rectus femoris, and triceps surae all need to be addressed in concert to keep the body balanced in the sagittal plane. At my hospital, gait analysis is usually performed to determine the degree of imbalance at each of the major lower extremity joints, and appropriate lengthenings are done of all contracted and/or dysfunctional musculature at hips, knees, and ankles during the course of a single

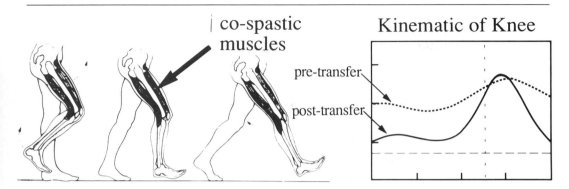

Fig. 10 *Hamstring lengthening and rectus femoris transfer. In cerebral palsy, the firing time of both the hamstrings and rectus femoris are prolonged. Therefore, in midswing, both muscle groups are active at a time when neither should be. As a result, the knee remains in flexion throughout stance and its range of motion is greatly diminished. Lengthening of the hamstrings in conjunction with transfer of the distal end of the rectus femoris back to the sartorius or gracilis will usually significantly improve function and range.*

surgical procedure in order to establish and maintain appropriate balance between joints. In most cases, a posterior transfer of the distal end of the rectus femoris is also required to balance the weakened hamstrings and unlock the knee in swing.

Rectus Femoris Transfer

As described above, the rectus femoris works principally in preswing and initial swing to augment hip flexion and prevent excessive knee flexion during rapid gait. However, in the child with cerebral palsy, the period of action of the rectus femoris is prolonged, and the muscle tends to fire continuously during the gait cycle or at least throughout the duration of swing phase. Furthermore, in a child with cerebral palsy, augmentation of swing phase knee flexion is usually required because these children tend to have inadequate acceleration forces at the hip and knee. Sutherland and associates[6] found some benefit in cerebral palsy gait by releasing the proximal end of the rectus femoris. However, Perry was the first to suggest posterior transfer of the distal end of the rectus femoris so that the muscle can actually augment knee flexion during swing.[7] My first rectus femoris transfer was carried out in 1982 with excellent results (Fig. 10). Between Newington and Gillett Children's Hospitals, I have now done several hundred.

In a recent paper presented at the American Academy of Cerebral Palsy and Developmental Medicine, the results of three different surgical approaches to the knee in cerebral palsy were compared: (1) simple hamstring lengthening; (2) hamstring lengthening with distal rectus femoris release; and (3) hamstring lengthening with rectus femoris transfer.[7] Of the three methods, hamstring lengthening in conjunction

Table 1 Comparison of results of surgical approaches to the knee in cerebral palsy

Type of Procedure	Number	Mean Increased Range of Motion (degrees)	Significance
Hamstring lengthening only	19	9	p < 0.01
Hamstring lengthening + rectus femoris release	21	9	not significant
Hamstring lengthening + lateral rectus femoris transfer	12	7	not significant
Hamstring lengthening + medial rectus femoris transfer	64	17	p < 0.01

with rectus femoris transfer was far superior, providing all the prerequisites to the procedure were met (Table 1). Not only did the rectus femoris transfer increase the range of knee motion during swing, it also improved the timing of knee flexion. In normal gait, peak knee flexion occurs in initial swing when the foot is still in equinus and maximum toe clearance is needed. In cerebral palsy gait, peak knee flexion is later, usually occurring in midswing. This results in loss of foot clearance in initial swing. Rectus femoris transfer tends to restore the timing of knee flexion in swing, whereas simple hamstring lengthening and/or distal rectus release does not. Thus, when the rectus femoris transfer is performed there is improved foot clearance during walking, which comes about as result of the improvements in both the range and the timing of knee flexion in swing. During analysis of results, however, it became clear that transfer medially to the sartorius or gracilis was superior to lateral transfer into the iliotibial band. Furthermore, the procedure was effective only if the following prerequisites either were present or could be established: (1) Hamstring contractures must be corrected, and the knee must be able to come to full extension in midstance. (2) The foot must be plantargrade and stable in stance. Valgus and/or varus deformities of the foot must be correctable either through bracing or surgery. (3) The foot must be in the line of progression or else a moment arm adequate to maintain knee extension in midstance and terminal stance cannot be generated (Fig. 11). Minor malrotation of 10 degrees or less, particularly if it is dynamic, can be accepted, but greater magnitudes of malrotation must be corrected surgically with bony osteotomies.

Initially, I believed that dynamic deformities could be corrected by transferring the rectus femoris to an insertion that would provide a corrective torque in the transverse plane, that is, either laterally to the biceps femoris or medially and posteriorly to the stump of the semitendinosus. However, a recent review of all rectus femoris interventions at Newington Children's Hospital revealed that the insertion site of the rectus femoris has no statistical effect on the rotation of the limb in gait.[8] However, major malrotations of the femur or tibia must be corrected with osteotomy to get the foot into the line of progression so that an adequate plantarflexion/knee extension couple can be generated

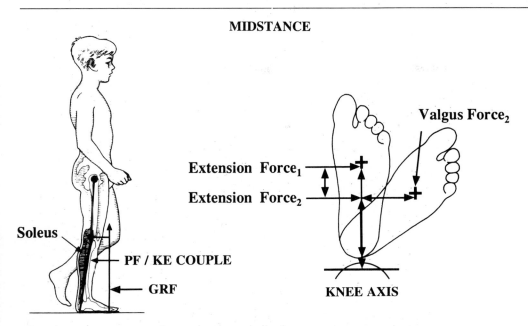

Fig. 11 *Lever arm deficiency. Muscles always work as part of a force-couple (force x distance to the center of the axis of motion). Therefore, the plantarflexion/knee extension (PF/KE) couple depends on the appropriate alignment and rigidity of the foot. If this is not present, the extension moment against the knee will be inadequate even with adequate strength of the triceps surae.*

against the hamstrings. (4) In the case of an overlengthened or weak posterior calf, an adequate plantarflexion/knee extension couple must be restored through the use of a floor-reaction type of ankle-foot orthosis to prevent excessive ankle dorsiflexion and secondary excessive knee flexion in midstance (Fig. 12). (5) Adequate acceleration forces must be present to flex the hip and propel the limb through swing.

Surgical Technique

In the ambulating patient, rectus femoris transfer is indicated if the Duncan-Ely test is positive. The Duncan-Ely test is based on the fact that the rectus femoris spans both the knee and the hip. With the patient lying prone, the knee is flexed quickly, and the examiner looks for a rise of the buttocks and feels for increased tone within the limb. Dynamic electromyography is very useful in addition to the rectus femoris test, because it will prove that the rectus femoris is overactive if the electromyogram is continuously active throughout swing. Because overactvity of the rectus femoris produces limitation of knee flexion in swing, in the Gillette Children's Hospital laboratory, we like to see that the total range of knee flexion during swing is diminished by 15 degrees or more before doing the procedure. Ideally, then, the decision is best made using a combination of the clinical evaluation

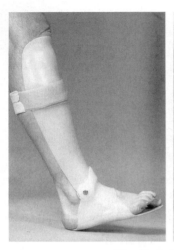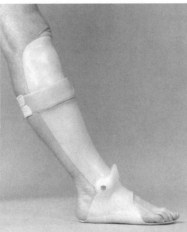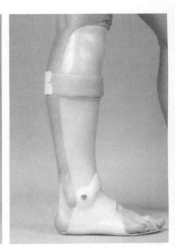

Fig. 12 *A floor reaction ankle-foot orthosis. A rear entry, hinged, floor reaction, ankle-foot orthosis will allow free ankle movement in plantarflexion during first and third rockers, but will restrict dorsiflexion in second rocker. Therefore, the forward motion of the tibia is restricted in second rocker and as a result, the extension moment generated at the knee is increased as the ground reaction moves further anterior to the knee. (Reproduced with permission from Gage JR:* Gait Analysis in Cerebral Palsy. *London, MacKeith Press with Blackwell Scientific Publications, 1991, p 140.)*

plus gait analysis. However, if gait analysis is not available it would be necessary to rely on slow motion video of the patient's gait to prove that the total range of knee motion is diminished and on the clinical evaluation alone (positive Duncan-Ely sign) to prove that the muscle is spastic and the patient would benefit from rectus femoris transfer.

In performing the transfer, separation of the rectus femoris from the rest of the quadriceps is usually best done at least 4 to 5 cm proximal to the patella. The tendon is wide but quite flat in its anteroposterior diameter, and an inexperienced surgeon is likely to take the central portion of the vastus intermedius with the rectus femoris if it is not carefully identified. Once the rectus femoris has been separated from the underlying vasti, the proper interval can be determined by inserting a finger proximally and palpating the underside of the muscle belly of the rectus femoris. At a point about 3 cm above the patella, the rectus femoris blends into the common quadriceps tendon and further separation is impossible. It must be tenotomized at this point or the suprapatellar pouch will be entered. Once the rectus is isolated and released from its insertion, it should be freed proximally along its medial and lateral edges so that the muscle can follow the line of transfer.

The distal end of the rectus femoris has been transferred into any of several locations: the sartorius, the gracilis, the distal stump of the semitendinosus, or the iliotibial band. Following a recent study of all of the rectus femoris transfers I performed since I started doing the transfer in 1982, I have discarded the lateral transfer into the iliotibial band and the medial transfer to the stump of the semitendinosus.[8] The former was discarded because in this larger, more recent study, it did not statistically change transverse rotation, nor was it as effective in increasing sagittal plane motion as were the transfers to the other sites. The later transfer, to the distal stump of the semitendinosus, was also discarded because it necessitated sacrificing the semitendinosus which, in the postoperative gait studies, frequently resulted in excessive lumbar lordosis. Thus, the distal end of the rectus femoris is now being transferred medially to either the sartorius or the gracilis.

For transfer to the sartorius, the medial intramuscular septum is opened as far proximally and distally as possible, the sartorius is brought up into the anterior compartment in continuity, and the rectus femoris is wrapped around the sartorius and sutured back to itself so that it encircles the muscle like a napkin ring. The repair is done with the knee flexed to about 35 degrees.

For transfer to the gracilis, the medial intramuscular septum is opened in the same manner and the gracilis is brought up into the anterior compartment in continuity. If the transfer were performed in the same manner as that described for the sartorius, the tension on the gracilis would increase considerably and would probably create an adduction contracture. Therefore, if the intramuscular tendon of the gracilis is large enough, it is tenotomized as far proximally as possible; the distal portion is stripped out of the gracilis, leaving the muscle intact; and the distal stump of the gracilis tendon is sutured directly to the distal end of the rectus femoris using a Pulvertaft anastomosis. If the tendon is not large enough to permit this, the transfer is performed in a manner similar to that described for the sartorius and then an intramuscular tenotomy of the gracilis tendon is done as close to the anastomosis as possible. In either event, the entire transfer can be done from the anterior thigh approach by opening the medial intramuscular septum; locating the sartorius posteriorly, taking care not to damage the vessels in the subsartorial canal; and then bringing the muscle into the anterior compartment in continuity. However, it is somewhat easier to free the gracilis and/or sartorius of their investing soft tissues through a posterior approach. If, as is usually the case, the hamstrings are to be lengthened as part of the procedure, both wounds are left open until after the completion of the rectus femoris transfer to facilitate exposure.

Transfer of the distal end of the rectus femoris to either the sartorius or the gracilis converts the rectus femoris from a hip flexor-knee extensor to a hip flexor-knee flexor during late stance and swing. Furthermore, prolonged action of the muscle, which almost always occurs in cerebral palsy, is no longer as critical because the muscle can now continue to act into terminal swing without interfering with gait. Thus, when the rectus femoris acts to augment hip flexion during preswing and initial swing, it will also flex the lower limb, which, in turn, will have the effect of facilitating swing phase foot clearance.

Techniques of hamstring lengthenings are well known and the specifics of lengthening will not be discussed here. However, it is important to remember that the hamstrings serve an important function in gait both as knee flexors and as hip extensors. As discussed earlier, because a hip flexion deformity tends to predominate in cerebral palsy, a person with spastic diplegia or quadriplegia will attempt to stabilize the knee with the quadriceps and then will call on the hamstrings to assist in hip extension during the first half of stance (Fig. 2). Weakening of the hamstrings by surgical lengthening allows more complete knee extension but invariably leads to weakening of hip extension, which may manifest itself either as excessive hip flexion or increased lumbar lordosis. For this reason, I no longer sacrifice the semitendinosus. If only the medial hamstrings are to be lengthened, I perform a Z-lengthening of the semitendinosus. In this event, the gracilis is usually used for the insertion point of the rectus femoris transfer, and the method I use to deal with it has already been described. The semimembranosus is lengthened by cutting its investing aponeurotic fascia at a 45-degree angle to the long axis of the muscle. Two or three such cuts can be made about 1 cm apart, taking care not to cut the underlying muscle fibers and stretching the muscle before making the next cut.

However, if both the medial and lateral hamstrings are to be lengthened, postoperative lordosis will invariably be a problem even if the hip flexors are also lengthened and the semitendinosus is lengthened rather than sacrificed. Eggers[9] tried to solve this dilemma by converting the hamstrings into pure hip extensors. He accomplished this by transferring their distal ends into the back of the femur, with disastrous results—many children lost knee flexion.

It recently occurred to me that Eggers may have had the right idea, but pursued it with too much enthusiasm. Therefore, if lengthening of both the medial and lateral hamstrings is required, I have started to transfer just the semitendinosus to the femur in conjunction with a judicious lengthening of the remaining hamstrings. The new insertion point of the semitendinosus is usually into the adductor magnus insertion, into the medial or lateral gastrocnemius origins, or directly into the femur. Although the transfer is done with the patient in a prone position and the hip in extension, I do not insert the semitendinosus under much tension, and I make a concerted attempt to preserve as much of the length of its tendon as possible. I take these precautions because in some of the first transfers, in which the semitendinosus was put directly into the femur under tension with sacrifice of much of the distal tendon, a loss of hip flexion in initial swing, with concomitant loss of step length, was apparent. Nevertheless, if this complication can be avoided, the conversion of the semitendinosus to a monoarticular muscle has the potential to accomplish two things: weakening the hamstrings as knee flexors while still preserving their power as hip extensors, and converting the semitendinosus from an internal to an external rotator if the insertion point of the transfer is taken lateral to the longitudinal axis of the femur.

After hamstring lengthening is performed, it should be possible to straight-leg raise the patient to 70 degrees. If the hamstrings are lengthened beyond this point, the patient may have recurvatum after surgery, during the stance phase of gait. In addition, if both medial and lateral hamstrings are lengthened, it is usually necessary to perform an intramuscular tenotomy of the psoas tendon as described by Salter[10] in order to maintain balance between the hip flexors and extensors.

Children who have had long-standing hamstring contractures may have fixed flexion deformity of the knee even after hamstring lengthening. My personal experience is that this disorder usually responds to serial casting in the postoperative period, although Bleck[3] recommends posterior capsulotomy or, if necessary, extension osteotomy of the distal femur. At any rate, if ambulation is the goal, then full knee extension is mandatory. Even for children who are nonambulatory, full knee extension is usually required for adequate transfers. Therefore, in the nonambulatory patient, I usually perform a distal rectus femoris release in conjunction with the hamstring lengthening to prevent the fixed extension that can occasionally occur in these children secondary to cospasticity of quadriceps and hamstrings. This is particularly likely to occur in a very spastic or mixed spastic-athetoid child who undergoes hamstring lengthening.

Stages of Recovery

Surgical recovery can be divided into three stages: (1) healing of soft tissues and bone (approximately 6 weeks); (2) strengthening (approximately 12 weeks); and (3) retraining of gait (approximately 12 months).

The Period of Healing

During the healing period, the child has pain and is vulnerable to injury. Traditional wisdom has dictated that the best way to deal with this is by immobilization. Unfortunately, byproducts of immobilization are weakness, osteopenia, and fibrosis with loss of motion. Dr. Michael Sussman, an orthopaedist then in Charlottesville, Virginia, was one of the first to suggest that these children should be rapidly mobilized after surgery (personal communication, 1978). After more than ten years of using early mobility in the rehabilitation of these children, I am convinced that the benefits of early mobility far outweigh the risks.

With the single stage approach, many of these children will have up to 12 incisions combined with muscle lengthenings and transfers, osteotomies, and arthrodeses. Therefore, pain is the major problem during the first three days after surgery. I believe that there are three major components to the pain: tissue injury from the surgery itself; muscle spasms secondary to pain and the child's spasticity; and anxiety. Furthermore, each of the three components seems to augment or magnify the others. Thus, reduction of any one of the three components reduces them all. After I started doing selective dorsal rhizotomy, I soon noticed that the children who had had rhizotomy seemed to have far less pain and spasm during convalescence from subsequent orthopaedic procedures. Obviously that could be related to the diminished sensation produced by the rhizotomy of sensory rootlets. However, I believe that it is secondary to the normalized muscle tone, ie, the diminished spasticity. Good physiologic preparation before surgery is useful in reducing patient anxiety. However, despite the best efforts of psychologists, physicians, and parents, many children are still anxious. Therefore, because diazepam is a mild sedative, a good antianxiety agent, and one of the best acute muscle relaxants available, I believe it should be used routinely on these children for 48 to 72 hours. If the child is in an intensive care or good surgical support unit for the first 24 hours, I prefer to use the drug intravenously in small doses at three- to four-hour intervals. After 24 hours, diazepam can be given orally.

During the first eight years of the one-stage surgical approach, a variety of pain medications were tested, with generally poor results. Following surgery, the children (and their parents) would experience three very unpleasant days. However, in the past two years, caudal catheters have been used to deliver continuous bupivacaine hydrochloride or fentanyl infusion. In my hospital, the catheter is inserted at the beginning of the surgical procedure by the anesthesiologist, and the medications that are administered in the first 72 hours are ordered and monitored by the anesthesiologist. Bupivacaine hydrochloride is usually used during the surgery and fentanyl after surgery. However, with the combination of caudal fentanyl and small doses of oral or intravenous diazepam, postoperative pain can now be controlled very adequately. A Foley catheter is generally used during the first 36 to 48 hours to avoid having to move the patient excessively, for comfort, and to facilitate collection of accurate intake and output data. Because of the multiple surgical incisions, the long operating time, and the need for indwelling catheters, prophylactic antibiotics are routinely used for 24 to 48 hours. The usual choice is intravenous cefazolin at a daily dosage of 25 to 50 mg/kg.

Mobilization is generally started on the third day after surgery, after the Foley and caudal catheters have been removed. Casting above the knee is rarely done, because even if femoral osteotomies were done in conjunction with the procedures described for the knee, the AO hip plates provide adequate internal fixation. When I am not comfortable with the internal fixation, the two short leg casts are tied together with a bar, controlling transverse rotation of the lower extremities while still allowing flexion-extension mobility of the hips and knees. Knee immobilizers can be used over the casts to keep the knees in relative extension and to reduce risk of injury to the hamstring lengthenings and/or rectus femoris transfers. If transfer of the distal end of the semitendinosus to the femur has been done, the hips are not permitted to be flexed more than 45 degrees for the first 14 days after surgery. This means that the child must sit in a reclining back wheelchair. It does not, however, prevent the child from standing and/or walking during that time, as long as a standing position can be assumed without excessive hip flexion. On or about the third day after surgery, the knee immobilizers are removed by the physical therapist in order to begin gentle, passive, range of motion exercise of the hips and knee. At the end of the therapy session, the knee immobilizers are reapplied.

If no long bone osteotomies or subtalar arthrodeses have been done, standing can begin on the fourth or fifth day after surgery and walking in parallel bars begins as soon thereafter as the patient can tolerate it. If osteotomies or arthrodeses have been done, weightbearing is not allowed on that side for three weeks. Once the patient is comfortable and afebrile, he/she is discharged and given a reclining back wheelchair for home use. This usually occurs on the fifth to seventh day after surgery. The physical therapist teaches the range of motion program to the parents so the child may continue the joint exercises three times daily at home. If the child uses a walker while in the hospital, a walker is also provided for home use. Knee immobilizers can be removed as soon as the child can adequately control the knee and prevent buckling when walking. As the walking program begins, the knee immobilizers are generally removed one at a time, starting with the strongest or least involved side. During subsequent sessions, they are alternated from side to side until both knees are stable enough that the immobilizers can be removed without fear of collapse while walking. Usually, the child is able to walk without the knee immobilizers, using a walker, in 14 to 21 days after surgery. By that time the child is alternating the daytime sitting position between knees extended (long sit position) and knees flexed and is sitting erect. To range the hips into extension, the patient is also spending several hours in each 24-hour period in the prone position.

The Period of Strengthening

Four weeks after surgery, the muscles are considered healed and physical therapy is shifted from walking and passive range of motion to vigorous stretching, muscle strengthening, and gait training. A stationary bicycle and swimming therapy are both very useful during this period. Although full healing and strengthening are usually complete by three months after surgery, gait usually continues to improve for a full year as the child learns to incorporate the new muscle lengths into his/her walking patterns. Postoperative gait analysis is then performed to assess the results of surgery and, if necessary, to fine-tune bracing and/or surgery.

References

1. Hicks R, Tashman S, Cary JM, et al: Swing phase control with knee friction in juvenile amputees. *J Orthop Res* 1985;3:198–201.
2. Ziv I, Blackburn N, Rang M: Muscle growth in normal and spastic mice. *Dev Med Child Neurol* 1984;15:94–99.
3. Bleck EE: *Orthopaedic Management in Cerebral Palsy.* Philadelphia, JB Lippincott, 1987, pp 351–354.
4. Rang M, Silver R, de la Garza J: Cerebral palsy, in Lovell WW, Winter RB (eds): *Pediatric Orthopaedics*, ed 2. Philadelphia, JB Lippincott, 1986, p 365.
5. Baumann JU, Ruetsch H, Schurmann K: Distal hamstring lengthening in cerebral palsy. An evaluation by gait analysis. *Int Orthop* 1980;3:305–309.

6. Sutherland DH, Larsen LJ, Mann R: Rectus femoris release in selected patients with cerebral palsy: A preliminary report. *Dev Med Child Neurol* 1975;17:26–34.

7. Gage JR, Perry J, Hicks RR, et al: Rectus femoris transfer to improve knee function of children with cerebral palsy. *Dev Med Child Neurol* 1987;29:159–166.

8. Muik E, Ounpuu S, Gage JR, et al: The effects of rectus femoris transfers on sagittal plane kinematics. *Dev Med Child Neurol* 1990;31(suppl 62):8.

9. Eggers GWN: Transplantaton of hamstring tendons to femoral condyles in order to improve hip extension and to decrease knee flexion in cerebral spastic paralysis. *J Bone Joint Surg* 1952;34A:827–830.

10. Salter RB: Role of innominate osteotomy in the treatment of congenital dislocation and subluxation of the hip in the older child. *J Bone Joint Surg* 1966;48A:1413–1439.

Consensus

Definition of Crouched Gait

Crouched gait is commonly recognizable, but has not always been specifically defined. In crouched gait, the knee lacks normal dynamic extension during stance phase; the ankles may be plantarflexed, neutral, or dorsiflexed; and the hips generally are flexed, and often are internally rotated and adducted.

The issue of walking with or without aids appears to have little to do with the specific definition of crouched gait. Younger children or those with weakness or more severe neurologic involvement may use aids and still exhibit crouch.

Causes of Crouched Gait

Despite the persistent knee flexion of crouched gait, it should be emphasized that quadriceps weakness is not a factor in this condition. The hamstrings frequently exhibit static contractures and/or dynamic overactivity leading to relative shortening. High-riding patella (patella tendon elongation) may occur in long-standing crouched gait during growth and may cause knee pain or quadriceps dysfunction.

At the hip, there is a relative functional imbalance of the hip flexors and extensors that can lead to anterior pelvic tilt associated with dynamic or static hip flexion deformities. The hip flexors, which are contracted, may include iliopsoas, tensor fasciae latae, adductors, and gluteus minimus muscles; some or all of these might be involved. The role of weak hip extensors is unclear, but there may be relative gluteus maximus insufficiency in the face of flexor spasticity.

At the ankle, isolated iatrogenic overlength-ening of the gastrocnemius-soleus complex may exaggerate crouch. Equinus deformities (static or dynamic) may occur in isolation, but the most common cause of heel rise seems to be persistent knee flexion during stance.

At the foot, hindfoot valgus and midfoot abduction may lead to an ankle/foot leverage that is inadequate to encourage knee extension. Extensive external tibial rotation or midfoot breakdown would have the same adverse effect.

Balance and other central nervous system disorders may also play a role in the generation of crouch. This issue is covered elsewhere in this publication but should be taken into account by the surgeon evaluating patients with crouched gait for surgery, because nonmusculoskeletal causes might limit the success of surgical intervention.

Indications for Hamstring Surgery

Surgery is generally indicated for children who have spastic diplegia with crouched gait sufficient to cause knee symptoms or to lead to a realistic expectation of problems in later childhood. Although there is no absolute cookbook approach for such surgery, the following represent typical indications: (1) persistent knee flexion angle of 20 to 30 degrees during stance; (2) popliteal angle greater than 40 to 45 degrees or straight leg raise less than 45 degrees; and (3) when gait analysis is available, presence of hamstring overactivity (prolongation or premature activity) with the presence of persistent knee flexion of 20 to 30 degrees or inadequate knee extension in terminal swing. A dynamic quick-stretch test technique should be used to get a better idea of dynamic hamstring tightness. This surgery should be done when the child reaches relative maturity of gait (4 to 8 years of age).

In patients with crouched gait, if ankle surgery (gastrocnemius-soleus release) is contemplated, then hamstring tightness should be evaluated and, generally, should be treated at the same time. In addition, the hip should be examined and appropriately treated.

When there are significant variations from routine crouched gait, consultation with other experienced orthopaedists and/or three-dimensional gait analysis is recommended.

Other Indications for Hamstring Lengthening

If hip flexion deformity (contracture of 20 to 30 degrees) or excessive pelvic tilt is present, lengthening of the iliopsoas mechanism should be considered. The most popular method is aponeurotic lengthening at the pelvic brim. Permanent weakness may result if the iliopsoas tendon is released from the lesser trochanter in an ambulatory patient.

If dynamic adduction or static adduction contracture exists, percutaneous adductor longus tenotomy may be indicated. However, aggressive release may lead to hip weakness or pelvic instability in the ambulatory patient. In general, the surgeon should attempt to balance pelvic deformities (static or dynamic) without overweakening the muscles required to control the pelvis during stance and to accelerate the limb during swing.

Specific Techniques of Hamstring Lengthening

Distal hamstring surgery is performed most commonly in this country. Surgery may be done in the prone or supine position. However, if surgery is to be done in the prone position, a thorough examination must be done in the supine position after the patient is under anesthesia, including palpation of the medial and lateral hamstrings, so the surgeon will have a specific surgical plan before the patient is turned.

Medial hamstring lengthening may be done alone or in combination with lateral hamstring lengthening. Lateral hamstring lengthening must be performed along with medial in the older child. Isolated lateral hamstring lengthening alone is not indicated.

Specific management of individual muscles is outlined in the following guidelines: (1) semitendinosus, tenotomy or Z-lengthening; (2) gracilis, tenotomy, intramuscular tenotomy, or Z-lengthening; (3) semimembranosus, aponeurotomy without lengthening so much at any individual aponeurotomy that the muscle underneath is torn; performing several aponeurotomies or using a spiral aponeurotomy technique is preferred; and (4) lateral hamstrings, aponeurotomy. Recent electromyographic (EMG) evidence suggests that the biceps femoris short head is rarely spastic, and only the longus needs to be surgically lengthened.

The presence of knee flexion contracture in the younger child with crouched gait does not need to be addressed surgically if hamstring lengthening is performed. The residual contracture can be treated with casts or will gradually stretch out without the need to do capsulotomies.

Postoperative immobilization is generally brief, either with casts or splints. After that, management is variable. Some surgeons use night splints for 3 months, some use night splints for a long time if hamstrings are tight.

Rectus Femoris Transfer

Distal rectus femoris transfer to the sartorius, gracilis, or lateral knee structures has become an important procedure for patients undergoing hamstring lengthening, because of the frequent development of a stiff-knee gait following the improved knee extension seen after the lengthening. The specific indications have been worked out in the gait analysis laboratory, and include stiff-knee gait (prevention of adequate knee flexion during swing) and EMG evidence of prolonged swing-phase activity in the rectus femoris. Guidelines for rectus transfer in the absence of a gait analysis laboratory include a positive quick Duncan-Ely test preoperatively. Some surgeons feel that rectus transfer is indicated in nearly all patients with spastic diplegia who undergo hamstring lengthening for crouched gait. Rectus transfer may be indicated after rehabilitation from hamstring lengthening if a stiff-knee gait is present. The transfer itself may be medial to the gracilis or sartorius or lateral to the iliotibial band, although interference with the iliotibial band knee extensor function may occur.

Value of Gait Analysis

Gait analysis laboratories are not available to evaluate every patient with crouched gait. When adequate facilities for accurate gait analysis are present, and when knowledgeable individuals are available to interpret the studies, gait analysis is useful in determining the preoperative knee motion, presence of overactivity of individual hamstring muscles, presence of swing-phase rectus EMG activity, and documentation of stiff-knee gait. The laboratory might be particularly useful for complex cases that do not seem to follow routine patterns of movement or for patients for whom multiple complex combined procedures are being contemplated.

Suggested Research

There are numerous areas for research on treatment of the diplegic patient with crouched gait. The actual causes of crouched gait are unknown and the roles of hip flexor spasticity, gluteus maximus weakness, adductor tightness, foot and ankle deformities, and torsional deformities need to be clarified. The relationship between postoperative hamstring weakness and lumbar lordosis requires further elucidation. How central nervous system and balance dysfunction relates to crouched gait is unknown. The question of whether prolonged activity of hamstrings is due to spasticity or is a functional adaptation to help extend the hip or to compensate for a forward flexed posture needs investigation. The relationship of external tibial rotation as a late complication of medial hamstring lengthening alone needs to be defined. The role of anteversion in crouched/internal rotation gait, and the timing of its correction are areas of great concern and require investigation.

Section Eight
Tight Achilles Tendon

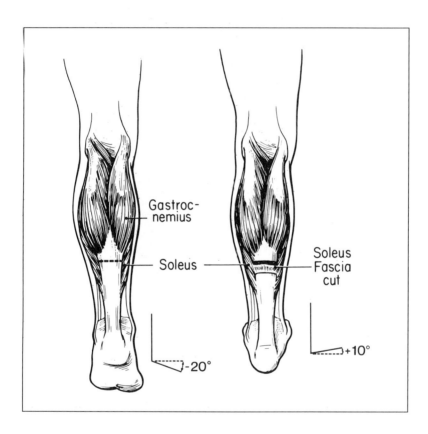

Chapter 26

Nonsurgical Treatment of Tight Achilles Tendon

John M. Mazur, MD
Daniel E. Shanks, MD
R. Jay Cummings, MD
William P. McCluskey, MD
Lisa Federico, PT
Melinda Goins, PT

Tight Achilles tendons in patients with spastic diplegia may be treated by both surgical and nonsurgical techniques. Current approaches include passive and active stretching, positioning, strengthening, the development of balance and coordination of movement, and the use of casts and ankle-foot orthoses to prevent secondary deformities and to improve function. Surgery is reserved for patients in whom physical therapy and bracing have not been successful. Lengthening the Achilles tendon in children who walk and stand with their knees flexed may result in severe knee flexion deformities with dorsiflexion of the ankles. Excessive dorsiflexion of the ankle from Achilles tendon surgery may, in turn, lead to a severely crouched position, making walking very difficult (Fig. 1).

Despite many years of experience with various therapeutic measures, the medical community is still divided as to the best treatment for tight Achilles tendon in cerebral palsy patients. Many of the approaches to the problem have been unsuccessful, and they may be lengthy, expensive, and even detrimental. In this chapter, we will review the advantages and disadvantages of the various nonsurgical treatments for tight Achilles tendons. These treatments will be discussed in terms of the cause and pathophysiology of a tight Achilles tendon. We will present available data that support the success or failure of the various treatment plans.

Pathophysiology

The gastrocnemius and soleus both insert into the os calcis via the Achilles tendon, but they have separate origins. The soleus comes from the posterior tibia and the gastrocnemius from the posterior distal femur. Electromyographic studies of normal walking show that both muscles act simultaneously during the stance phase of gait, beginning soon after heel strike and stopping just before toe off. Essentially, the two muscles function as one triceps surae muscle. The triceps surae muscle crosses and, therefore, helps control the movements of knee,

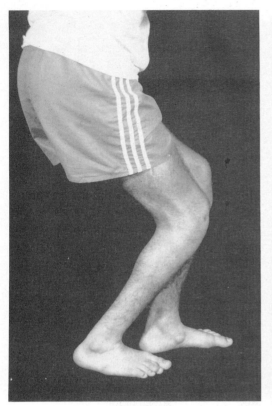 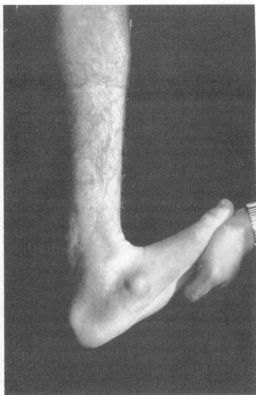

Fig. 1 *Left*, *16-year-old patient with spastic diplegia 2 years after bilateral heel-cord lengthening. The ankles are collapsing into dorsiflexion, and the knees and hips into flexion.* ***Right***, *Passive dorsiflexion of the ankle in the same patient. Note the excessive dorsiflexion secondary to the overlengthened heel cord.*

ankle, and subtalar joints. The coordinated, harmonious actions of the triceps surae, its antagonists (tibialis anterior, extensor digitorum longus, and extensor hallucis longus), and its synergists (flexor digitorum longus, flexor hallucis longus, peroneal, and tibial posterior) make it possible to have a normal heel-to-toe gait. In normal walking, the main function of the triceps surae is to prevent gravity from dorsiflexing the ankle in stance.

In normal individuals, the prevention of ankle dorsiflexion is important to the biomechanics of the knee in stance. If the triceps surae were absent or nonfunctional, the ankle would collapse into dorsiflexion, creating a force vector behind the knee axis of rotation, and lead to excessive knee flexion. The quadriceps would then have to work harder to prevent the knee from collapsing into flexion.

In the majority of children with spastic cerebral palsy, equinus deformity of the ankle and foot greatly disrupts walking and disturbs the normal biomechanics of the body. The triceps surae is hyperactive and may contract out of sequence, even into the swing phase of gait. The equinus deformity results from this spasticity and the exaggerated stretch reflex or it may be fixed because of permanent muscle and tendon shortening. A tight Achilles tendon usually will cause the patient to walk in a toe to toe or a toe to heel gait pattern, depending on the severity of the deformity and the body weight available to overcome the exaggerated stretch reflex of the calf muscle.

A taut Achilles tendon may also lead to genu recurvatum because of the biomechanical forces affecting the knee. If dorsiflexion of the ankle is prevented, the tibia becomes a lever that thrusts the knee into hyperextension when the foot touches the floor. If the hamstrings are also spastic, they may overcome the extension force vector that would produce recurvatum, and the knee will remain flexed in stance. Although the gastrocnemius crosses the knee posteriorly, it plays an insignificant role in producing a knee flexion deformity. Therefore, when a knee flexion contracture is present, it is likely to be caused by spastic hamstrings and not a spastic gastrocnemius.

Foot deformities are commonly associated with tight heel cords. With resistance to dorsiflexion, the calcaneus tends to rotate under the talus and become displaced laterally, and the talus drops into plantarflexion. The talus becomes very prominent, and the weightbearing forces become centered over the head of the talus, leading to painful callosities. If the peroneal muscles are spastic, the planovalgus deformity becomes even more accentuated. A spastic anterior tibial muscle can produce a varus force leading to an equinovarus foot and painful callosities over the fifth metatarsal. If the posterior tibial and toe flexors are spastic, a varus heel and forefoot will result. Thus, a tight heel cord is often only one factor of a multifactorial problem. The foot deformities resulting from a tight heel cord vary depending on the influence of associated spastic muscles and other biomechanical factors that may exist in the individual patient.

Rationale for Nonsurgical Treatment

Orthopaedic surgeons need to be open to all forms of treatment for tight Achilles tendons in children with spastic diplegia. Initially, nonsurgical treatment should be tried in all children, at least until the age of 4 years, because passive stretching, active exercises to strengthen the anterior tibial muscle, serial casting, inhibitive casts, and ankle-foot orthoses may be successful. If so, such potential risks of surgery as overlengthening, anesthesia, infection, and hypertrophic scars can be avoided. Surgical lengthening of the Achilles tendon can be deleterious to the triceps surae. Experimental studies in cats have shown that muscle mass is lost after surgical elongation of the Achilles tendon.[1] This loss of muscle mass and strength in the triceps surae may inhibit walking and lead to a calcaneal crouched gait pattern (Fig. 1).

Medication

Medical therapy for movement disorders in cerebral palsy is discussed in Chapter 18. The most commonly used agents for the medical treatment of spasticity are diazepam, baclofen, and dantrolene. Diazepam and baclofen act at GABA sites; dantrolene acts directly on skeletal muscle. However, medical management of spasticity has been disappointing. Few studies exist that can be used to evaluate objectively the effects of medications. They are limited by the small numbers of patients studied, the variability of the populations studied, the parameters used to measure spasticity, and the short duration of therapy. Medical management of spasticity appears helpful in a small number of patients, especially where muscle spasms either interfere with activity or cause discomfort. Functional improvement, however, is difficult to establish. For some patients, there is a subjective improvement reported by caregivers and therapists, which allows passive exercises to be more easily accomplished. Although medical management alone is ineffective for treating tight Achilles tendons in children with spastic diplegia, it may be a useful adjunct to other forms of treatment.

Chemical Neurectomy

Theoretically, selective neurectomy, either chemical or surgical, can decrease or eliminate gastrocnemius and soleus spasticity. Historically, surgical neurectomy predates chemical neurectomy as indicated by Stoffel's[2] description of selective motor neurectomies for cerebral palsy. Several authors have advocated combining an Achilles tendon lengthening with a partial gastrocnemius denervation, a soleus denervation, or some combination of the two.[3–5]

The results of isolated surgical neurectomies have been reported by several investigators.[6–9] Neurectomy alone was felt to be uniformly unsuccessful when there was a fixed contracture of the triceps surae. In the absence of contracture, if pure spasticity resulted in clonus (or a dynamic plantar thrust), a neurectomy could be useful. If the gastrocnemius was the source of the clonus, the ankle clonus would decrease on examination with the knee flexed, and a selective motor neurectomy could be performed on one or two branches of the tibial nerve to the gastrocnemius-soleus.[8] However, many of these patients ultimately underwent a heel-cord lengthening. Phelps[7] concluded, in 1967, that neurectomies were "temporarily good, but in the long run they accomplish nothing, because in spite of everything, the nerve will grow back,... the clonus in an ankle will come back after a period of years." In 1988, Tolo and Sponseller[9] reported on 15 children who underwent bilateral selective soleus neurectomies for ankle clonus. This subgroup represented less than 5% of their clinic's cerebral palsy population. Eleven had a concomitant heel-cord lengthening. With a 2- to 8-year follow-up, 12 had no recurrence of clonus, one had a repeat neurectomy, and two had mild clonus with improved gait. Evans[10] felt that this procedure, with heel-cord lengthening, gave permanent correction of equinus. The isolated neurectomy helped clonus, although, in some cases, the heel cord needed to be lengthened later.

A chemical neurolysis can be done at many levels. The tibial nerve may be blocked, using a closed technique, with either 5% phenol, 45% ethyl alcohol (ethanol), or local anesthetic. The technique for the block is demanding. Peripheral nerves,[11–13] the large motor branches,[14,15] and the endplate areas[16] can be identified with electrical nerve conduction equipment and selectively blocked. The more proximal blocks are easier to perform. The more proximal portions of the nerve contain both sensory and motor fibers, and more dysesthetic complications are likely to occur following injections in this region. The more distal branches are motor and injections in this region are less likely to result in dysesthesias. To do a complete block, all branches must be blocked. A total block may be useful if one wishes to determine the effect of a paralyzed gastrocnemius-soleus muscle.

With an intramuscular block, the stimulating electrode approaches the nerve through the muscle belly. The injection is made in the neighborhood of the motor nerve endings or near the endplates, with 1 to 5 ml of 45% ethanol or 5% phenol injected at each point.[15–19] O'Hanlan and associates[17] used an intramuscular ethanol wash technique that does not require electrical guidance. Although it is quick, it still requires anesthesia. For the gastrocnemius-soleus muscle, a total of 30 to 40 ml of 45% ethanol is injected into six to eight sites (5 ml per injection) divided evenly throughout the muscle.

In general, phenol blocks (duration: 1 month to 3 years)[11–13] last longer than ethanol blocks (duration: 7 days to 6 months),[17–19] which last longer than local anesthetic blocks (duration: 1 to 7 hours).[12] Higher concentrations of ethanol and phenol give better results than lower concentrations (the difference between axon destruction and demyelination), with respect to completeness of block and duration of effect. Within limits, the precision of the injection also affects the completeness and duration of the block. An open tibial nerve block is no better than a well done closed tibial nerve block.[20] The alcohol wash technique, in which no effort is made to locate a motor branch precisely, gives the least consistent effects.[17,18]

No permanent eradication of equinus gait through use of these techniques has been reported. Clonus may be eradicated temporarily, but there are no studies documenting the duration of the effect in cerebral palsy. Repeat blocks appear to do little good because a second attempt rarely works. Children with mild spasticity do better than those with more severe spasticity. Therefore, those with severe spasticity and those with recurrence of spasticity after an initial block are not candidates for repeated injections.

Most authors regard blocks as a therapeutic test to be used before surgical lengthening or neurectomy although there may be other indications. For example, a block may be indicated to manage a 4-year-old child with dynamic equinus and no contracture who will not wear an ankle-foot orthosis or otherwise participate in nonsurgical care.[21] A block may also be useful to uncover a dystonia or athetosis. Dramatic improvement of these patients with a block may indicate that a neurectomy may be efficacious. The block can uncover an unbalanced antagonist or help surgeons and therapists evaluate the child to determine whether surgery might be effective.

Blocks are not completely problem-free and may result in complications. Gastrocnemius-soleus injections and tibial nerve blocks can cause a local reaction to the medication, mimicking phlebitis.[14] The tibial nerve is also a sensory nerve, and, therefore, dysesthesias occur frequently.[13] Pain of injection has forced most practitioners to use general anesthesia.[22] If a block includes branches to the posterior tibialis, an unopposed peroneal muscle may cause a valgus deformity. Fortunately, the above complications are usually temporary and controllable.

Physical Therapy

The primary objective of physical therapy in the treatment of tight Achilles tendons is to maintain or regain range of motion in order to prevent or reduce contracture and maximize functional mobility.[23] In cerebral palsy, the spastic triceps surae becomes contracted because of the constant muscle stimulation. Eventually, the muscle shortens sufficiently to prevent complete range of motion of the tibial-talar and subtalar joints.

The shortening can be accentuated by intrinsic adaptive changes in response to a prolonged equinus ankle posture. Experimental studies have shown that the equinus position allows the triceps surae to shorten, and, with time, the muscle fibers can lose 40% of their sarcomeres.[24] A deleterious cycle is set into motion with triceps surae spasticity: The plantarflexed ankle shortens the triceps surae, then the shortened muscle leads to more equinus and brings the ankle into increasing fixed plantarflexion. This cycle may be prevented or broken with physical therapy, which should include range of motion and stretching exercises with the muscle relaxed.[25]

Passive stretching and joint mobilization techniques restore normal range of motion when this range is limited by muscle shortening and loss of soft-tissue elasticity.[26] These techniques lengthen the elastic portion of the muscle, passively providing greater range of motion. However, any increase in range obtained by forced motion will be lost unless maintained by active motion of the ankle dorsiflexors or by holding the ankle in dorsiflexion with supportive devices, eg, night splints, ankle-foot orthoses, or casts.

The ankle dorsiflexors working in opposition to a contracted triceps surae muscle are mechanically disadvantaged because of excess length. Adaptation by changing their spindle bias may further reduce their action. Many children with spastic diplegia have no voluntary control of their ankle dorsiflexors, and the plantarflexors contract unopposed. Therefore, therapy uses strengthening techniques to improve tibialis anterior function to oppose the triceps surae. Additional facilitation techniques include vibration, quick icing, brushing, and lapping. Other neuromuscular facilitation includes such techniques as topical anesthesia (benzocaine),[27] manual contacts, traction, approximation, repeated contractions, quick stretch, resistance, and tilt table-wedge board standing.[28] Electromyographic feedback has also been used to improve control in muscles opposing spasticity.[23]

Rolfing is contraindicated in the treatment of tight Achilles tendons.[29] Rolfing involves a 10-hour cycle of deep manual manipulation of the myofascial tissues of the body. Manual pressure is applied to areas in which muscle tendons are felt to adhere to each other rather than slide over one another in normal fashion. This technique has been shown to increase the tightness of the plantarflexors, which worsens the equinus deformity.[29]

When instituted early, physical therapy is useful in the prevention of severe equinus deformities. If severe contractures occur, however, other modalities, described below, will be needed in conjunction with the treatments thus far described.

Serial Inhibitive Casting

Serial inhibitive casting has been effectively used to treat tight Achilles tendons.[30–38] Its success may result from elongation of the muscle by the addition of sarcomeres.[32–38] In addition, however, there is evidence that inhibitive casting can reduce the tone of the triceps surae by stimulating reflexogenous areas in the foot.[38]

The technique described by Sussman and Cusick[37] is used most commonly for applying the tone-reducing inhibitive cast. The child is relaxed in a prone position with the hip extended and knee flexed to relax the ankle plantarflexors. The skin is protected by stockinette and a thin layer of cast padding. Felt strips are placed medially and laterally to the calcaneus tendon to improve contact and afford rigid immobilization. Felt is also placed under the toes to extend them at the metatarsophalangeal joints and prevent plantar grasping. Plaster or fiberglass is then applied with the ankle and foot held in a neutral position with calcaneal congruency. Full weightbearing is encouraged. The casts are worn for one to two weeks and then bivalved; the two halves are held together with straps to allow removal for bathing and range of motion exercises. The length of time the inhibitive casts are used varies with the patient's individualized functional problems, the severity of equinus deformity, and the improvement noted at the time of cast change. The cast should be changed weekly, gradually increasing dorsiflexion of the ankle. Stabilizing the ankle and reducing spasticity will improve the child's standing and walking.

Proving the efficacy of inhibitive casting has been difficult. Collection of objective data to document the benefit of treatment depends on the ability to measure overall functional change. Before independent walking begins, there is no objective technique for measuring the efficacy of cast treatment. Sussman and Cusick[37] reported improvement of patients' functional status over time in a physical therapy program that

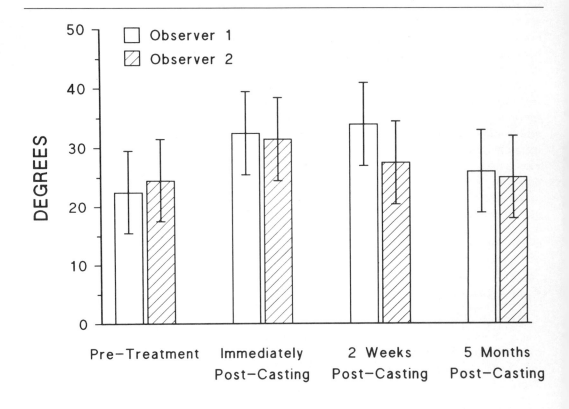

Fig. 2 *Average passive ankle dorsiflexion ± one standard deviation before and after inhibitive casting for tight Achilles tendons in children with spastic diplegia. (Redrawn with permission from Watt et al.[32])*

included casting. However, the study did not include a control group. Watt and associates[32] studied 28 children with spastic cerebral palsy who were treated with inhibitive casts for three weeks as part of their physical therapy program. The changes observed in passive ankle motion are summarized in Figure 2. These results indicate a temporary improvement in passive range of ankle dorsiflexion, which supports the use of an ankle-foot orthosis after a period of inhibitive cast treatment to maintain the desired results. A tight Achilles tendon is likely to recur, because the triceps surae may not grow appropriately with the bone. Therefore, it may be necessary to repeat the casting several times during the growing years.

Ankle-Foot Orthoses

Ankle-foot orthoses are of no value for a fixed deformity. However, once the equinus is corrected, an ankle-foot orthosis can help prevent a recurrent deformity. Ankle-foot orthoses in slight dorsiflexion are also used to treat children with genu recurvatum.[39]

Lightweight plastic ankle-foot orthoses have largely replaced the conventional short leg double upright metal braces. These plastic ankle-foot orthoses are strong, cosmetically acceptable, and can be fitted precisely to the patient. They are secured with velcro straps in regular shoes without outside attachments. Ankle-foot orthoses are comfortable and can be worn as night splints to maintain the correction of an equinus deformity obtained by some other treatment modality such as inhibitive casting.[40]

The most valuable use of ankle-foot orthoses in spastic diplegia is to improve standing balance by inhibiting extensor tone. Controlling a spastic gastrocnemius-soleus muscle group and holding the ankle in neutral position with calcaneal congruency will allow the child to stand and walk more efficiently. Mossberg and associates[41] studied energy expenditure during gait with and without ankle-foot orthoses in children with spastic diplegia. They found that energy expenditure during ambulation at self-selected speeds was reduced by the application of ankle-foot orthoses in these children.

The principles of tone reduction on which inhibitive casting was based have been transferred to the fabrication of ankle-foot orthoses.[42] The tone-reducing ankle-foot orthosis takes advantage of the reflexogenous points in the foot to facilitate dorsiflexion and inhibit plantarflexion. It is designed to dorsiflex the toes at the metatarsophalangeal joint and to reduce spasticity in the gastrocnemius and soleus. The tone-reducing ankle-foot orthosis has not been objectively shown to be more effective than a conventional ankle-foot orthosis.

Recently, the custom-molded plastic hinged ankle-foot orthosis with a plantarflexion stop (Fig. 3) has been introduced. The advantage of this device is that it allows some range of normal dorsiflexion to occur at the ankle joint, but still inhibits unwanted plantarflexion. The potential for ankle dorsiflexion allows stretching of the Achilles tendon and may reduce spasticity of the triceps surae. Bracing with a hinged ankle-foot orthosis theoretically might produce a more normal gait pattern; however, little data exist that support the efficacy of a hinged ankle-foot orthosis. Middleton and associates[43] compared the gait of a 4.5-year-old child with spastic diplegia wearing a rigid ankle-foot orthosis with the gait of the same child wearing a hinged ankle-foot orthosis. Walking in a hinged ankle-foot orthosis resulted in more natural ankle motion during stance phase, greater symmetry of lower extremity motion, and more normal knee motion than walking in a rigid ankle-foot orthosis.

Summary

A logical therapeutic approach to a tight Achilles tendon in children with spastic diplegia requires an understanding of the pathophysiology of spasticity and the biomechanical complications of spastic gastroc-

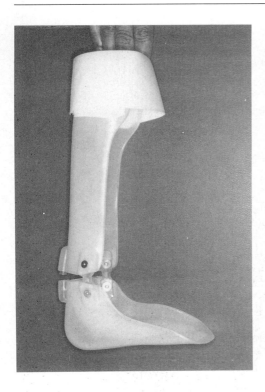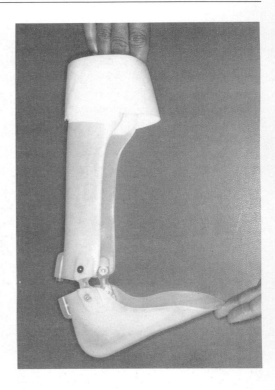

Fig. 3 *Ankle-foot orthosis with hinge joint for ankle motion.*

nemius and soleus muscles. Nonsurgical treatment of tight Achilles tendons can be beneficial. Medications to relax the triceps surae have limited value alone, but may be useful in conjunction with other forms of treatment. Local nerve and muscle blocks can be temporarily effective, but because they are painful, they are difficult to do in young children without general anesthesia.

Physical therapy techniques to elongate the triceps surae in the relaxed state may increase the length of the muscle through the addition of more sarcomeres. Painful stretching of a spastic muscle can be detrimental. Rolfing should be avoided, because it can increase plantarflexion tightness and make an equinus deformity worse.

Serial inhibitive casting effectively increases ankle dorsiflexion, but the effect is transient if no further measures are taken. Ankle-foot orthoses are recommended to prevent recurrence of equinus deformity after fixed contractures are corrected, and these should be worn as long as there is a chance for relative growth inhibition in the triceps surae while the tibia is growing normally. Nonsurgical treatments of tight Achilles tendons may not always be successful, but the risk of complications are few and surgery is still an option if the nonsurgical means fail.

References

1. Blanchard O, Cohen-Solal L, Tardieu C, et al: Tendon adaptation to different long term stresses and collagen reticulation in soleus muscle. *Connect Tissue Res* 1985;13:261–267.
2. Stoffel A: The treatment of spastic contractures. *Am J Orthop Surg* 1913;10: 611–644.
3. Eggers GWN, Evans EB: Surgery in cerebral palsy. *J Bone Joint Surg* 1963; 45A:1275–1305.
4. Silver CM, Simon SD: Gastrocnemius-muscle recession (Silfverskiöld operation) for spastic equinus deformity in cerebral palsy. *J Bone Joint Surg* 1959;41A:1021–1028.
5. Eggers GWN: Transplantation of hamstring tendons to femoral condyles in order to improve hip extension and to decrease knee flexion in cerebral spastic paralysis. *J Bone Joint Surg* 1952;234A:827–830.
6. Banks HH, Green WT: The correction of equinus deformity in cerebral palsy. *J Bone Joint Surg* 1958;40A:1359–1379.
7. Phelps M: Complications in treatment of cerebral palsy. *Clin Orthop* 1967;53: 44–45.
8. Baker LD, Hill LM: Foot alignment in the cerebral palsy patient. *J Bone Joint Surg* 1964;46A:1–15.
9. Tolo V, Sponseller P: Soleus neurectomy: An effective procedure in cerebral palsy. *Orthop Trans* 1988;12:696.
10. Evans E: The status of surgery in cerebral palsy. *Clin Orthop* 1966;47:130–131.
11. Spira R: Management of spasticity in cerebral palsied children by peripheral nerve block with phenol. *Dev Med Child Neurol* 1971;13:164–173.
12. Khalili A, Benton J: A physiologic approach to the evaluation and the management of spasticity with procaine and phenol nerve block. *Clin Orthop* 1966;47:97–104.
13. Petrillo C, Chu D, Sanders W: Phenol block of the tibial nerve in the hemiplegic patient. *Orthopedics* 1980;3:871–874.
14. Easton J, Ozel T, Halpern D: Intramuscular neurolysis for spasticity in children. *Arch Phys Med Rehabil* 1979;60:155–158.
15. Tardieu G, Tardieu C, Hariga J, et al: Treatment of spasticity by injection of dilute alcohol at the motor point or by epidural route. Clinical extension of an experiment on the decerebrate cat. *Dev Med Child Neurol* 1968;10:555–568.
16. DeLateur B: A new technique of intramuscular phenol neurolysis. *Arch Phys Med Rehabil* 1972;53:179–185.
17. O'Hanlan J, Galford H, Bosley J: The use of 45% alcohol to control spasticity. *Va Med Mo* 1969;96:429–436.
18. Carpenter EB, Seitz DG: Intramuscular alcohol as an aid in management of spastic cerebral palsy. *Dev Med Child Neurol* 1980;22:497–501.
19. Carpenter E: Role of nerve blocks in the foot and ankle in cerebral palsy: Therapeutic and diagnostic. *Foot Ankle* 1983;4:164–166.
20. Garland D, Lucie R, Waters R: Current uses of open phenol nerve block for adult acquired spasticity. *Clin Orthop* 1982;165:217–222.
21. Bleck E: *Special Assessments and Investigations in Orthopaedic Management in Cerebral Palsy*, Clinics in Developmental Medicine. Philadelphia, Blackwell Scientific Publications, 1987, no 99/100, pp 97–100.
22. Griffith E, Melampy C: General anesthesia use in phenol intramuscular neurolysis in children with spasticity. *Arch Phys Med Rehabil* 1977;58:154–157.
23. Cherry D: Review of physical therapy alternatives for reducing muscle contracture. *Phys Ther* 1980;60:877–881.
24. Tardieu C, Tardieu G, Colbeau-Justin P, et al: Trophic muscle regulation in children with congenital cerebral lesions. *J Neurol Sci* 1979;42:357–364.

25. Odeen I: Reduction of muscular hypertonus by long-term muscle stretch. *Scand J Rehab Med* 1981;13:93–99.
26. Kanda T, Yuge M, Yamori Y, et al: Early physiotherapy in the treatment of spastic diplegia. *Dev Med Child Neurol* 1984;26:438–444.
27. Sabbahi M, DeLuca C, Powers W: Topical anesthesia: A possible treatment method for spasticity. *Arch Phys Med Rehabil* 1981;62:310–314.
28. Bohannon R, Larkin P: Passive ankle dorsiflexion increases in patients after a regimen of tilt table-wedge board standing. *Phys Ther* 1985;65:1676–1678.
29. Perry J, Jones MH, Thomas L: Functional evaluation of rolfing in cerebral palsy. *Dev Med Child Neurol* 1981;23:717–729.
30. Zachazewski J, Eberle E, Jefferies M: Effect of tone-inhibiting casts and orthoses on gait: A case report. *Phys Ther* 1982;62:453–454.
31. Bertoti D: Effect of short leg casting on ambulation in children with cerebral palsy. *Phys Ther* 1986;66:1522–1529.
32. Watt J, Sims D, Harckham F, et al: A prospective study of inhibitive casting as an adjunct to physiotherapy for cerebral-palsied children. *Dev Med Child Neurol* 1986;28:480–488.
33. Sussman MD: Casting as an adjunct to neurodevelopmental therapy for cerebral palsy. *Dev Med Child Neurol* 1983:25:804–805.
34. Hinderer KA, Harris SR, Purdy AH, et al: Effects of 'tone-reducing' vs. standard plaster-casts on gait improvement of children with cerebral palsy. *Dev Med Child Neurol* 1988;30:370–377.
35. Hanson C, Jones L: Gait abnormalities and inhibitive casts in cerebral palsy. *J Am Podiatr Med Assoc* 1989;79:53–59.
36. Booth B, Doyle M, Montgomery J: Serial casting for the management of spasticity in the head-injured adult. *Phys Ther* 1983;363:1960–1966.
37. Sussman M, Cusick B: Preliminary report: The role of short-leg tone-reducing casts as an adjunct to physical therapy of patients with cerebral palsy. *Johns Hopkins Med J* 1979;145:112–114.
38. Duncan W, Mott D: Foot reflexes and the use of the "inhibitive cast." *Foot Ankle* 1983;4:145–148.
39. Simon SR, Deutsch SD, Nuzzo RM, et al: Genu recurvatum in spastic cerebral palsy: Report on findings on gait analysis. *J Bone Joint Surg* 1978;60A:882–894.
40. Rosenthal R: The use of orthotics in foot and ankle problems in cerebral palsy. *Foot Ankle* 1984;4:195–200.
41. Mossberg K, Linton K, Friske K: Ankle-foot orthoses: Effect on energy expenditure of gait in spastic diplegic children. *Arch Phys Med Rehabil* 1990;71:490–494.
42. Jordan R: Therapeutic considerations of the feet and lower extremities in the cerebral palsied child. *Clin Podiatr Med Surg* 1984;1:547–561.
43. Middleton E, Hurley G, McIlwain J: The role of rigid and hinged polypropylene ankle-foot-orthoses in the management of cerebral palsy: A case study. *Prosthet Orthot Int* 1988;12:129–135.

Chapter 27

The Vulpius Gastrocnemius-Soleus Lengthening

Robert K. Rosenthal, MD
Sheldon R. Simon, MD

Introduction

The most common deformity in children with spastic cerebral palsy is equinus of the ankle.[1] This deformity may be secondary to a fixed contracture or to dynamic overactivity of the gastrocnemius-soleus complex, either alone or in combination with other abnormal muscles about the ankle.

Banks and Green[2] and Green and McDermott[3] were early advocates of surgical treatment of deformities associated with spastic cerebral palsy. Their conclusions that orthopaedic procedures for the correction of a fixed equinus deformity were effective became an important guideline for others. Along with Phelps,[4] they stressed the importance of postoperative management, physical therapy, and bracing. More recently, Bleck[5] also supported the concept that surgery remains the preferred method of correcting spastic equinus deformity. While the relative merits of physical therapy and bracing are being debated, the surgeon has the opportunity to truly correct the deformity. Banks and Green[2] focused on a sliding lengthening of the heel cord. In contrast, the Vulpius aponeurotic lengthening of the gastrocnemius-soleus muscles[6] was considered by many to give more reliable results than many of the alternatives currently being used. The value of the Vulpius procedure was recently confirmed by Javors and Klaaren.[7]

We believe a number of important concepts should be reviewed and discussed before performance of what is technically a simple orthopaedic procedure. Perry and Hoffer[8] noted that the Silfverskiöld test, which is more valid if done while the patient is anesthetized, will assist in identifying whether equinus deformities are caused by a contracture of either the gastrocnemius or soleus muscle, or both. The gastrocnemius is tested by applying a dorsiflexion force to the foot, first with the knee extended, then with the knee flexed; if the equinus primarily results from a gastrocnemius contracture, it will disappear with the knee flexed. Any residual equinus deformity can then be attributed to a soleus contracture.

Sutherland[9] outlined the importance of calf muscle function for the stability of the weightbearing lower extremity. He also emphasized the very great potential force that can be produced by the gastrocnemius and soleus muscles. Thus, any lengthening should try to preserve as much of the strength of that muscle complex as is possible.

Gage and associates[10] reviewed preoperative and postoperative gait analysis data from patients with spastic diplegia. Based on this material, he promoted the concept that simultaneous correction of deformities at multiple joints is effective and produces less morbidity than when the surgery is done in stages.

In their article on Achilles tendon lengthening, Gaines and Ford[11] correlated factors of spasticity and voluntary control in setting operative ankle position and, thus, determining the amount of lengthening required. Segal and associates[12] reported that gait analysis indicated a high prevalence of calcaneus gait as a result of overlengthening of the Achilles tendon in patients who had a ''Z''-type lengthening.

This chapter focuses on our experience with the original Vulpius/ Stoffel aponeurotic lengthening of the gastrocnemius and soleus muscles.

Patients

Eighty-seven patients with spastic diparesis underwent Vulpius gastrocnemius-soleus fascial lengthenings from January 1, 1977, through June 30, 1991. The patients ranged in age from 2 years 8 months to 19 years 9 months with a mean age of 5 years 10 months.

Indications for Surgery

A progressive equinus deformity of five degrees or greater with a deteriorating gait pattern was the basic criterion for lengthening. Many patients wearing orthoses began to develop pressure sores because the orthosis could no longer contain the deformity. Usually, the patient was allowed no more than 15 degrees of equinus. Gait studies were obtained when gait measurement facilities were available. The uniqueness of this study results from the large number of patients examined and their long-term follow-up. Also these spastic diparetic patients, all of whom were moderately spastic and ambulatory (with or without assistive devices), were closely followed.

Surgical Technique

The surgery was performed with the patient in the supine position under general anesthesia. Sometimes concomitant hamstring surgery was performed, and the patient was placed in the prone position. A tourniquet was used, set at twice the child's systolic blood pressure. A longitudinal incision was made in the lower middle region of the calf on the medial side to avoid the sural nerve. This usually corresponded

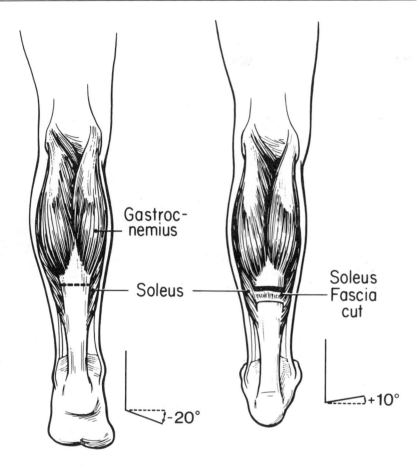

Fig. 1 *Original Vulpius technique.*

to the palpable lower border of the gastrocnemius muscle. The fascia over the gastrocnemius muscle was incised, revealing its aponeurosis. Dissection to the medial and lateral margins defined the boundaries of the aponeurosis. A sharp transverse horizontal incision was made in the aponeurosis of the gastrocnemius muscle. The ankle was dorsiflexed enough to reveal the aponeurosis of the soleus muscle, which was then also incised horizontally (Fig. 1). In most cases, one or two aponeurotic bands in the soleus were encountered and were cut. The ankle was then dorsiflexed five to ten degrees in all cases. If resistance was met at neutral, a second aponeurotic cut (Fig. 2) was made in a similar fashion.

The wound was closed with absorbable sutures at all layers and reinforced with steri-strips. If surgery was limited to the calf, the foot was immobilized in a short leg cast with the ankle dorsiflexed five degrees for three to four weeks. If dynamic hamstring spasticity, hamstring tendon contractures, and/or the adductor tendon were also lengthened,

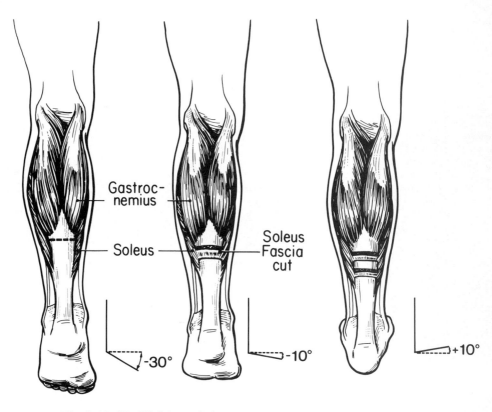

Fig. 2 *Modified Vulpius technique.*

the foot and knee were immobilized in a long leg cast for the same period of time. All patients were ambulatory within one to three days after surgery, whenever possible. All casts were bivalved for night use for at least 6 months. Intravenous antibiotics were administered to all patients preoperatively and for 24 hours postoperatively.

Results

Of the 87 patients, 74 required only one bilateral Vulpius procedure and 13 (15%) required a repeat procedure (Table 1). In addition, two children had a Vulpius procedure on one side and an Achilles tendon lengthening on the other. There were 41 boys and 46 girls, all of whom were ambulatory at the time of surgery. Average age at the time of surgery was 5 years 10 months. Average follow-up was 8 years 2 months. Additional surgery required at the time of the heel cord lengthening is listed in Table 2.

The average age of the 13 patients requiring a second procedure was 4 years 0 months at the time of the first procedure and 10 years 7 months

Table 1 Vulpius gastrocnemius-soleus lengthening

First Surgery Age (Yrs)	(Mos)	Additional Surgery	Second Surgery Age (Yrs)	(Mos)	Surgery Performed	Third Surgery Age (Yrs)	(Mos)	Surgery Performed
2	8		10	7	Bilateral Vulpius			
4	0		12	4	Bilateral Vulpius			
5	7	Bilateral medial hamstring tendon lengthening	19	9	Bilateral Vulpius			
2	8	Bilateral adductor myotomy	6	5	Bilateral Vulpius; Bilateral hamstring tendon lengthening			
3	0	Bilateral medial hamstring tendon lengthening	7	3	R Vulpius; R posterior tibial tendon lengthening			
4	4		11	5	Bilateral Vulpius; Bilateral hamstring tendon lengthening			
3	1	Bilateral adductor myotomy	9	11	Bilateral Vulpius; Bilateral medial hamstring tendon lengthening	13	7	L Vulpius; L posterior tibial tendon lengthening
6	5		13	2	Bilateral Vulpius; Bilateral calcaneal osteotomy			
3	5	Bilateral adductor myotomy	14	3	Bilateral Vulpius; Remove fem plates			
3	1		10	8	L Vulpius	14	2	L Vulpius; L bunion
3	9		11	0	Bilateral Vulpius			
3	8	Bilateral adductor myotomy	10	4	Bilateral Vulpius			
6	0		9	9	Bilateral Vulpius	14	5	R Vulpius; R anterior tibial plication
Averages								
4	0		11	3		14	1	

at the time of the second procedure. During a final growth spurt, three patients required a third procedure at an average age of 14 years 1 month. There were no postoperative infections and no problems with the location of any incision. The children who had a repeat lengthening also provided us with the opportunity to evaluate the original operative site. In a number of cases, small metal neuro-clips were attached to the cut ends of the gastrocnemius fascia. At the time of reoperation it was noted that the previous operative gap was filled in with scar tissue and,

Table 2 Additional surgery required at heel-cord lengthening

Procedure	No. of Patients
Bilateral adductor myotomy and superficial obturator neurectomy	33
Bilateral iliopsoas tendon lengthening	4
Bilateral femoral osteotomy	1
Bilateral hamstring tendon lengthening	25
Posterior tibial tendon lengthening	3
Peroneal tendon lengthening	7
Plantar fasciotomy	3
Subtalar arthrodesis	1

at times, was indistinguishable from the normal. When neuro-clips were in place, they were monitored with roentgenograms and their gap distance did not change from immediately after surgery to long-term follow-up.

By clinical assessment, all patients benefited from the basic procedure. Gait analysis was available for a select group of 26 patients. Unpublished force-plate data gathered in the gait laboratory revealed that equinus gait caused a high torque around the ankle during the stance phase of gait because of the powerful contraction and deformity of the gastrocnemius-soleus complex. Gastrocnemius-soleus lengthening improved the position of the ankle and reduced the torque around the ankle in stance phase. This lengthening did not weaken the gastrocnemius-soleus muscles; the force of contraction was lessened as a result of better ankle position at heel strike. If weakness in the anterior tibia was noted, the patient's improved gait could easily be maintained with use of an ankle-foot orthosis.

Using gait analysis, we were able to document three types of motion patterns at the ankle after surgery: normal or near normal throughout the cycle, corrected equinus in stance but not during swing, and lack of full correction about the ankle during the entire gait cycle. A consistent finding in the eight patients who demonstrated a normal motion pattern after surgery was normal firing of ankle dorsiflexors during swing phase (Fig. 3). Lack of normal dorsiflexion activity during swing phase was a consistent finding in the 14 patients who had corrected equinus in stance but not during swing phase (Fig. 4). In these patients, control of ankle equinus with bracing, through use of an ankle-foot orthosis, led to a uniform increase in stride length by providing a stable "roll-over" mechanism at the ankle. The third pattern was seen in four patients whose ankle dorsiflexors and plantarflexors fired during most of the gait cycle (Fig. 5). This group demonstrated a tendency towards calcaneus during late stance and a "drop foot" in swing.

In general, changes in velocity, cadence, and stride length were related to the child's preoperative condition. The younger patients or those with slower preoperative cadence and shorter stride length appeared to benefit most from the surgery, as demonstrated by an increase in their velocity. The length of time after surgery at which the child was observed also had an effect on the outcome. Improvement in

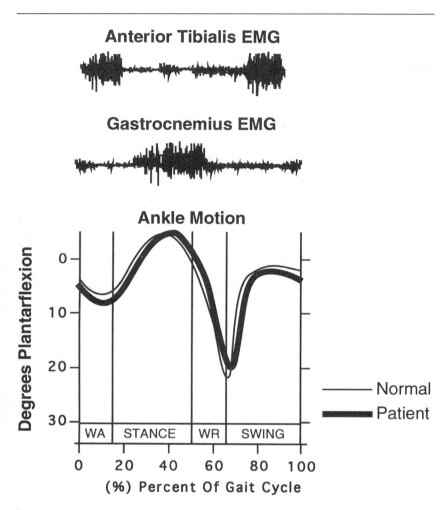

Fig. 3 *Gait analysis: Normal or near normal group.*

velocity was noted in the most normal group in less than one year; but after one year, improvement in velocity was noted in 22 out of 26 patients.

Discussion

In his original article, Vulpius[6] described a "lengthening of up to 3 cm to the gastrocnemius-soleus complex," but surgeons in that era were operating on older children. The dilemma of what to do for the younger child is still being debated. Clearly, if indications warrant, appropriate surgery, including the Vulpius procedure, can be performed, however it must be recognized that a repeat procedure may be required at least once, as this series indicates. However, the procedure

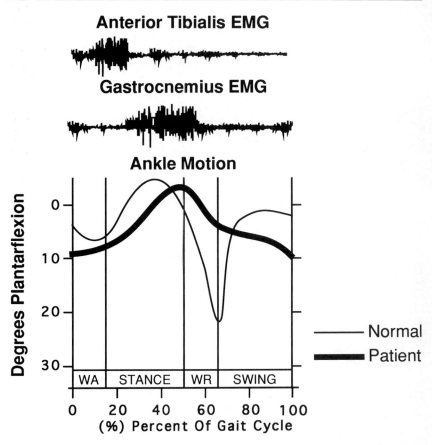

Fig. 4 *Gait analysis: Second pattern. Equinus corrected in stance but not during swing.*

is simple enough and produces such favorable results that it is worth performing on young children. This procedure is also preferable to an alternate technique that could result in overlengthening. In this series, the Vulpius procedure did not produce excessive overlengthening that could not be controlled in an ankle-foot orthosis.

Sage[13] indicated that the benefits of early surgery may not always be maintained throughout the period of growth and repeat surgery may become necessary in the future. This was the case for only 13 of our patients, who then required second Vulpius procedures. However, after the first procedure they had improved, and except for three patients were stable and ambulatory for at least six years before the second procedure. We also observed that, in general, this early Vulpius gastrocnemius-soleus muscle lengthening procedure virtually eliminated the need for bony ankle and foot reconstructive surgery in later years; the foot muscles were balanced early and bony malformations rarely

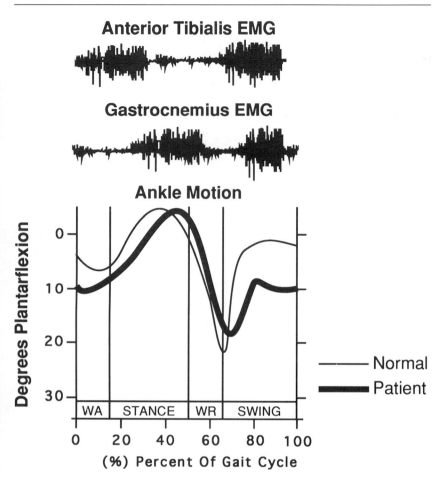

Fig. 5 *Gait analysis: Third pattern. Ankle dorsiflexors and plantarflexors fire during most of the gait cycle.*

occurred. There does not seem to be any correlation between simultaneous hamstring tendon or hip adductor surgery and avoidance of a second Vulpius procedure.

In summary, the advantages of the Vulpius aponeurotic gastrocnemius-soleus lengthening are numerous. The procedure is technically easy. A predictable result is achieved with virtually no complications; overlengthening is rare and can be controlled with an ankle-foot orthosis if it occurs. In children 6 years of age or younger, if a lengthening is necessary, a repeat procedure can be anticipated in 6 to 7 years. A recurrence rate of 14% of total patients is acceptable, considering the nature of the condition. In children older than 6 years, the recurrence rate is only 1%.

Conclusion

In conclusion, for patients with spastic diplegia, the Vulpius gastrocnemius-soleus fascial lengthening offers a safe, reliable, and predictable method of correcting an equinus problem of the ankle when a contracture is found in both muscles of the complex.

References

1. Banks H: The foot and ankle in cerebral palsy, in Samilson R (ed): *Orthopedic Aspects of Cerebral Palsy*. Philadelphia, JB Lippincott, 1975, pp 195–220.
2. Banks H, Green W: The correction of equinus deformity in cerebral palsy. *J Bone Joint Surg* 1958;40A:1359–1379.
3. Green W, McDermott L: Operative treatment of cerebral palsy of spastic type. *JAMA* 1942;118:434–439.
4. Phelps WM: Long-term results of orthopaedic surgery in cerebral palsy. *J Bone Joint Surg* 1957;39A:53–59.
5. Bleck EE: Management of the lower extremities in children who have cerebral palsy. *J Bone Joint Surg* 1990;72A:140–144.
6. Vulpius O, Stoffel A: Tenotomie der endschnen der Mm. gastrocnemius et soleus, in *Orthopadische Operationslehre*. Stuttgart, Ferdinand Enke, 1913, pp 29–31.
7. Javors JR, Klaaren HE: The Vulpius procedure for correction of equinus deformity in cerebral palsy. *J Pediatr Orthop* 1987;7:191–193.
8. Perry J, Hoffer MM: Gait analysis of the triceps surae in cerebral palsy: A preoperative and postoperative clinical and electromyographic study. *J Bone Joint Surg* 1974;56A:511–520.
9. Sutherland DH: An electromyographic study of the plantar flexors of the ankle in normal walking on the level. *J Bone Joint Surg* 1966;48A:66–71.
10. Gage JR, Fabian D, Hicks R, et al: Pre- and postoperative gait analysis in patients with spastic diplegia: A preliminary report. *J Pediatr Orthop* 1984;4:715–725.
11. Gaines RW, Ford TB: A systematic approach to the amount of Achilles tendon lengthening in cerebral palsy. *J Pediatr Orthop* 1984;4:448–451.
12. Segal L, Thomas SE, Mazur JM, et al: Calcaneal gait in spastic diplegia after heel cord lengthening: A study with gait analysis. *J Pediatr Orthop* 1989;9:697–701.
13. Sage F: Cerebral palsy, in Crenshaw A (ed): *Campbell's Operative Orthopaedics*. St. Louis, CV Mosby, 1986, pp 2854–2864.

Chapter 28

Biomechanical/Neurophysiologic Factors Related to Surgical Correction of Equinus Deformity

Sheldon R. Simon, MD
Andrew W. Ryan, MD

Introduction

Equinus deformity is one of the most common indications for surgical treatment in patients with cerebral palsy. Since the early 1900s, many different procedures have been done to correct this deformity. However, until the 1970s all these procedures could be classified into two categories: (1) lengthening of the Achilles tendon (TAL) and (2) recession or lengthening of the gastrocnemius portion of the muscle-tendon complex (Vulpius procedure). In 1974, Pierrot and Murphy[1] proposed "heel cord advancement" (HCA). Instead of changing the muscle-tendon length, HCA shortens the lever arm through which the triceps surae generates torque about the ankle.

All three types of procedures can eliminate the equinus deformity; however, opinions differ as to how the procedures alter ankle mechanics and allow a normal gait pattern to be restored. Suggested reasons include: "the muscle is weakened"; "atrophy of the muscle occurs secondary to postoperative casting"; and "the correction of the deformity allows the antagonist to work and oppose the ankle plantarflexors." Murphy suggested that reducing the lever arm by HCA weakens the gastrocnemius-soleus muscle complex during the initial phases of single limb stance but allows near-normal strength to remain at "push off" (the end of stance).[1]

Good to excellent results have been reported with each type of procedure.[1-6] Follow-up studies of patients undergoing lengthening of the Achilles tendon have shown that some patients will develop a calcaneus gait, while in others the deformity may recur.[3,7] Gastrocnemius recession (see Chapter 27) may also be associated with excessive dynamic plantarflexion with or without genu recurvatum and subsequent recurrence of the equinus contracture. Although fewer results have been reported for HCA than for the other two procedures, poor gait results reported for HCA include calcaneus gait as well as recurrent or persistent equinus.[1,5,6]

Because cerebral palsy affects not just the ankle joint, but the coordination and magnitude of muscle control at other joints as well, it must be considered in a global fashion. Thus, some of the problems arising from surgical procedures to correct equinus deformity relate to the "proper selection of patients." Because there are no strict criteria for determining which procedure is most efficacious, the decision is left to the individual physician to determine which procedure to use and when to use it based on his/her own experiences and preferences.

This chapter examines the theoretical biomechanical and physiologic factors about the ankle that may play a role in explaining the outcomes of these procedures and, thus, influence the choice and timing of procedures for correction of the equinus deformity.

Basic Biomechanical Considerations

Ankle Motion

The axis of the ankle joint may be considered to be in a plane almost perpendicular to the sagittal plane, which allows dorsiflexion/plantarflexion motion. The ankle is considered to be in neutral position when the long axis of the foot is at a 90-degree angle to the long axis of the leg. The ankle has approximately 45 degrees of motion, from about 20 degrees of dorsiflexion to about 25 degrees of plantarflexion, with significant variation between individuals.[8] Only part of this motion is used during gait, in which the ankle's arc of motion ranges from 5 to 10 degrees dorsiflexion in the second half of single-limb stance to maximum plantarflexion of 20 to 25 degrees at the end of stance-beginning of swing.

A normal gait cycle begins with heel strike, which takes place with the ankle in neutral position and the forefoot off the ground. During weight acceptance, ankle plantarflexion of 10 degrees occurs first, and by midweight acceptance (double-limb stance) the foot is planted flat on the ground (Fig. 1, *top*). The tibia then rotates forward over the planted foot during the next 0.2 seconds, and the ankle's angle changes rapidly to 5 degrees of dorsiflexion by mid single-limb stance. The ankle holds this angle through the rest of single-limb stance, even though the heel comes off the ground shortly after maximum dorsiflexion is reached. After the other heel lands, push-off is initiated and the ankle goes into 20- to 25-degree plantarflexion during the last part of stance (weight release).

External Torque

The forward motion of the tibia during stance arises from body weight and momentum becoming directed anterior to the ankle joint. Because the forces of forward momentum and body weight are external to the ankle, they create an external torque that tends to dorsiflex the ankle. It has been calculated that during a normal gait cycle the external dorsiflexing torque for a 150-lb individual at the initiation of single-limb stance phase is -25 ft-lb. This steadily rises to a value of $+75$

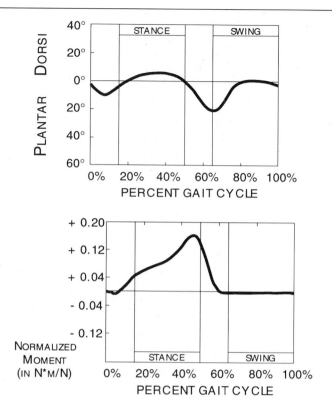

Fig. 1 *Top, Normal ankle motion and (**bottom**) normal external ankle dorsiflexion moments. In other diagrams these curves are shown for comparison. Note that external moments are negative during weight acceptance; markedly positive during single-limb stance (stance); and zero during swing.*

ft-lb by the end of single-limb stance.[9] The initial negative dorsiflexion torque is actually a positive plantarflexion torque resulting from the application of the force of body weight to the foot behind the heel, posterior to the ankle joint axis. As body weight manifested in the foot's center of pressure moves forward toward the toes, the lever arm to the ankle axis steadily lengthens and the external torque causing dorsiflexion increases correspondingly (Fig. 1, *bottom*). Although the body's momentum might decrease slightly during the first half of single-limb stance, momentum increases during the second half of single-limb stance, as the body's weight starts falling forward over the foot. Therefore, the external ankle dorsiflexion torque steadily increases throughout single-limb stance as the magnitude of the force as well as its lever arm increase. During weight release (push off) this torque decreases as more weight is shifted to the opposite leg. This pattern remains the same regardless of speed, but its magnitude increases with fast walking and decreases as the subject slows down.

Internal Torque

If there were no muscle activity affecting the ankle, then the torque generated by the body's weight and momentum would cause continuous dorsiflexion throughout single-limb stance (calcaneus gait). However, in the normal limb the changing activity of muscles acting through a relatively constant lever arm during the gait cycle opposes this external torque. By creating internal torques, the muscles act to restrain and control the amount of ankle motion allowed. The result is a pattern of ankle motion during stance that is relatively constant regardless of walking speed. Dynamic electromyographic analysis of the plantarflexors, including the gastrocnemius, soleus, peroneals, posterior tibialis, and toe flexors demonstrates that all of these muscles are active during single-limb stance, although they are not active during double-limb stance (weight acceptance and weight release).[10,11] The gastrocnemius-soleus complex (triceps surae) is the primary contributor to the internal torque generated.[11–13] If the large mass of these muscles and their conjoined, longer lever arm are considered in comparison to those of the other plantarflexors, the gastrocnemius and soleus each can be assumed to contribute approximately 40% to the total plantarflexion torque generated; combined, they supply 80% of the torque.[11,12] In the absence of the triceps surae, the secondary plantarflexors can provide only up to 40% of the normal total effort.[12] Although activity of these secondary plantarflexors may have some influence on preoperative ankle function and postoperative outcome of ankle function in a child with cerebral palsy, for clarity of discussion, we will assume that all of the internal plantarflexion torque comes from the triceps surae, and we will not consider the contribution of the secondary plantarflexors.

Whether the ankle remains at a constant angle or rotates smoothly into dorsiflexion, the internal torque generated by the triceps surae must resist the external reaction torques of body weight and momentum in a prescribed manner. Thus, the torque developed by the triceps surae (force of the muscle multiplied by its tendon's perpendicular distance to the axis of the ankle joint) increases as stance phase progresses. Because there is little change in the lever arm of the Achilles tendon, this increase in torque is generated by increased activity in the triceps surae.

Eccentric and Concentric Contraction by Triceps Surae

Because the gastrocnemius produces motion at two different joints, analysis of gastrocnemius activity must consider motion at both knee and ankle joints. The soleus produces motion at only one joint, so analysis of its activity during gait considers only ankle motion.

In normal gait during early stance, as the ankle begins to plantarflex and while the knee is slightly flexed, both the gastrocnemius and the soleus are at one of the shortest lengths they achieve during stance. In late weight acceptance and early single-limb stance, as the ankle undergoes rapid dorsiflexion (15 degrees in 0.2 seconds), the soleus contracts eccentrically. Then, as the ankle maintains a near-neutral position in the second half of single-limb stance, it contracts isometrically. Just before the push-off phase, the soleus shortens, acting concentrically for a brief period of time.

Early in stance, because the knee is extending while the ankle is dorsiflexing, the gastrocnemius is being stretched at both ends and must contract eccentrically along with the soleus. However, during the second half of single-limb stance, knee flexion is initiated earlier than ankle plantarflexion. The gastrocnemius thus begins to contract concentrically even though the soleus is contracting isometrically. This difference may necessitate different afferent neural input from stretch receptors as well as eliciting different efferent or motor output.

Basic Neurophysiologic Considerations

The biomechanical considerations above relate to how external torques are created and how the mechanical relationships between the muscles, joints, and bone change during gait. Neurophysiologic considerations primarily involve the regulation of the internal torques in their reaction to the external torques.

Length-Tension Relationships and Motor Nerve Recruitment

For a given amount of neurologic stimulus, the contractile force produced by the muscle increases in proportion to its length, up to a maximum level. The muscle length at which this force is at a maximum is called its resting length. Beyond the resting length, active tension generated by the muscle decreases as length increases. However, when the muscle is beyond its resting length, the passive resistance of the muscle produces tension, which increases with increased length (Fig. 2, *top left*). To date, no evidence exists to show that this inherent length-tension property of muscle (in the absence of contracture) is altered in cerebral palsy.

It is presumed that the resting length for the triceps surae exists at a neutral ankle position with the knee in full extension. Although there is a paucity of supporting data, the above statement will be assumed to be valid for this discussion. During gait, as the ankle position progresses from plantarflexion to neutral position early in stance, both gastrocnemius and soleus muscles should be capable of developing greater contractile tension to resist the increasing external torques (noted during stance) regardless of whether an increase in nerve stimulation supplements this activity. However, if the ankle remains at a neutral position during late single-limb stance, at the time when the external torques are increasing, triceps force would be considered near its maximum contractile output ability according to the length tension diagram, and the muscle could not actively increase force merely by changing length. To balance this increasing external torque and maintain the ankle at neutral position (isometric activity) requires a greater contribution from the passive elements and/or efferent neural stimulation, ie, an increase in firing rate and motor group recruitment (Fig. 2, *bottom*). The fact

369

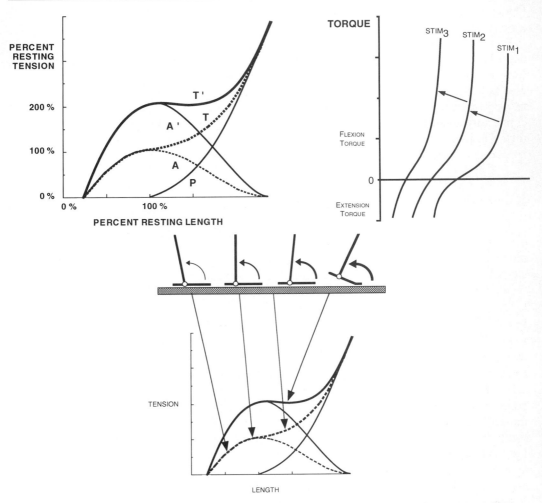

Fig. 2 *Top left, Idealized muscle length-tension (Blix) curves. Passive curve (P) is unchanged by neural stimulation. At baseline stimulation level, active curve (A) has peak tension at resting length, and total curve is (T'). With a higher neural stimulation level, active curve (A') can be attained, and total curve (T') will result. **Top right**, Shape of torque-angle curves is similar to the shape of Blix curves. Increasing stimulation makes the curves steeper and shifts them to the left. **Bottom**, Position of the ankle is shown during weight acceptance, early, mid, and late stance. External torque increases progressively, as designated by the arrows. Points on Blix curves for the triceps surae are indicated.*

that dynamic electromyographic activity of these muscles is amplified as stance phase progresses[11] suggests that an increase in nerve stimulation occurs in normal gait and that at least the contractile elements increase their contribution.

Afferent Organs and Feedback Control

Multiple types of afferent organs found in and around the muscle-tendon complexes include the Golgi tendon organs, muscle spindles, and stretch-sensitive free nerve endings. These respond to the length, tension, and velocity of the muscle by altering the firing rates and recruitment of efferent nerves.[14-18] During early single-limb stance, as the muscles contract eccentrically in response to the increasing external torque, stimulation of both displacement and velocity receptors seems to exist.[17] During the second half of single-limb stance, as the muscles contract isometrically with an increasing external torque demand, the predominant stimulant to these organs would be the increasing tension. The afferent stimulus thereby produced provides an additional regulatory mechanism, which influences the central nervous system in the production of the final efferent stimulus to each muscle.

Controversy exists as to whether efferent stimulus to muscle is pre-programmed or generated by learned feedback in a higher-order spinal or brain center response. There also is controversy as to which, how much, and by what mechanism each sensory organ detects the changes and contributes to the final control by such centers. Also, because both sensory innervation and muscle fiber type appear to differ somewhat between gastrocnemius and soleus muscles, the control of these two muscles might differ inherently.

Regardless of the relative contribution of each aspect of the neuromuscular system, examination of the intact system in animals and in humans shows that force-length curves obtained in the static condition resemble the torque-angle curves obtained during gait more closely than they do the Blix curves.[19] These curves can be used to characterize the static properties of the elbow musculature under reflex control. If external load as a reflection of external static force or torque is compared to muscle length or angular position of the joint, the curve produced is steep and rises rapidly (Fig. 2, *top right*). The existence of these elements in an intact individual alters the behavior of the force-length relationship of muscles from that seen in the typical Blix curves. For example, it has been shown that at the elbow joint under static equilibrium conditions with reflex control intact, when the external force or torque is compared to muscle length or angular joint position, the curve produced is steep and rises rapidly. These curves indicate a spring-like resistance to stretch and release of the neuromuscular system, whether it be from functionally isolated muscles or sets of several synergistic and antagonistic muscles operating to control joint rotation. Increased tone increases the resistance of the spring to produce the same tension at a different muscle length or joint rotation. Thus, with greater neurostimulation, this curve is slightly steeper in shape, and it shifts in a way that indicates that the same load can be resisted statically at shorter muscle lengths or lower joint angles. The torque-angle curves obtained during gait seem to resemble these curves more closely than Blix curves.

Pathologic Changes Due to Cerebral Palsy

Abnormal External Torques of Equinus Deformity

The typical gait of a child with cerebral palsy who has an equinus deformity is toe walking. Whether a dynamic or a fixed passive muscular contracture exists, the ankle with an equinus deformity has a range of motion that never allows a neutral dorsiflexed position. At best, 0 to 5 degrees of plantarflexion is seen during weight acceptance, and joint angles up to 30 degrees or more of plantarflexion can be seen during single-limb stance.

It should first be noted that children with cerebral palsy having an equinus deformity end the swing phase with the ankle in plantarflexion. This may be caused by abnormal activity of plantarflexor muscles in swing phase, an equinus contracture, lack of activity of ankle extensor muscles, or any combination thereof. When the child strikes the floor, then, with the toes first, foot-floor contact is initiated at the metatarsal heads, and the foot's center of pressure will, therefore, be located far anteriorly. Clearly, the external torque is not normal from the onset of stance: Body weight is anterior to the ankle and the lever arm acting on the ankle joint is long and located anterior to the center of rotation of the ankle joint, rather than posterior where it is in the normal child. Instead of starting as a plantarflexion torque, the external moment is initiated as a dorsiflexion torque equal to what might be seen at about mid single-limb stance in normal gait.

Abnormal Internal Torques

The equinus position at the end of swing causes toe strike at the initiation of stance and leads to abnormal external torque. Activity of plantarflexor muscles early in stance responds to this torque, creating internal torques that could be abnormally high for this phase of the gait cycle. What subsequently happens to ankle position as stance progresses depends on the interaction between the higher-than-normal external torque and the triceps surae internally generated torque.

In the absence of contracture, all evidence indicates that the sensory organs behave in a normal fashion in cerebral palsy. Differences in responses among children who have cerebral palsy are caused by variable problems in central control; ie, in a child with cerebral palsy, there is sufficient stimulus to affect the afferent system, but the response of the system is abnormal. All children with cerebral palsy do not respond alike. For example, if a clasp-knife response existed, an externally produced dorsiflexion torque might cause increased muscle force up to a certain position of ankle rotation; but, subsequently, even if the force were maintained, inhibition could reduce the internal muscle force and allow further dorsiflexion. In other children, if the system generated increased tone, the afferent stimuli could be abnormally amplified and produce a steadily rising muscle force that resists further dorsiflexion[4,14,15] and even causes a clonic response of increased plantarflexion. Alternatively, the central nervous system independently could generate high enough muscle forces to make changes from afferent stimuli a minor contribution, and marked resistance could occur even from the start of movement (rigidity). Thus, even without a true contracture or deformity, the dynamic response of the muscle to the elevated external torques in different children who have cerebral palsy produces different responses during the stance phase of gait. It is this dynamic feature that produces the abnormal features of the ankle in gait in young children even before a true contracture is present.

Pathophysiologic Effect of Contractures

Up to this point, only the dynamic force of the gastrocnemius-soleus muscle group has been presumed to be altered by cerebral palsy. However, when a contracture exists, there is increased thickness and shortening of the passive elements surrounding each muscle fiber.[4,17]

These changes alter the mechanical properties of the passive elements, stiffening the muscle and causing it to generate higher tension per unit increase in length. As growth occurs, the muscle stays shorter compared to the bone(s) on which it inserts and, with time, causes limitation in the ability to dorsiflex the ankle. The normal pattern of load sharing between the dynamic and the static elements is thereby shifted, relying more heavily on the static elements within the physiologic range seen in gait.

Alterations in passive components could also reduce the response of the afferent sensory organs and, consequently, decrease the response of contractile elements. Being in parallel (rather than "in series") with the passive elements as well as the muscle fibers, for a given tension, velocity, or length change, the afferent sensory organs could feel less of the response to change and provide less input to the central nervous system. The contracture then, because of its greater stiffness, its reduction in range of dorsiflexion allowed, and its dulling of the sensory organs, could become the major feature of the neuromuscular system relied upon to resist external torques.

The neurologic lesion in a child with cerebral palsy is not progressive. However, the passive stiffening, shortening, and perhaps dulling phenomenon of the muscle progresses as the child with cerebral palsy grows older, and may be the major factor causing gait deterioration with time. Depending on the severity of central nervous system involvement, the age of the child, and/or the degree of permanent contracture present, the pattern, as well as the magnitude of ankle equinus motion in stance, varies among children with cerebral palsy. In some children, internal torque, however generated, just balances the external torques, and the equinus at the initiation of stance may not change throughout the remainder of stance phase. In younger children, internal torque is generated primarily by the contractile muscle fibers while in older children a larger portion of this torque is generated by the passive elements of the contractile system as fixed contractures develop.

When the internal torque generated exceeds the external torque, progressive plantarflexion occurs; in the reverse situation, dorsiflexion occurs. Because the balance of passive versus active elements contributing to internal torque depends not only on age but also on length, the relationship of internal to external torque during the stance phase can change at any given age. This change alters the simple pattern of dorsiflexion/plantarflexion during stance. For example, early in stance with the ankle in plantarflexion, the dynamic contractile elements contribute the most force. If that force is less than the external torque, dorsiflexion proceeds to a point where either the contractile elements or the passive elements generate sufficient torque to balance the external torque. Thus, the pattern of dorsiflexion/plantarflexion during stance varies with changes in load sharing between the contractile and passive elements of the muscle system and with each element's relation to the magnitude of the external torque and the position of the ankle.

Physical examination of a child with cerebral palsy should provide data on the range of ankle motion and on ankle plantarflexor tone, including the degree, if any, of clasp-knife response, clonus, and rigidity. Quantitative gait analysis should provide data on ankle motion and external torque during the stance phase of gait. This knowledge will help the clinician to understand the dynamics of the process and, thus, result in the selection of the proper treatment.

Analysis of Equinus Correction Procedures

The Common Endpoint of Surgical Correction

In all three approaches to surgical correction of equinus deformity, the muscle itself is unchanged by the procedure. That is, the dynamic properties of the muscle's contractile and passive elements are the same after surgery as they were before the surgery. The three surgical procedures act only on the tendon, thereby lengthening the entire muscle-tendon complex and/or altering its lever arm.

Surgeons differ with regard to the exact amount of dorsiflexion allowed after surgery for correction of equinus deformity. However, one feature that is common to all three operations is the criterion that all surgeons use to judge the result obtained: Does the arc of motion of the ankle joint, with the knee extended, allow approximately 10 degrees of dorsiflexion beyond neutral? This affects both the external torque against which the internal torque must act and the position of the ankle at which the internal torque responds.

A surgical procedure that allows the ankle to initiate stance phase in a neutral position brings the center of pressure back toward the ankle and reduces the lever arm of body weight. This surgery, thus, reduces the abnormally high external torque in early stance phase, returning it closer to normal values. The external torque and the stimulus to generate internal torques early in stance are reduced.

Regardless of the neurological system's ability to preset the internal torque, the muscle has an inherent ability to initiate force in stance with an ankle at neutral. When the ankle's position changes from plantarflexion to neutral, the internal torque is resisted by an external torque with a lever arm that will progressively rise to the end of single limb stance. This situation would look more normal. Differences in how the muscle responds after heel strike then depend on the particular procedure performed.

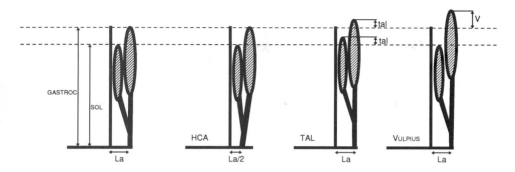

Fig. 3 *Schematic drawings of the equinus correcting procedures.* **Left,** *In preoperative condition, gastrocnemius and soleus lengths are shown, as well as the length of the Achilles tendon lever arm (La).* **Left center,** *HCA shortens lever arm by one-half (La/2).* **Right center,** *TAL lengthens the gastrocnemius and soleus equally, but leaves the lever arm unchanged.* **Right,** *Vulpius procedure lengthens the gastrocnemius, but alters neither soleus length nor lever arm.*

How Lengthening the Achilles Tendon (TAL) Achieves Correction

TAL changes the length of the tendinous portion of the triceps surae to allow dorsiflexion of 5 to 10 degrees. No change is made in the lever arm (Fig. 3, *right center*). Tendon lengthening alters neither the muscle's intrinsic properties nor its behavior; the tension developed after surgery is the same for a given inherent muscle length and external torque as it was preoperatively. The Achilles tendon is, however, longer after surgery, and the same muscle length causing a given muscle response will be present at a more normal ankle angle and external dorsiflexion torque (Fig. 4). The response that was present at about 10 degrees of plantarflexion, at the start of single-limb stance when the external dorsiflexion torque was high, will now occur later in stance. The result of a properly performed TAL is ankle motion of 5 degrees dorsiflexion in mid to late stance before internal torque balances or exceeds external torque. Overlengthening results in a delay in the development of balance of the external torque by the internal torque until mid to late stance; that is, dorsiflexion greater than 5 to 10 degrees will be seen in late stance (calcaneus gait). In contrast, lengthening too little causes muscle tension to be developed at too small a degree of dorsiflexion and to balance or be greater than the external torque too early in stance; that is, recurrent equinus will be seen.

How the Vulpius-Type Procedure Achieves Correction

Analysis of the Vulpius procedure is similar to that of the TAL, except that the torque-angle curves for the soleus and gastrocnemius must be considered separately. This procedure is usually used when there is no clinically significant contracture of the soleus. The gastroc-

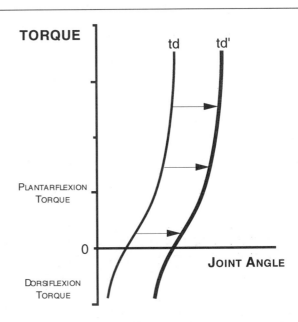

Fig. 4 *Effect of TAL on the torque-angle curve. The curve relating torque and angle is shifted to the right, allowing a greater joint angle to be achieved at any torque level.*

nemius recession procedure temporarily uncouples the gastrocnemius from the soleus portion of the triceps surae complex, but, after about six weeks, scar tissue reconnects the two ends. The net result is a tendon lengthening of only the gastrocnemius (Fig. 3, *right*).

The Vulpius procedure alters the resulting torque-angle curve for the triceps surae so that the gastrocnemius contributes less to internal torque at shorter displacements (less dorsiflexion), although its contribution remains high for higher displacements (more dorsiflexion). Because the soleus remains intact, its contractile ability should provide enough internal plantarflexion torque to oppose the reduced external dorsiflexion torque at low dorsiflexion angles. With the gastrocnemius contributing at higher angles of dorsiflexion, there should be sufficient resistance to higher external torques later in stance. Thus, a calcaneus gait should be a rare result.

However, it is still possible for recurrent equinus deformity to develop from the soleus if its dynamic properties are strong, because, early in stance, the external torque will not be excessively high. If the gastrocnemius is weakened by the Vulpius procedure and an equinus contracture develops in the soleus, knee hyperextension can occur.[20] Thus, success of the Vulpius procedure may be seen as correcting the set point of only one component of the system.

How the Heel Cord Advancement (HCA) Achieves Correction

Correcting equinus deformity by means of either a gastrocnemius recession or a TAL produces no change in the Achilles tendon's lever arm. In contrast, HCA reduces the lever arm of the triceps surae by approximately 50%. To maintain the same level of preoperative internal torque after reduction of the lever arm in HCA requires double the amount of triceps surae force produced preoperatively. This double force would have to be present during each interval of the entire single-limb stance phase for equinus to recur. If the triceps surae is unable to provide this force, internal torque will be reduced and the equinus position will be eliminated. If the muscle is able to respond to the higher demand, ankle motion will be in the normal range and produce a near normal gait.

The HCA makes a simple change in the structure of the ankle system: It alters the ability of the triceps surae to generate internal torque. Therefore, the ultimate success of HCA lies with the capacity of the muscle system to generate higher forces postoperatively than preoperatively. The higher forces may be generated dynamically as a result of the contractile elements' tonic response; statically as a result of the stiffened passive elements; and/or more responsively as a result of greater stimulation from afferent receptors increasing motor recruitment. Except in this last situation, it seems that the muscle would not respond with increased capacity. If, before surgery, the muscle had been able to respond with such increased capacity, greater plantarflexion would have been seen. However, the one feature that could change after HCA relates to the stimuli to the afferent sensory system. Because the lever arm is reduced by 50%, the excursion of the Achilles tendon is reduced by 50%. This, in turn, reduces the change in displacement and velocity sensed by afferent neural receptors traversed by the muscle tendon complex as it goes from plantarflexion to dorsiflexion. The reduced tendon excursion would result in reduced afferent velocity or displacement signals. However, the stimulus to afferent receptors responsive to tension would increase. How the afferent receptors adapt to their altered input and just how much these afferent signals add to more control over the active muscle tone in any child with cerebral palsy is not clear enough at this time to permit determination in any individual case of whether either possibility will occur.

In Murphy's[1] original article, the explanation given for the effectiveness of HCA is that at the end of single-limb stance, the lever arm of the Achilles tendon has shifted to the metatarsal heads, and the 50% reduction in torque in early stance becomes only a 15% reduction late in stance; thus, push off is maintained. This argument is faulty from a biomechanical standpoint. The success of this procedure can best be described in biomechanical and physiologic terms: A reduction in the lever arm of the triceps surae reduces its capacity to respond to external torques and will be successful if the triceps surae responds with properly increased forces to the relatively normal torques produced by better ankle position.

This new explanation of the surgical success of HCA appears to be of utmost importance and explains the results seen after HCA. It would also help determine, prior to surgery, which child should be specifically selected for this operation. Previous studies report from 9% to 18% excellent results: heel-toe gait, good push off, and no hyperextension of the knee, and approximately 65% to 73% good results: flat-foot strike with or without push off and no hyperextension of the knee.[1,5,6] The excellent group may incorporate individuals who have the inherent capacity postoperatively to generate sufficient force for the high demands at the end of single-limb stance to counter the reduction in the lever arm produced. Groups with good and poor results did not incorporate those individuals.

Predicting Success of Equinus Correction

Together with the information relating to range of motion and tone that is provided preoperatively from physical examination, information gained through preoperative gait analysis should enable the surgeon to decide whether HCA, TAL, or gastrocnemius recession is indicated for a child with cerebral palsy and equinus deformity. Regardless of the neurologic involvement and/or speed of gait and/or use of assistive devices, gait evaluation can now estimate torques at a given joint as well as provide data on the functional range of motion.[10] Electromyographic (EMG) data obtained with the motion data could be used to separate soleus activity from gastrocnemius activity and to determine the relative contribution of active and passive components in order to help select those patients best suited for each type of procedure.

Gait studies reveal that during single-limb stance all equinus deformities may yield not only different magnitudes but also different patterns of equinus. Some children show a fixed amount of equinus of variable magnitude. In these children the ankle motion curve is relatively flat during all of single-limb stance (type I, Fig. 5, *top left*). Other children show a greater degree of equinus at the initiation of single-limb stance than at the end (type II, Fig. 5, *top right*), whereas in still others, the reverse is the case (type III, Fig. 5, *center left*). Torques calculated in such children show patterns similar to those of ankle motion (Fig. 5, *center right*). In any of these motion patterns, an abrupt shift in the magnitude or rate of change can occur during single-limb stance, perhaps reflecting clonus or a clasp-knife type of response (Fig. 5, *bottom*). The pattern of EMG activity also can differ not only with regard to soleus versus gastrocnemius activity but also as to when in stance and at what ankle angle activity is seen in each. Because HCA increases muscle demand, this procedure would produce the best results in a child with a type III motion pattern and EMG activity present throughout stance. A good result could also be expected in a child with type I motion pattern. TAL would also be expected to work well in a child with a type I motion pattern. However, HCA or TAL will prob-

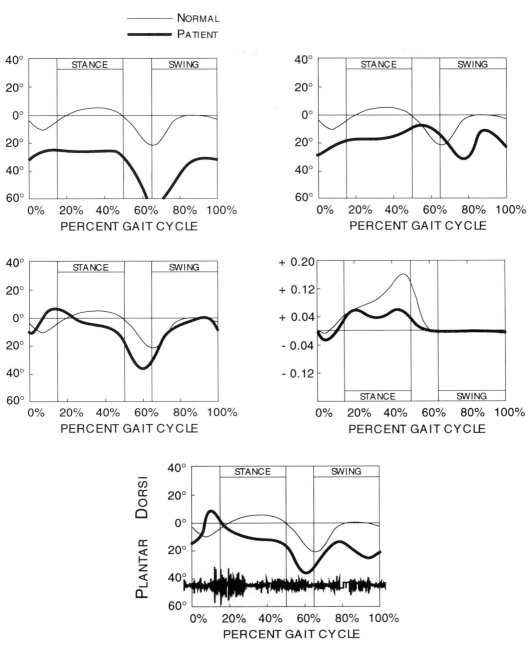

Fig. 5 *Patient data showing the three basic equinus patterns.* ***Top left,*** *Type I pattern holds ankle angle essentially unchanged throughout single-limb stance (stance).* ***Top right,*** *Type II pattern has increasing dorsiflexion during single-limb stance.* ***Center left,*** *Type III pattern has increasing plantarflexion during single-limb stance.* ***Center right,*** *Normalized external ankle torques, from patient data shown in Figure 5, center left, show a pattern similar to the ankle motion pattern.* ***Bottom,*** *Type III pattern shown with gastrocnemius EMG.*

ably produce only a fair or poor result (calcaneus gait at the end of single-limb stance) when performed on a child with a type II pattern, whereas a Vulpius procedure might prove best for that pattern, and poorest for a type III pattern.

Summary

A theoretical approach is made to the biomechanical and neurophysiologic considerations of the three procedures available to correct equinus deformity in children with cerebral palsy. The biomechanical rationale for success of each of the three procedures is given. This analysis also led to the original explanation for success of HCA being discarded and a new explanation offered.

Biomechanical considerations include the external torques caused by body weight and momentum and the internal torques generated by the muscles. These torques must be appropriately balanced during gait. However, the child with cerebral palsy creates abnormal torques, both external and internal, and the challenge to the surgeon is to correct these to the greatest extent possible without causing compensatory abnormalities. Neurophysiologic considerations include the influence of afferent receptors as well as the length-tension relationship of muscle in vitro, which can be expanded to the torque-angle relationship in vivo.

The surgeon must take this knowledge into consideration when planning surgical correction of equinus deformity. The endpoint for all three procedures is the same: Ankle motion that allows dorsiflexion to 5 to 10 degrees and plantarflexion to only 20 to 25 degrees. All three procedures achieve this endpoint with varying degrees of success, but overcorrection or recurrence can result. TAL works by shifting the torque-angle curve, but has a tendency to allow postoperative calcaneal gait. The Vulpius procedure works by shifting the torque-angle curve of the gastrocnemius, but leaves the soleus unchanged. This procedure can thus allow recurrence of equinus. Previous studies of HCA show the possibility for either recurrence or calcaneus gait. Its success results from decreasing the torque produced by the triceps surae and, possibly, from decreasing the Achilles tendon excursion, as well. None of the procedures changes the intrinsic properties of the muscle with or without contracture.

Preoperative gait analysis provides angular displacement and joint torque estimations that should be useful in deciding among the procedures. Three groups of patients are suggested: those who maintain ankle position; those with decreasing plantarflexion (dorsiflexion); and those with increasing plantarflexion during single-limb stance. Variations in the pattern are present in each. The third type of patient would appear to have the best results from HCA, the first type of patient might benefit best from TAL or HCA, and the second type might be served best by a Vulpius procedure.

References

1. Pierrot AH, Murphy OB: Albert E. Klinkicht Award, 1972. Heel cord advancement: A new approach to the spastic equinus deformity. *Orthop Clin North Am* 1974;5:117–126.
2. Banks HH: The management of spastic deformities of the foot and ankle. *Clin Orthop* 1977;122:70–76.
3. Gaines RW, Ford TB: A systematic approach to the amount of Achilles tendon lengthening in cerebral palsy. *J Pediatr Orthop* 1984;4:448–451.
4. Rang M: Cerebral palsy, in Morrissy RT (ed): *Pediatric Orthopaedics*, ed 3. Philadelphia, JB Lippincott, 1990, chap 13, pp 465–506.
5. Strecker WB, Via MW, Oliver SK, et al: Heel cord advancement for treatment of equinus deformity in cerebral palsy. *J Pediatr Orthop* 1990;10:105–108.
6. Throop FB, DeRosa GP, Reeck C, et al: Correction of equinus in cerebral palsy by the Murphy procedure of tendo calcaneus advancement: A preliminary communication. *Dev Med Child Neurol* 1975;17:182–185
7. Segal LS, Thomas SE, Mazur JM, et al: Calcaneal gait in spastic diplegia after heel cord lengthening: A study with gait analysis. *J Pediatr Orthop* 1989;9: 697–701.
8. Frankel VH, Nordin M: Biomechanics of the ankle, in Nordin M, Frankel V (eds): *Basic Biomechanics of the Musculoskeletal System*, ed 2. Philadelphia, Lea & Febiger, 1989, chap 8, pp 153–161.
9. Bresler B, Frankel JP: The forces and moments in the leg during level walking. *Trans ASME* 1950;72:27–36.
10. Procter P, Paul JP: Ankle joint biomechanics. *J Biomech* 1982;15:627–634.
11. Sutherland DH: An electromyographic study of the plantar flexors of the ankle in normal walking on the level. *J Bone Joint Surg* 1966;48A:66–71.
12. Murray MP, Guren GN, Baldwin JM, et al: A comparison of plantar flexion torque with and without the triceps surae. *Acta Orthop Scand* 1976;47:122–124.
13. Murray MP, Guten GN, Sepic SB, et al: Function of the triceps surae during gait: Compensatory mechanisms for unilateral loss. *J Bone Joint Surg* 1978;60A:473–476.
14. Cleland CL, Rymer WZ: Neural mechanisms underlying the clasp-knife reflex in the cat: I. Characteristics of the Reflex. *J Neurophysiol* 1990;64:1303–1318.
15. Cleland CL, Hayward L, Rymer WZ: Neural mechanisms underlying the clasp-knife reflex in the cat: II. Stretch-sensitive muscular-free nerve endings. *J Neurophysiol* 1990;64:1319–1330.
16. Houk JC, Cargo PE, Rymer WZ: Functional properties of the Golgi tendon organs in spinal and supraspinal mechanisms of voluntary motor control and locomotion, in Desmedt JE (ed): *Prog Clin Neurophysiol*. Basel, Karger, 1980, vol 8, pp 33–43.
17. Pitman MI, Peterson L: Biomechanics of skeletal muscle, in Nordin M, Frankel (eds): *Basic Biomechanics of the Musculoskeletal System*, ed 2. Philadelphia, Lea & Febiger, 1989, chap 5, pp 89–111.
18. Rymer WZ, Houk JC, Crago PE: Mechanisms of the clasp-knife reflex studied in an animal model *Exp Brain Res* 1979;37:93–113.
19. Houk JC, Rymer WZ: Neural control of muscle length and tension, in Brooks VB (ed): *Handbook of Physiology, Section 1: The Nervous System*. Bethesda, MD, American Physiological Society, 1981, vol 2, pp 292–294.
20. Simon SR, Deutsch SD, Nuzzo RM, et al: Genu recurvatum in spastic cerebral palsy: Report on findings by gait analysis. *J Bone Joint Surg* 1978;60A:882–894.

Chapter 29

Treatment of Equinus Deformity in Children With Cerebral Palsy at Moscow Children's Hospital No. 18

Evgeny G. Sologubov, MD

Foot deformities are very common in children with spastic diplegia, and up to 90% of them have valgus posture. Prior to surgery, bracing, gymnastic therapy, massage therapy, underwater massage, swimming, acupuncture, and magnetic therapy are used. In addition, occasional blocks with either alcohol or novocaine followed by serial casts and orthotics may be used.

When nonoperative treatment is unsuccessful, surgery is indicated to provide full correction. Preoperative assessment includes standing weightbearing radiographs, as well as plantography, which demonstrates weightbearing on the forefoot only, in most cases. The most common surgical procedure for treatment of equinus is the Strayer procedure, which has been used 66.5% of the time. There is somewhat of an abnormal gait for the first six months after surgery, which is resolved by the end of the first postoperative year. In this series of patients, there were no complications, relapses, or calcaneus deformities. It is felt that postoperative rehabilitation is important to prevent weakness of the triceps surae.

The Vulpius procedure was done in 21.1% of the cases. This procedure was used most frequently in children over 10 years of age; it accounted for 73.5% of the operations in this age group, whereas it was used in only 25% of the operations on children under ten. This procedure is never used for children less than 5 years of age, because it resulted in calcaneus deformity in 27% of patients in this age group.

The author feels that the Strayer procedure is the safest and most effective procedure for treatment of the equinus deformity in children 3 years of age and older.

Consensus

Equinus is the most common deformity in patients with cerebral palsy. It is caused by spasticity, primarily of the triceps surae muscle, with or without weakness of the ankle dorsiflexors. Not every equinus deformity requires treatment, but equinus posture of the foot and ankle increases the instability of already compromised balance. This also necessitates an increase in knee and hip flexion during swing or circumduction of the leg if sagittal flexion cannot be increased. If the triceps surae is spastic and contracted, it frequently is associated with a valgus deformity in patents with spastic diplegia. Toe-walkers with hip and knee flexion (crouched gait) may not have a true equinus contracture, and any dynamic knee flexion deformity must be evaluated as to its relationship to the equinus. If placing the knee in extension in a cylinder cast or immobilizer causes the ankle equinus or toe-toe gait to disappear, lengthening of the Achilles tendon will not correct the equinus. True ankle equinus also must be distinguished from midfoot equinus.

Equinus deformity is preferable to calcaneus deformity. The jump position of flexed hips and knees and equinus ankles is better tolerated than the crouched position of flexed hips and knees and calcaneus feet that lowers the buttocks closer to the walking surface and affords no push-off in walking.

A logical therapeutic approach to a spastic triceps surae in a child with spastic diplegia depends on an understanding of the pathophysiology and biomechanical considerations of spasticity of the gastrocnemius-soleus complex. It should be emphasized that treatment of patients with diplegia is signifi-cantly different from that of hemiparetic patients, for whom a more aggressive surgical approach usually is required.

Nonoperative Treatment

Nonoperative treatment of a spastic triceps surae can be beneficial in patients with spastic diplegia. Medications to relax the gastrocnemius-soleus complex have limited value alone, but they may be helpful in conjunction with other forms of treatment to reduce spasticity systematically. Local nerve and muscle blocks can be effective temporarily, but these are painful and difficult to do in young children without general anesthesia. Stretching exercises are beneficial primarily to prevent contractures, and they may lead to increased muscle length by stimulating muscle growth by addition of sarcomeres. Painful stretching of a spastic muscle, however, can be detrimental. Serial and inhibitive casting have proven beneficial, most often for increasing ankle dorsiflexion in children 2 to 6 years of age, but the effect is transient if no further measures are taken. After fixed contractures are corrected, ankle-foot orthoses may be used to minimize recurrence of equinus deformity, but the morbidity of long-term orthosis wear and the possibility of the development of a rocker-bottom deformity must be weighed against the morbidity of a repeat lengthening of the triceps apparatus.

Nonoperative treatment of a tight triceps surae may not always be successful, but the risk of complications is slight and surgery can be done if nonoperative methods fail. One nonoperative treatment method appropriate for further research is night-time, low-intensity, electrical stimulation, which may prove beneficial for mild to moderate diplegia.

Surgical correction is indicated for true contracture of the triceps surae or significant equinus during gait, for which other means, such as bracing, are not successful. If the child does not demonstrate good sitting and standing balance, correction of the equinus deformity will not aid ambulation. If possible, surgery should be delayed until the child is 5 to 7 years of age, at which time there is a low risk of recurrence of the contracture. The Achilles tendon should never be overlengthened. No more than 5 degrees of ankle dorsiflexion should be attempted at casting when surgically correcting equinus and spastic paralysis.

Surgical Treatment

Many different surgical procedures have been described for lengthening the triceps surae, but they are of three basic types: (1) lengthening of the gastrocnemius alone (Strayer), with or without soleus recession (Vulpius); (2) anterior translocation of the Achilles tendon (Throop); and (3) lengthening of the Achilles tendon.

Lengthening of the gastrocnemius was first described by Vulpius and Stoffel. Muscle-tendon length correction is restored by scar tissue, which fills in the recessed area and reduces spasticity. The basis for gastrocnemius lengthening is the Silfverskiöld test, which evaluates the amount of ankle dorsi-flexion with the knee in both flexion and extension. This test must be performed with the patient under general anesthesia.

Excellent to poor results have been reported after both the Vulpius and Strayer procedures. A recurrence rate of 1% in children older than 5 years has been reported after the Vulpius procedure. In younger children, a repeat procedure usually is required within 6 to 7 years. A recurrence rate of 12% has been reported in younger children, but this is considered acceptable considering the nature of the condition for which the procedure is performed. Rarely is it associated with recurvatum deformity, and there is also a low incidence of calcaneus deformity after the procedure.

Anterior translocation of the Achilles tendon, as described by Throop and associates, involves detaching the Achilles tendon from the posterior aspect of the calcaneus and transferring it anteriorly to a new location on the calcaneus. Because results of this more complicated procedure have not been superior to other means of Achilles tendon lengthening, it generally is not recommended. Furthermore, frequent recurrence of the deformity has been reported after anterior translocation.

Achilles tendon lengthening by z-plasty or a sliding technique may be combined with posterior capsulotomy of the ankle and subtalar joints, but this is required rarely, usually in older patients.

Future research in quantitative gait analysis may provide more exact indications for each of these surgical procedures.

Section Nine
Varus Foot

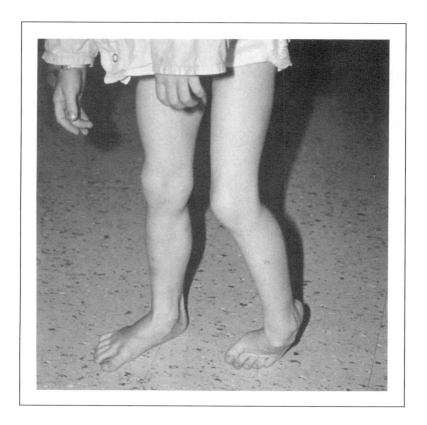

Chapter 30

Varus Foot in Cerebral Palsy: An Overview

David H. Sutherland, MD

Biomechanics of the Foot and Ankle

The sagittal plane movements of the foot and ankle during weight-bearing are quite familiar, but a brief review of the movements in the coronal and transverse planes, pertinent muscle actions, and floor reaction forces will provide background for the chapters on varus foot.

The subtalar joint has an oblique axis, measuring 42 degrees superiorly in the inferolateral to superomedial direction (Figs. 1 and 2).[1] With foot strike, the calcaneus falls into valgus, and as indicated by the initial medial shear recorded by the force plate, valgus thrust is generated. This medial shear is transmitted to the subtalar joint, leading to internal rotation of the talus and subsequent pronation of the forefoot.[2]

The main objective of the first period of stance, initial double-limb support, is to accept the body weight from the opposite foot. In single-limb support, the next period in stance, body weight is transferred over the planted foot. The eccentric action of the plantarflexor muscles decelerates the forward rotation of the tibia, thereby moving the force line in front of the knee joint and contributing to knee extension in stance phase. The alignment of the posterior compartment muscles influences the mechanics of the foot. The concentric contraction of the muscles medial to the subtalar axis generates an inverting force on the heel. The combination of heel inversion and supination of the forefoot creates a rigid lever arm to help slow the fall of the body's center of gravity during the push-off phase.[3] As the calcaneus inverts, the talus externally rotates through linkage, and an external torque is recorded by the force plate.

The muscles aligned to produce inversion of the hind foot are the triceps surae, tibialis posterior, flexor hallucis longus, flexor digitorum longus, tibialis anterior, and extensor hallucis longus (Fig. 3). Of these, the three most important are the tibialis anterior, the tibialis posterior, and the triceps surae. The tibialis anterior dorsiflexes and supinates the foot while the tibialis posterior inverts (adduction movement) and plantarflexes it, mimicking to some degree the action of the triceps surae. Moreover, the tibialis anterior is predominantly a swing phase muscle

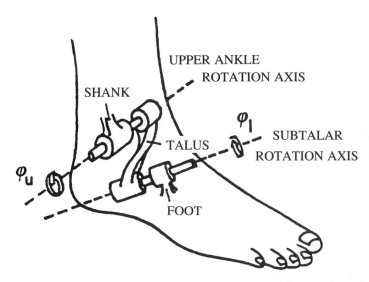

Fig. 1 *The rotational axis of the ankie joint and the rotational axis of the subtalar joint modeled as a system of three rigid links connected by ankle and subtalar hinge joints. (Reproduced with permission from Dul J: Development of a minimum fatigue optimization technique for predicting individual muscle forces during human posture and movement with application to the ankle musculature during standing and walking. DAI 1983;44(10B).)*

while the tibialis posterior and the triceps surae normally are stance phase muscles.

The muscles aligned to produce eversion are the extensor digitorum longus, peroneus longus, and peroneus brevis (Fig. 3). In swing phase, the extensor digitorum longus and the tibialis anterior act to balance the lift of the foot, preventing supination and inversion. During single-limb support, the peronei, acting with the other plantarflexor muscles, help balance the forces acting across the subtalar joint during stance phase.

Functional Deficit

In addition to problems in shoe fitting and wear and a cosmetically objectionable foot, varus alignment also results in weightbearing instability and/or difficulty in swing-phase foot clearance, which are the significant functional problems.

Gait Parameters

The results of gait analysis studies have been inconclusive and confusing.[4-8] Abnormalities in both tibialis anterior and tibialis posterior

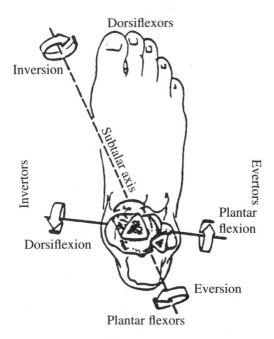

Fig. 2 *Transverse plane alignment of axis of ankle joint and axis of subtalar joint. (Reproduced with permission from Mann.[1])*

muscle activity have been identified, and many subjects demonstrate overactivity in both muscles. In my laboratory, helpful information is obtained through use of all the primary gait analysis tools, ie, dynamic electromyography (EMG), force, and movement measurements. For example, if dynamic early swing-phase inversion of the foot occurs during activity of the tibialis anterior while the tibialis posterior is silent, a split anterior tibialis tendon transfer is selected as the treatment. Thus, it is possible to come closer to establishing cause and effect relationships by correlating motion curves and dynamic EMG than by relying on EMG alone.

Tibialis posterior overactivity is more likely to interfere with stance phase stability, contributing to equinus, deficient loading, and deficient lateral shear. Again, correlating EMG with motion and force measurements improves the odds for a successful treatment plan. It is important to ask if the varus foot occurs in swing or stance phase, or both, and if there is fixed deformity that will require bony procedures for correction. The treatment plan may include lengthening of the tibialis posterior and split transfer of the tibialis anterior or it may include a single muscle transfer or lengthening. In all cases, the plan should be based on objective analysis and not on playing the odds. The outcome must be analyzed by a repeat gait analysis to ensure improvement in treatment.

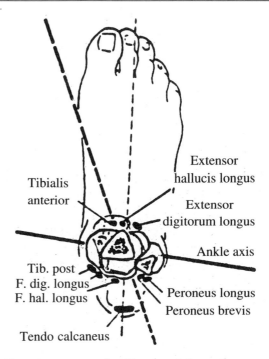

Tibialis
anterior

Extensor
hallucis longus

Extensor
digitorum longus

Ankle axis

Tib. post
F. dig. longus
F. hal. longus

Peroneus longus
Peroneus brevis

Tendo calcaneus

Fig. 3 *Position of invertor, evertor, dorsiflexor, and plantarflexor muscles with respect to the axis of the ankle joint and the axis of the subtalar joint. (Reproduced with permission from Mann.[1])*

Technologic Advances

One hindrance in application of movement measurements to the study of foot problems has been the difficulty in separating tibiotalar, subtalar, and forefoot movements. A method for making such measurements with a commercially available system has been described, and when this technique or similar techniques have been validated by other investigators, the methods can be used in other laboratories and data can be gathered from many sources. Another breakthrough in the field of gait analysis, which offers great promise for improving the yield from force measurements, has been the development of systems for measuring dynamic foot pressure. These systems measure the pressure on the plantar surface of the foot throughout stance phase. The pressure is displayed graphically by a color code that gives the pressure in force per unit area or by a three-dimensional contour map.

Case Example

This 8-year-old boy was delivered by Caesarean section because of fetal distress at the end of a full-term pregnancy. In his first year of

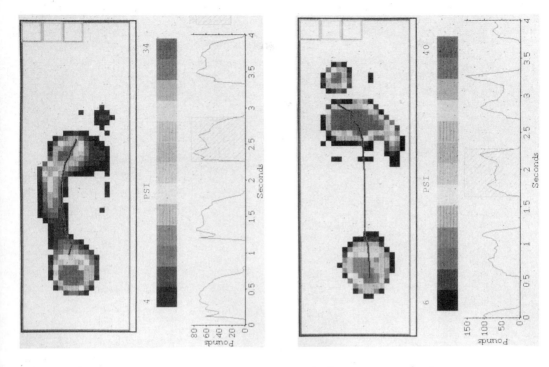

Fig. 4 *Tekscan recording of dynamic pressure distribution of the left and right foot of a patient with left spastic hemiparesis.*

life, a diagnosis of left mild hemiparesis, secondary to a porencephalic cyst, was established. His developmental milestones were within the normal range, and functional impairment was minimal. His orthopaedic surgeon referred him to the Motion Analysis Laboratory for further study of the isolated finding of dynamic varus deformity of the left foot. This finding may have been related to a recent growth spurt because his parents had not noted the foot abnormality until the year preceding the gait study.

A gait study was performed using movement measurement, dynamic EMG, and force measurement. In addition, a study of the dynamic foot pressure was carried out. The most cogent measurements from the total study have been extracted to show how gait analysis contributes to selection of the most appropriate treatment.

The dynamic foot pressure distribution of the left (hemiparetic side) and right feet is shown in Figure 4. The vertical force curves next to the foot pressure illustrations indicate the time of dynamic pressure sampling. In Figure 4, *left*, the sampling time coincides with first peak vertical pressure (loading), while Figure 4, *right*, shows the pressure distribution at second peak (push off). Left foot pressure is concentrated on the lateral portion of the midfoot and forefoot. Dynamic EMG of

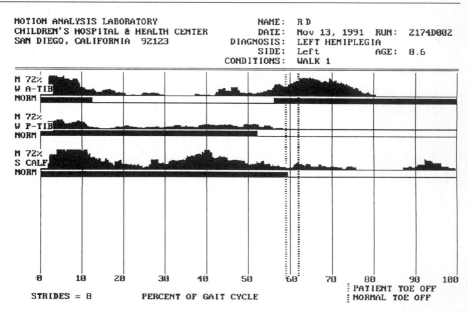

MOTION ANALYSIS LABORATORY
CHILDREN'S HOSPITAL & HEALTH CENTER
SAN DIEGO, CALIFORNIA 92123

NAME: R D
DATE: Nov 13, 1991 RUN: 2174D002
DIAGNOSIS: LEFT HEMIPLEGIA
SIDE: Left   AGE: 8.6
CONDITIONS: WALK 1

STRIDES = 8   PERCENT OF GAIT CYCLE

PATIENT TOE OFF
NORMAL TOE OFF

Fig. 5 *Dynamic EMG of left tibialis anterior, tibialis posterior, and gastrocnemius-soleus muscles in patients with varus foot resulting from spastic hemiparesis.*

the tibialis posterior, obtained with fine-wire electrodes, reveals normal phasic activity, while that of the tibialis anterior, obtained with surface electrodes, reveals normal stance-phase activity and intense initial swing-phase activity with early cessation at 80% of the gait cycle (Fig. 5). The gastrocnemius-soleus EMG, obtained with surface electrodes, shows some abnormal low level activity in swing phase with normal activity in stance phase.

This EMG information is most useful when the phasic activity of the tibialis anterior, tibialis posterior, and gastrocnemius-soleus are correlated with the movements of the ankle and foot. In this patient, sagittal plane ankle motion is abnormal with increased dorsiflexion in late stance phase (Fig. 6). This abnormal curve is more likely to occur with spasticity of the tibialis anterior than the tibialis posterior. Foot rotation is also abnormal with a sharp internal rotation movement in swing phase, from toe-off to approximately 80% of the gait cycle (Fig. 7). The tibialis anterior is very active during this period while the tibialis posterior shows no activity (Fig. 5); therefore, it is reasonable to select the tibialis anterior and exclude the tibialis posterior as the principle cause of the movement abnormality. The surgical plan for this patient, based on the gait analysis, is to perform a split anterior tibial transfer.[5] It would be unwise to lengthen the heel cord because ankle dorsiflexion in stance phase is already excessive.

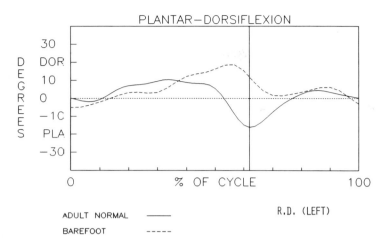

Fig. 6 *Sagittal plane motion curve of left ankle of patient with varus foot resulting from spastic hemiparesis.*

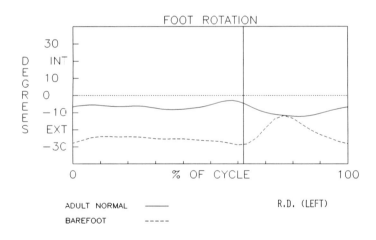

Fig. 7 *Transverse plane motion curve of left foot rotation of patient with varus foot resulting from spastic hemiparesis.*

Summary

In cerebral palsy, imbalance of the invertor and evertor muscles can result in varus alignment of the foot. The primary functional problems of varus foot are weightbearing instability and/or difficulty in foot clearance in swing phase. Additional problems include difficulties in shoe fitting, abnormal shoe wear, and unacceptable cosmesis. Gait studies have shed some light on alterations of muscle activity that can cause varus foot but have fallen short of providing clear guidelines for treatment of this common problem. Confusion exists because dynamic EMG does not give definitive information about the quantity of muscle tension and because the analyses have not included motion measurements that distinguish between the movements occurring in the hindfoot and forefoot. Until recently, tools did not exist for making these measurements; however, biomechanical studies of foot and ankle function, which are now possible, will allow greater precision in the selection of operative treatment for varus foot.

References

1. Mann RA: Biomechanics of the foot. *Atlas of Orthotics: Biomechanical Principles and Application.* St. Louis, CV Mosby, 1975, pp 257–266.
2. Mann R: Biomechanics of the foot and ankle in Mann R (ed): *Surgery of the Foot.* St. Louis, CV Mosby, 1989.
3. Sutherland D, Valencia F: Normal and abnormal gait, in Drennan J (ed): *The Child's Foot and Ankle.* New York, Raven Press, 1992, pp 19–35.
4. Barto PS, Supinski RS, Skinner SR: Dynamic EMG findings in the varus hindfoot deformity and spastic cerebral palsy. *Dev Med Child Neurol* 1984;26: 88–93.
5. Green NE, Griffin PP, Shiavi R: Split posterior tibial-tendon transfer in spastic cerebral palsy. *J Bone Joint Surg* 1983;65A:748–754.
6. Hoffer MM, Barakat G, Koffman M: 10-year follow-up of split anterior tibial tendon transfer in cerebral palsied patients with spastic equinovarus deformity. *J Ped Orthop* 1985;5:432–434.
7. Wills CA, Hoffer MM, Perry J: A comparison of foot-switch and EMG analysis of varus deformities of the feet of children with cerebral palsy. *Develop Med Child Neurol* 1988;30:227–231.
8. Barnes MJ, Herring JA: Combined split anterior tibial-tendon transfer and intramuscular lengthening of the posterior tibial tendon: Results in patients who have varus deformity of the foot due to spastic cerebral palsy. *J Bone Joint Surg* 1991;73A:734–738.
9. Alexander I, DeLozier G. Integrated three-dimensional motion analysis and dynamic foot pressure assessment in the evaluation of foot and ankle mechanics. Presented at Seventh Annual Summer Meeting of the American Orthopaedic Foot and Ankle Society, Boston, MA, July 25–28, 1991.

Chapter 31

What is the Normal Function of Tibialis Posterior in Human Gait?

Christopher L. Vaughan, PhD
Jodi H. Nashman, BS
M. Susan Murr, RPT

Introduction

Children who have cerebral palsy with spastic hemiplegia, a disorder that involves the upper and lower extremities on the same side, tend to have a plantarflexed ankle and varus foot position.[1] These positions are most evident during the swing phase of the gait cycle (Fig. 1). While the triceps surae muscle is clearly the deforming force responsible for equinus deformity, the deforming forces causing the varus deformity of the hindfoot are less obvious. The two muscles that are normally implicated are the tibialis posterior (an invertor and weak plantarflexor) and the tibialis anterior (an invertor and dorsiflexor). The anatomy and action of these muscles are seen in Figure 2. One of the challenges in pediatric orthopaedics is to plan the best surgical strategy for managing the child with spastic hemiplegia who has an equinovarus deformity. However, agreement on the correct strategy is far from unanimous.[2]

Efforts to identify the deforming muscle have focused on the use of dynamic electromyography (EMG).[3] The following recommendations have been summarized from the literature: (1) If the tibialis anterior fires continuously or out of phase (that is, during the whole stance phase), then its tendon is split and transferred medially to the cuboid.[4] (2) If the tibialis posterior fires continuously, the available procedures are: (a) lengthening of the tendon,[3] (b) tendon release or tenotomy,[4] and (c) split tendon transfer to the peroneus brevis.[5] (3) If the tibialis posterior fires out of phase, its tendon is transferred either anterior to the medial malleolus or through the interosseous membrane to the dorsum of the foot.[3] While all of these authors used EMG analysis to plan their surgery, very few made any effort to characterize the outcome in an objective manner. Kinematics, the movement of body segments, and kinetics or dynamics, the forces causing these movements, have essentially been ignored. Furthermore, while the activity of the tibialis anterior has been well-established through use of both fine-wire and surface EMG,[6] the normal activity of the tibialis posterior is much less certain.

There are very few studies in the literature that actually present data for the tibialis posterior. Bowker and Hall[7] presented a figure that sum-

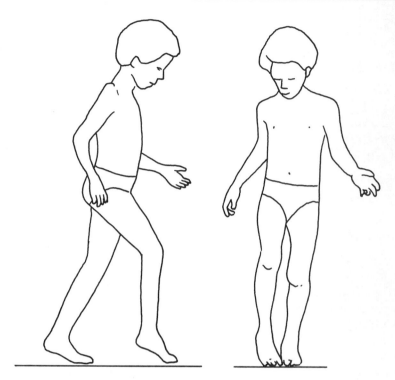

Fig. 1 *Two views of a child with spastic hemiplegia during the latter part of the swing phase in gait: sagittal plane (**left**) and frontal plane (**right**). (Adapted with permission from Sutherland.[1])*

marized the EMGs of 28 lower extremity muscles, one of which was the tibialis posterior. This figure showed the muscle to be active exclusively in stance, having a biphasic pattern with an eccentric peak at 20% of the gait cycle and a concentric peak at 45%. These data would tend to suggest that the tibialis posterior's action is almost identical to that of the triceps surae, providing active plantarflexion during late stance. The authors cited Dr. Charles Bechtol of Los Angeles as their source, but we can find no publication to verify their data. Houtz and Walsh[8] presented raw EMG signals that were similar to the envelopes of Bowker and Hall,[7] but all their data were based on surface EMG electrodes. As can be seen in the cross-sectional diagram of calf musculature in Figure 3, any effort to measure tibialis posterior with surface electrodes would almost certainly result in considerable cross-talk from superficial muscles. Sutherland,[9] however, did use fine-wire electrodes, and he confirmed the placement of the wires with electrical stimulation. His data were based on just four subjects and were presented in binary format: The muscle was either ''on'' or ''off.'' He showed that the tibialis posterior was active only in stance phase, from 6% to 48% of the gait cycle. More recently, Perry[10] has presented fine-wire data for

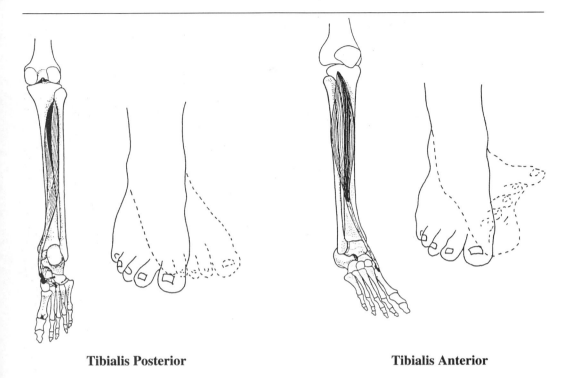

Tibialis Posterior   **Tibialis Anterior**

Fig. 2 *The two primary invertors of the foot, tibialis posterior and tibialis anterior, showing their origins and insertions, plus their actions. Note that the anatomic illustration of tibialis posterior (**left**) is a posterior view, while the other views are anterior. (Adapted with permission from Daniels et al.[19])*

25 subjects, which showed considerable variability, although tibialis activity was confined to the stance phase.

In a preliminary study, based on six subjects, we found that the action of the tibialis posterior was consistent within subjects, but there was less consistency between subjects.[11] In fact it was not unusual to find a subject whose muscle was always active for part of the swing phase. This led us to ask the question that is the title of this chapter: What is the normal function of the tibialis posterior in human gait? Our purpose is, therefore, to try to answer this question.

Subjects and Methodology

A group of 10 normal healthy adults between the ages of 21 and 38 were studied. There were five men and five women. All subjects were neurologically normal and volunteered willingly. Each subject performed four trials at a freely-selected pace, walking barefoot on a level carpeted walkway. During each trial, the positions of the calf and foot in three-dimensional (3-D) space were collected simultaneously with EMG recordings.

399

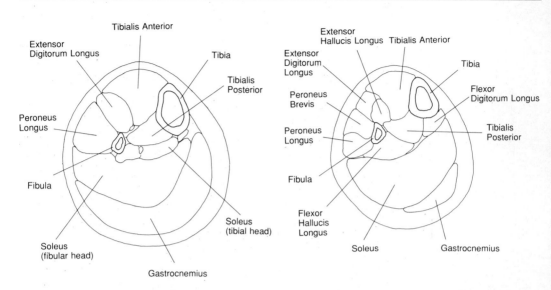

Fig. 3 *Transverse section of the leg showing the primary musculoskeletal structures: **Left**, through the bellies of the gastrocnemius and soleus, about 2 cm distal to the tibial tubercle; **Right**, about 12 cm distal to the tibial tubercle. (Adapted with permission from photographic cryosections in Von Hagens et al.[20])*

The kinematic data were captured at 60 Hz for 3 seconds using a 3-D recording system and a body-surface-marker set developed by Kadaba and associates.[12] The markers consisted of five small plastic balls (2 to 3 cm in diameter) covered with retroreflective material. These were attached with double-sided tape, to the right knee joint line (posterior to the lateral femoral condyle), right lateral malleolus, right heel, and over the second metatarsal head of the right foot. The final marker was attached to a 7.5-cm wand that was strapped onto the middle of the right calf in the frontal plane. The primary purpose of these markers was to determine the gait events (eg, heel-strike and toe-off), although we were also able to determine the 3-D angles at the ankle joint.[13]

The EMG signals from five muscles on the right side were captured: tibialis anterior, peroneus longus, lateral gastrocnemius, soleus, and tibialis posterior. Surface electrodes were used for the first four muscles, while in-dwelling wire electrodes were necessary to isolate the tibialis posterior. The bipolar fine-wire electrodes were fabricated from 50-μm Stablohm wire and 25 gauge hypodermic needles using the technique described by Basmajian and DeLuca.[14] The location of the electrodes was according to Winter,[15] while the fine-wire electrode was inserted in the tibialis posterior according to Sutherland (unpublished course notes, 1989) (Table 1). Location of the wires in the tibialis posterior (Fig. 3) was confirmed by electrical stimulation. The stimu-

Table 1 Electrode placement for collection of EMG signals

Muscle	Electrode Placement
Tibialis anterior	Over the area of greatest muscle bulk just lateral to the tibial tubercle on the proximal part of the leg
Peroneus longus	Midway along the line between the head of the fibula and the lateral malleolus
Lateral gastrocnemius	Over the area of greatest muscle bulk on the lateral calf
Soleus	Proximal electrode was placed 1 cm distal to the medial head of the gastrocnemius, distal electrode 2 cm away.
Tibialis posterior	With the calf externally rotated, the needle was inserted 12 cm distal to the tibial tubercle and 2 cm medial to the tibia in a posterolateral direction.

lation parameters included a pulse width of 300 μsecond, rate of 50 pulses per second, and on-ramp time of 2 seconds for a gradual build-up to maximum strength. Intensity was generally in the range of 10 to 20 mA and was sufficient to generate either a palpable tendon contraction (posterior to the medial malleolus) or an observable movement of the foot (Fig. 2). It is important to report that we performed the stimulation prior to and following the walking trials. In each case, the fine-wire electrodes were still located in the tibialis posterior after data capture.

The EMG signals were captured via an 8-channel telemetry unit, which meant that the subject was not encumbered with an umbilical cord of trailing wires. There were seven main components: pregelled silver/silver chloride surface electrodes and fine-wire electrodes; light-weight preamplifiers (45 g including cable and connector) with a gain of 8,000; a transmitter unit (less than 0.6 kg) carried on the subject's back with a halter vest; a receiver unit; a high-pass filter (greater than 30 Hz) to remove any motion artifact; a 12-bit analog-to-digital converter sampling at 1,000 Hz; and an IBM-compatible personal computer. The raw EMG data were processed through a program that performed full-wave rectification and low-pass filtering with a cut-off frequency of 3 Hz, using a standard linear envelope detector.[16] One gait cycle per trial was extracted using two consecutive heel-strikes from the synchronized video data. Normalization in the time domain was accomplished by expressing the data as a percentage of the gait cycle (0% to 100%) in 1% increments. Finally, the magnitudes of the EMG signals were expressed as a percentage of the maximum signal during the gait cycle in accordance with the work of others in this field.[17]

To evaluate the repeatability of EMG patterns, a variety of techniques have been proposed in the past. Yang and Winter[16] proposed use of the coefficient of variation, which is the sum of the standard deviations divided by the sum of the means at each point in the cycle. However, we found this statistic to be inappropriate for evaluating signals that do not differ greatly from the cycle mean.[11] Instead, we have adopted the Variance Ratio (VR) statistic, first proposed by Hershler and Milner[18] and used more recently by Kadaba and associates[6] and Pierotti and associates.[17] The variance ratio is defined as follows:

$$VR = \frac{\sum\limits_{t=0}^{100} \sum\limits_{n=1}^{N} (\overline{E_{nt}} - \overline{E_t})^2 \ / \ 101(N-1)}{\sum\limits_{t=0}^{100} \sum\limits_{n=1}^{N} (\overline{E_{nt}} - \overline{E})^2 \ / \ (101N-1)} \qquad (1)$$

where

$$\overline{E_{nt}} = \frac{1}{C} \sum_{c=1}^{C} E_{cnt} \qquad (2)$$

$$\overline{E_t} = \frac{1}{N} \sum_{n=1}^{N} \overline{E_{nt}} \qquad (3)$$

$$\overline{E} = \frac{1}{101} \sum_{t=0}^{100} \overline{E_t} \qquad (4)$$

and t is the time in the gait cycle (0 ... 100), n is the subject number out of a total of N subjects (six in this study), c is the cycle number out of a total of C cycles (four in this study), and E_{cnt} is the EMG signal amplitude for cycle c, subject n, at time t.

Results and Discussion

Table 2 is a summary of the anthropometric and temporal-distance data for all the subjects. There are a number of points to make from this table. First, the average speed of 1.25 m/sec is less than what we would expect for normal adult gait.[12] Because cadence (114.8 steps/min) is within the normal range, a decreased stride length (1.31 m) has obviously contributed to the reduction in speed. We attribute this decrease to the likelihood that the subjects felt somewhat uncomfortable with the fine-wire electrodes in their tibialis posterior, and, thus, they walked in a tentative manner. Second, the proportion of the gait cycle spent in stance (61.2%) was within normal limits and was extremely consistent (indicated by a low standard deviation of 2.9%).

Figure 4 illustrates the raw EMG data for the tibialis posterior for a single trial by two subjects (numbers 1 and 5), while Figure 5 is an ensemble average of tibialis posterior for the same two subjects. Figures 4, *left*, and 5, *top*, present the classic biphasic patterns attributed to the tibialis posterior in the literature[7,9]: Two peaks in stance, at about 10% and 40% of the cycle, followed by a relatively quiescent period during swing. In contrast, Figures 4, *right*, and 5, *bottom*, demonstrate a quite different pattern: The tibialis posterior was relatively quiescent in stance (although there was some variability between 15% and 20% of the cycle), but exhibited a consistent peak in early swing phase at 70% of the cycle.

The variance ratio data are presented in Table 3, which contains the individual variance ratios for the five muscles, as well as the grand ensemble variance ratios. Note that the tibialis posterior, which has some low individual variance ratios, has the highest grand ensemble variance ratio. The mean EMG data for the tibialis posterior for all

Table 2 Mean anthropometric and temporal-distance data for all subjects

No.	Sex	Mass (kg)	Height (m)	Stride Length (m)	Cadence (steps per min)	Speed (m/sec)	Stance Phase (%)
1	M	78.2	1.79	1.45	109.5	1.33	62.0
2	M	86.4	1.98	1.51	110.2	1.39	62.7
3	M	80.5	1.80	1.42	106.3	1.25	65.0
4	F	56.4	1.65	1.16	113.5	1.10	64.6
5	F	72.7	1.73	1.25	107.6	1.12	63.5
6	M	78.2	1.79	1.28	121.5	1.29	62.4
7	F	52.3	1.55	1.04	119.6	1.04	63.5
8	M	70.5	1.65	1.34	108.7	1.22	58.9
9	F	54.6	1.66	1.38	129.2	1.49	56.0
10	F	56.8	1.63	1.26	122.1	1.29	57.6
Mean		68.6	1.27	1.31	114.82	1.25	61.6
s.d.		11.9	0.12	0.13	7.35	0.13	2.9

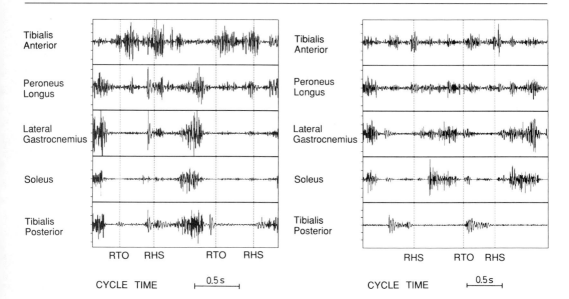

Fig. 4 *Raw EMG date for subject 1 (**left**) and subject 5 (**right**). The first four muscles were captured with surface electrodes and the tibialis posterior with fine wires. RHS = right heel strike. RTO = right toe-off.*

subjects is illustrated in Figure 6, which includes the biphasic pattern during stance as well as an increase in activity in early swing. Note, too, the relatively large standard deviation (indicated by the dashed lines above and below the mean) throughout the cycle. The tibialis anterior and lateral gastrocnemius have much lower grand ensemble variance ratios than the tibialis posterior (Table 3), and their curves have been plotted in Figures 7 and 8.

The tibialis anterior functions primarily as a dorsiflexor. It is active

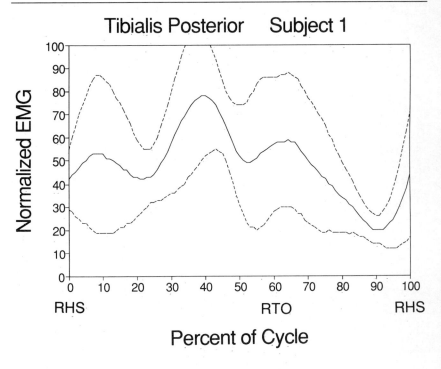

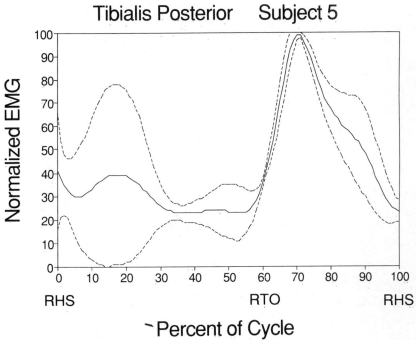

Fig. 5 *Ensemble averaged EMG data for the tibialis posterior for subject 1 (**top**) and subject 5 (**bottom**). The solid line is the mean while the dashed lines indicate plus and minus one standard deviation.*

Table 3 Variance ratios for tibialis anterior, peroneus longus, lateral gastrocnemius, soleus, and tibialis posterior for all subjects

No.	Tibialis Anterior	Peroneus Longus	Lateral Gastrocnemius	Soleus	Tibialis Posterior
1	0.16	0.22	0.14	0.18	0.54
2	0.12	0.37	0.10	0.08	0.46
3	0.16	0.08	0.07	0.21	0.58
4	0.11	0.36	0.33	0.16	0.71
5	0.36	0.48	0.13	0.24	0.22
6	0.37	0.52	0.30	0.75	0.79
7	0.25	0.18	0.02	0.05	0.85
8	0.12	0.11	0.57	0.10	0.89
9	0.17	0.33	0.67	0.11	0.67
10	0.11	0.14	0.33	0.28	1.23
Grand ensemble*	0.20	0.60	0.72	0.27	1.03

*Note that the grand ensemble variance ratios are not simply the average of the individual variance ratios. They are calculated using equations (1) through (4).

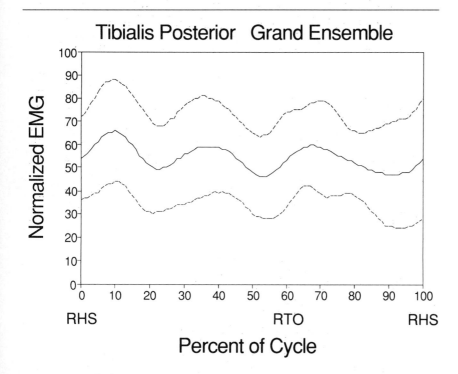

Fig. 6 *Grand ensemble averaged EMG data for the tibialis posterior for all subjects. The solid line is the mean, while the dashed lines indicate plus and minus one standard deviation.*

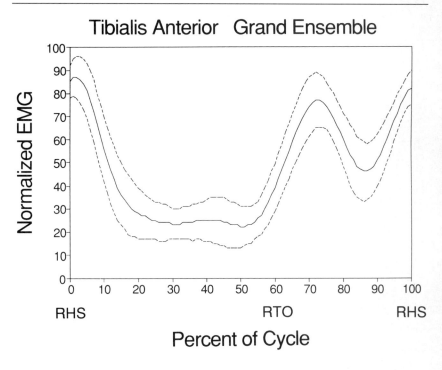

Fig. 7 *Grand ensemble averaged EMG data for the tibialis anterior for all subjects. The solid line is the mean, while the dashed lines indicate plus and minus one standard deviation.*

in early stance, preventing the foot from slapping on the ground, contracting eccentrically because the ankle is plantarflexing (Fig. 9). It is then relatively quiescent during the rest of stance (from 20% to 60% of the cycle), becoming active again in early swing to dorsiflex the foot and prevent toe drag. After a momentary decrease in late swing, the tibialis anterior's activity picks up from 90% to 100% in anticipation of heel-strike. The role of this muscle has been well established (and accepted) in the literature.[6,15] The gastrocnemius functions primarily as a plantarflexor. It provides some stability to the ankle joint at heel-strike, but increases substantially in midstance, peaking at 40% of the gait cycle and providing the plantarflexor torque needed during push-off. Thereafter it falls off rapidly and remains quiet during most of swing. The role of the gastrocnemius has also been well established by various researchers.[6,9,15] This bring us, then, to the question raised in the beginning: What is the normal function of the tibialis posterior?

As highlighted in Figure 2, the tibialis posterior has two primary actions: Inversion of the foot, and (weak) plantarflexion at the ankle. As seen in Figures 4–6, there are three distinct periods in the gait cycle when the tibialis posterior may be active: At 10% and 40% in stance, and at 70% in early swing. Note that individual subjects will not exhibit

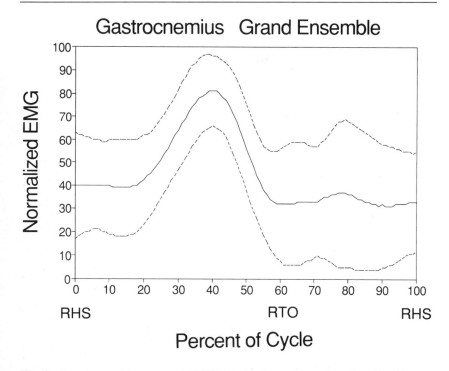

Gastrocnemius   Grand Ensemble

Fig. 8 *Grand ensemble averaged EMG data for the gastrocnemius for all subjects. The solid line is the mean, while the dashed lines indicate plus and minus one standard deviation.*

each of these features. In early stance, the tibialis posterior is acting concentrically as an inverter (Fig. 9), while in late stance (when the foot is being everted) it probably contributes to the active plantarflexion of the triceps surae. The activity of the tibialis posterior seen in early swing in some subjects (Fig. 4, *right*) probably contributes to the inversion of the foot (Fig. 9), thus assisting the tibialis anterior, which is also active at this time (Fig. 7). Perhaps the contribution of the peroneal muscles, which have the primary function of everting the foot, has been overlooked in the past. It seems likely that the tibialis posterior and, to a lesser extent, the tibialis anterior play an important role in balancing the peroneals. This is most evident in Figure 4, *right*, where both the peroneus longus and the tibialis posterior are active in early swing.

The variability seen in the activity of the tibialis posterior (Figs. 4–6, Table 3) suggests that each person has a strategy tailored to his/her own anatomy and neuromuscular control, that uses the tibialis posterior in a unique way. Because we have established that each subject must be considered as an individual, and that there is no single representative pattern for normal individuals, the insistence that dynamic EMG be used for planning surgeries[4] might be difficult to implement. In fact, as

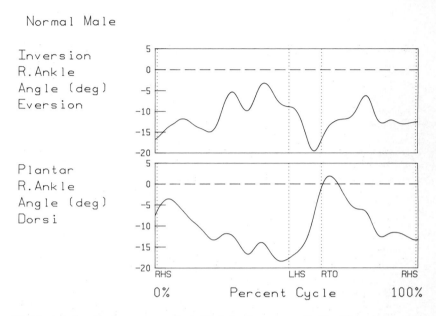

Normal Male

Inversion
R.Ankle
Angle (deg)
Eversion

Plantar
R.Ankle
Angle (deg)
Dorsi

RHS   LHS   RTO   RHS

0%   Percent Cycle   100%

Fig. 9 *Angular displacement at the ankle joint for a normal male. These curves were generated from the software in Vaughan and associates.[13]*

demonstrated recently by Barnes and Herring,[2] acceptable results can apparently be achieved without dynamic EMG.

Conclusions

Based on the data presented in Table 3 and Figures 4–6, the following conclusions may be drawn for normal adult subjects: (1) The tibialis posterior, while demonstrating low individual variance ratios, had the highest grand ensemble variance ratio of all muscles. (2) Some subjects exhibited EMG patterns for the tibialis posterior that agreed with the literature: Two peaks in stance, at 10% and 40% of the cycle. (3) Other subjects demonstrated a quite different EMG pattern for the tibialis posterior, one that had a peak in early swing at 70% of the gait cycle. (4) The activity of the tibialis posterior and the tibialis anterior (invertors of the foot) should be studied in conjunction with the activity of the foot evertors, peroneus longus and brevis. (5) The use of dynamic EMG to study tibialis posterior activity in children with spastic hemiplegia when planning tendon transfer surgery may need to be reconsidered.

Acknowledgments

This work was done with the financial support of the Kluge Research Fund, and the Orthopaedic Research and Education Foundation.

References

1. Sutherland DH: *Gait Disorders in Childhood and Adolescence*. Baltimore, MD, Williams & Wilkins, 1984.
2. Barnes MJ, Herring JH: Combined split anterior tibial-tendon transfer and intramuscular lengthening of the posterior tibial tendon. *J Bone Joint Surg* 1991;73A:734–738.
3. Bleck EE, Spastic hemiplegia, in *Orthopaedic Management in Cerebral Palsy*. Philadelphia, MacKeith Press, 1987.
4. Perry J, Hoffer MM: Preoperative and postoperative dynamic electromyography as an aid in planning tendon transfers in children with cerebral palsy. *J Bone Joint Surg* 1977;59A:531–537.
5. Green NE, Griffin PP, Shiavi R: Split posterior tibial-tendon transfer in spastic cerebral palsy. *J Bone Joint Surg* 1983;65A:748–754.
6. Kadaba MP, Wootten ME, Gainey J, et al: Repeatability of phasic muscle activity: Performance of surface and intramuscular wire electrodes in gait analysis. *J Orthop Res* 1985;3:350–359.
7. Bowker JH, Hall CB: Normal human gait, in American Academy of Orthopaedic Surgeons *Atlas of Orthotics: Biomechanical Principles and Application*. St. Louis, CV Mosby, 1975, pp 133–143.
8. Houtz SJ, Walsh FP: Electromyographic analysis of the function of the muscles acting on the ankle during weight-bearing with special reference to the triceps surae. *J Bone Joint Surg* 1959;41A:1469–1481.
9. Sutherland DH: An electromyographic study of the plantar flexors of the ankle in normal walking on the level. *J Bone Joint Surg* 1966;48A:66–71.
10. Perry J: *Gait Analysis. Normal and Pathological Function*. Thorofare, NJ, Slack Inc, 1992.
11. Murr SM, Vaughan CL, Bowsher K, et al: Repeatability of muscle activity in normals using fine wire EMG. Proceedings of Sixth Annual East Coast Clinical Gait Conference, East Lansing, MI, December 1990, pp 127–130.
12. Kadaba MP, Ramakrishnan HIK, Wootten ME, et al: Repeatability of kinematic, kinetic, and electromyographic data in normal adult gait. *J Orthop Res* 1990;7:849–860.
13. Vaughan CL, Davis BL, O'Connor J: *Dynamics of Human Gait*. Champaign, IL, Human Kinetics Publishers, 1992.
14. Basmajian JV, DeLuca CJ: *Muscles Alive*, ed 5. Baltimore, Williams & Wilkins, 1985.
15. Winter DA: *The Biomechanics and Motor Control of Human Gait*. Waterloo, ON, University of Waterloo Press, 1987.
16. Yang JF, Winter DA: Electromyographic amplitude normalization methods: Improving their sensitivity as diagnostic tools in gait analysis. *Arch Phys Med Rehabil* 1984;65:517–521.
17. Pierotti SE, Brand RA, Gabel RH, et al: Are leg electromyogram profiles symmetrical? *J Orthop Res* 1991;9:720–729.
18. Hershler C, Milner M: An optimality criterion for processing electromyographic (EMG) signals relating to human locomotion. *Trans Biomed Eng* 1978;25:413–420.
19. Daniels L, Worthingham C: *Muscle Testing. Techniques of Manual Examination*. Philadelphia, WB Saunders, 1972.
20. Von Hagens G, Romrell LJ, Ross MH, et al: *The Visible Body: An Atlas of Sectional Anatomy*. Philadelphia, Lea & Febiger, 1991.

Chapter 32

Split Anterior Tibial Tendon Transfer

Bernard Roehr, MD
E. Dennis Lyne, MD

The orthopaedic surgeon encounters several upper and lower extremity deformities while treating the patient with cerebral palsy, and the patients who benefit the most from surgical procedures are those with spastic or mixed involvement. Historically, four types of nonfixed deformities have been treated with tendon transfers. Hindfoot varus can be treated with procedures that address the spastic anterior or posterior tibialis muscles; hindfoot valgus is treated with peroneus brevis transfer; intoeing due to spastic medial hamstrings is treated with hamstring transfer; and elbow and wrist flexion deformities are treated with a flexor carpi ulnaris transfer.

At least one fourth of all patients with cerebral palsy will develop deformities of the foot and ankle.[1] A variety of deformities are seen, including equinus, calcaneus, equinovarus, equinovalgus, and pure hindfoot varus and valgus. The objective of this chapter is to describe the role of the split anterior tibial tendon transfer in the treatment of the patient with cerebral palsy.

When examining the patient with cerebral palsy, a thorough history should be obtained.[2] This should include identifying possible causes of the brain injury as well as the achievement and timing of developmental milestones. The history should also include a thorough description of the child's present functional level. In evaluating foot and ankle deformities, attention must be given to previous diagnostic studies and surgical and nonsurgical treatments. The presence of a progressive deformity calls for special consideration. Physical examination should include an assessment of the potential for independent ambulation as outlined by Bleck.[3] One must take care to evaluate the patient both statically on the examination table, and dynamically by observing the pattern of gait. With respect to the foot and ankle, it is important to determine whether the abnormality is the primary cause of the gait disturbance or secondary to a more proximal abnormality. Femoral anteversion and internal tibial torsion can give the appearance of a varus hindfoot, when the heel is not truly in varus.[4] Observing the position of the foot during both the swing and stance phases of gait is important in determining the muscle or muscles involved in a particular defor-

411

mity. It is particularly important to observe the child with cerebral palsy in as functional a situation as possible.

A varus hindfoot is one of the more common deformities seen in the foot and ankle of patients with cerebral palsy; it may be present with or without an associated equinus deformity. Seen most commonly in patients with hemiplegia, this deformity also is seen occasionally in spastic diplegic and quadriplegic patients. Five muscles can contribute to a varus deformity: the anterior tibialis, posterior tibialis, flexor hallucis longus, flexor digitorum longus, and soleus.[5] The contribution of the soleus to hindfoot varus can be corrected by lengthening the Achilles tendon. The flexor hallucis longus and flexor digitorum longus can be lengthened or transferred with few resulting problems. The key to appropriate treatment of the equinovarus foot is in determining the contribution of the anterior and posterior tibialis muscles to the deformity.

Several methods have been described to determine which of these muscles is the primary cause of the varus deformity. These include static and dynamic clinical examination, foot switch analysis, and dynamic electromyography (EMG). Clinical clues that point toward anterior tibialis spasticity include observing the presence of forefoot supination during active dorsiflexion. An increasing varus posture when the child stands on tiptoe indicates posterior tibialis spasticity. Foot switch analyses without concomitant EMG have been shown to be unreliable in distinguishing between anterior and posterior tibialis spasticity as a cause for varus deformity of the foot.[5] The most reliable approach, in addition to clinical examination, is the use of dynamic EMG.

Three patterns of spasticity are observed using dynamic EMG.[6] In the first pattern, the posterior tibial muscle displays a reverse phase action (action during swing phase). This can be effectively treated with posterior tibialis tendon transfer through the interosseous membrane. The second and most common pattern is caused by a continuous tibialis posterior muscle action and is frequently treated using a posterior tibial tendon lengthening or split posterior tibial tendon transfer. The third pattern shows continuous activity of the anterior tibialis muscle. This situation is best addressed using the split anterior tibial tendon transfer as described by Hoffer and associates.[7]

A variety of anterior tibial tendon transfers have been described. Sometimes a calcaneal varus deformity of the foot can result from overlengthening the Achilles tendon. In this situation, a lateral transfer of the anterior tibialis tendon may be beneficial. The entire tendon insertion may be transferred to the base of the second or third metatarsal to change the action of the anterior tibialis from varus dorsiflexion to pure dorsiflexion. Inserting the tendon further laterally must be avoided because an even more problematic calcaneal valgus foot may result. There are situations where one should consider anterior tibial tendon transfer or release in the nonwalking patient to assist with footwear and heel pressure sores. In selected nonwalking patients, the calcaneus deformity can be treated by anterior tibial tendon release alone. Failure to address the calcaneus deformity can lead to devastating heel prob-

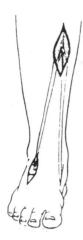

Fig. 1 *Incisions for split anterior tibial tendon transfer. (Reproduced with permission from Hoffer et al.[7])*

lems and shoe fit problems, which are concerns regardless of ambulatory capacity.

The major role of the anterior tibial tendon transfer is in the equinovarus foot, which is caused by continuous anterior tibialis muscle activity. It is important to distinguish between dynamic and fixed deformity, as this will determine the need for associated Achilles tendon and posterior tibial tendon lengthening at the time of anterior tibial tendon transfer. It is also important to note the presence of fixed deformity, because tendon transfers will not work in this situation, and this problem must be addressed by other methods. Tendon transfers can, however, assist in preventing further deformity and should be reserved for patients in whom nonsurgical measures, such as stretching, casts, bracing, and gait training, have failed.

The most popular anterior tibial tendon transfer used in such cases is the split anterior tibial tendon transfer as described by Hoffer and associates.[7] In this operation the lateral half of the anterior tibial tendon is moved to the cuboid, neutralizing the varus pull of the anterior tibial tendon and creating a balanced yoke on the foot. The first incision is dorsomedial over the medial cuneiform, at the base of the first metatarsal (Fig. 1). The tendon is identified, split in half, and then isolated using umbilical tape. A second incision is made at the musculotendinous junction of the anterior tibialis in the distal leg, and the lateral half of the tendon is released at its insertion and drawn up into this wound. A third incision is made longitudinally over the dorsum of the cuboid, and the lateral half of the anterior tibial tendon is passed subcutaneously into the third incision. Two drill holes are then made at converging angles into the cuboid with a 7/64-inch drill (Fig. 2). Care is taken to preserve the roof of bone between these holes. The lateral

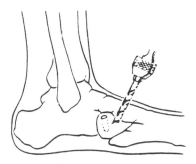

Fig. 2 *Method of placing drill holes. (Reproduced with permission from Hoffer et al.[7])*

slip of the tendon is passed through the holes and sutured to itself with the ankle in slight dorsiflexion and the hindfoot in eversion. Occasional modifications are necessary for fixation if the tendon does not have the desired length.

In our experience this procedure can be performed without making the second incision over the distal leg by subcutaneously tunneling the lateral half of the anterior tibial tendon into the incision over the cuboid. While this method has the theoretic possibility of jeopardizing the anterior tibial artery and deep branch of the peroneal nerve, this has not been our experience. In cases of fixed equinovarus deformity, lengthening of the Achilles and posterior tibial tendons is performed in conjunction with the transfer. A short leg walking cast is then applied with the foot and ankle in neutral, and weightbearing is allowed at the beginning of the third postoperative week. The cast is removed six weeks postoperatively, and the patient is then placed on protected weightbearing for at least two weeks when practical. Bracing may be necessary after removal of the cast.

In Hoffer and associates'[8] series, 21 feet had some fixed deformity and six had pure dynamic deformities. All patients had continuous activity of the anterior tibial muscle as documented by dynamic EMG, and, in addition, there was continuous activity of the posterior tibial muscle in eight feet. Six underwent split anterior tibial tendon transfer alone and 13 had concomitant Achilles tendon lengthening. The eight feet with continuous posterior tibial muscle spasticity also had myotendinous lengthening of the posterior tibialis. One patient later required a calcaneal osteotomy. Although all patients required orthoses preoperatively only one required an orthosis at ten-year follow-up. The operation improved gait and alleviated problems with footwear in the ambulatory patients and improved wheelchair positioning in the nonambulatory patients.[8]

In summary, careful identification of the functional deformity, as well as the spastic muscle or muscles, is essential in the planning of tendon transfers about the foot and ankle. Calcaneus, as well as varus, can be a progressive problem requiring surgical intervention. One must be aware of any fixed deformities, because these frequently require additional procedures, although anterior tibial transfer alone may prevent further progression. It is critical to identify the presence of a combination of abnormal muscle pulls, for instance, the anterior tibialis and Achilles tendon. As with most tendon procedures, these are not recommended in the athetoid or dystonic child. Overtightening of the transferred tendon or portion of tendon should be avoided, because a varus or equinovarus foot that is overcorrected can be worse than the original deformity. Surgery should be considered for children with spastic or mixed cerebral palsy with significant foot deformity regardless of their ambulatory capacity, because severe calcaneus can lead to heel ulcers, and equinovarus to inability to maintain the foot in a shoe, which can be especially troublesome in colder climates.

References

1. Bassett FH III, Baker LD: Equinus deformity in cerebral palsy, in Adams JP (ed): *Current Practice in Orthopaedic Surgery*. St. Louis, CV Mosby, 1966, vol. 3, pp 59–74.
2. Kasser JR, MacEwen GD: Examination of the cerebral palsy patient with foot and ankle problems. *Foot Ankle* 1983;4:135–144.
3. Bleck EE: Locomotor prognosis in cerebral palsy. *Dev Med Child Neurol* 1975;17:18–25.
4. Bennet GC, Rang M, Jones D: Varus and valgus deformities of the foot in cerebral palsy. *Dev Med Child Neurol* 1982;24:499–503.
5. Wills CA, Hoffer MM, Perry J: A comparison of foot-switch and EMG analysis of varus deformities of the feet of children with cerebral palsy. *Dev Med Child Neurol* 1988;30:227–231.
6. Perry J, Hoffer MM: Preoperative and postoperative dynamic electromyography as an aid in planning tendon transfers in children with cerebral palsy. *J Bone Joint Surg* 1977;59A:531–537.
7. Hoffer MM, Reiswig JA, Garrett AM, et al: The split anterior tibial tendon transfer in the treatment of spastic varus hindfoot of childhood. *Orthop Clin North Am* 1974;51:31–38.
8. Hoffer MM, Barakat G, Koffman M: 10-year follow-up of split anterior tibial tendon transfer in cerebral palsied patients with spastic equinovarus deformity. *J Pediatr Orthop* 1985;5:432–434.

Chapter 33

Split Posterior Tibial Tendon Transfer: The Universal Procedure

Neil E. Green, MD

Varus and equinovarus deformities of the hind part of the foot are seen relatively frequently in children with spastic hemiplegia and quadriplegia and infrequently in those with spastic diplegia, although many patients with hemiplegia have no identifiable injury. Many different procedures, directed at the posterior tibial tendon, have been advocated to correct this equinovarus posture.[1-10] Baker and Hill[1] removed the tendon from its sheath and rerouted it anterior to the medial malleolus, with good results in 27 feet. However, Bleck[3] noted poor results with this operation, often manifested by late deformities of the calcaneus, because the transferred spastic posterior tibial muscle acted continuously as a strong dorsiflexor of the ankle. Bisla and associates[2] reported no change in gait after this operation in most of the feet that they reviewed, and stated that none had complete correction of the varus deformity. Tenotomy of the posterior tibial tendon at its insertion has led to collapse of the talonavicular joint with significant valgus deformity,[3] but lengthening of the tendon has been favored and has produced good results.[3,11] Transfer of the posterior tibial tendon through the interosseous membrane has been popular,[2-4,7-10] but an unacceptable number of poor results have been reported.[2,3,7,8]

Hoffer and associates[5] postulated that the spastic anterior tibial muscle is an important cause of varus deformity of the hind part of the foot in spastic hemiplegic cerebral palsy. They reported good results in a series of patients in whom split anterior tibial tendon transfer (SPLATT) was used. In this procedure the anterior tibial tendon is split at its insertion, and then half of the tendon is moved laterally to the cuboid bone.

Kaufer,[6] in 1977, described the split posterior tibial transfer. He originally reported good results in 29 of 30 feet. Since 1976, his procedure has been used at Vanderbilt University Medical Center with excellent results. Forty-five children who underwent this procedure have been reviewed and constitute the study group for this report.

Materials and Methods

Since 1976 split posterior tibial tendon transfer has been performed on 45 children with spastic cerebral palsy. All but one of these children

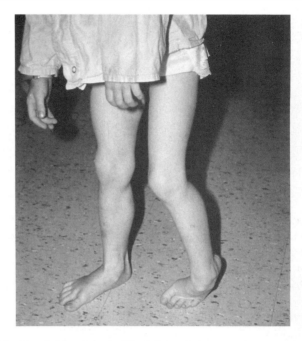

Fig. 1 *Child with a left hemiplegia. The left foot is in an equinovarus position, and the deformity is supple. (Reproduced with permission from Green NE, Griffin PP, Shiavi R: Split posterior tibial-tendon transfer in spastic cerebral palsy.* J Bone Joint Surg *1983;65A:749.)*

also underwent a simultaneous lengthening of the Achilles tendon. The patients ranged in age from 3 to 10 years, with a mean age of 6.0 years. Forty-two of the 45 children had a spastic hemiplegia that had been present since the neonatal period. The other three children had bilateral hemiplegia with asymmetric, bilateral involvement. None of the children had undergone previous surgical procedures on the leg that underwent the split posterior tibial tendon transfer. All of the children were spastic, and none had any evidence of athetosis.

All but one of the children had an equinovarus gait. During the swing phase of gait, the foot was in an equinovarus posture. The first portion of the foot to strike the ground at the end of swing was the head of the fifth metatarsal. The lateral border of the midfoot and sometimes the hindfoot next made contact with the ground (Fig. 1). In the children in whom the hindfoot was flexible, the medial border of the hindfoot made floor contact. In most patients, the heel did not strike because of the contracture of the heel cord, although one child did not have an associated equinus deformity. The varus deformity was flexible in 40 of the 45 feet. One of the children had a rigid varus deformity of the hind part of the foot without an equinus component.

The muscle activity of 30 of the children was studied electromyographically in the Vanderbilt University Medical Center gait laboratory. The studies were performed using surface electrodes for the anterior tibial, peroneus longus, gastrocnemius, and soleus muscles. A needle electrode was used to record the activity of the posterior tibial muscle. Pressure switches were placed at various locations on the plantar aspect of the foot so that the muscle activity could be correlated with the gait cycle. Video analysis was provided with dual television cameras. One camera recorded the gait from the front and then from the back, and the other camera provided a profile. These images were recorded on tape. A computer was used to average the duration of electromyographic activity throughout all of the gait cycles, and a printout of this average for each of the five muscles was generated.[12]

All 45 children underwent a split posterior tibial-tendon transfer, and 43 of the 45 also underwent a sliding heel-cord lengthening. Five children had fixed varus deformity of the hind part of the foot. Two children underwent a lateral closing-wedge osteotomy of the calcaneus 12 and 16 months after the split posterior tibial-tendon transfer; the other three children underwent osteotomy of the calcaneus at the time of the split tendon transfer.

Indications

A simple heel-cord lengthening was performed in hemiplegic children when a significant, isolated equinus deformity was present. The indication used for heel-cord lengthening in hemiplegic children was inability to passively dorsiflex the foot to the neutral position.[3] All of the children who underwent a heel-cord lengthening, therefore, had a true contracture of the triceps surae. In addition, the dynamic deformity was always more severe than the static deformity; therefore, the equinus posture during gait was greater than would be expected from evaluation of the static deformity alone.

Bleck[3] stated that surgical treatment is indicated in a child with a spastic pes varus deformity: ''When the deforming force of the spastic muscle persists, skeletal changes in the direction of the deforming force can be anticipated. Early surgery can prevent skeletal deformities.'' Therefore, all of the children who had a dynamic varus deformity of the hind part of the foot underwent split posterior tibial-tendon transfer. In three children the transfer was performed after the development of a skeletal deformity, and an osteotomy of the calcaneus had to be performed as well.

Technique

Three separate incisions are used. The first incision is 2 cm long and is positioned over the insertion of the posterior tibial tendon on the navicular bone. The distal end of the tendon is identified, and its sheath is opened as far proximally as possible. The tendon is split longitudinally, and the plantar half is sharply dissected from its insertion. The free end is then grasped, and the tendon is split longitudinally as far proximally as possible (Fig. 2, *top*).

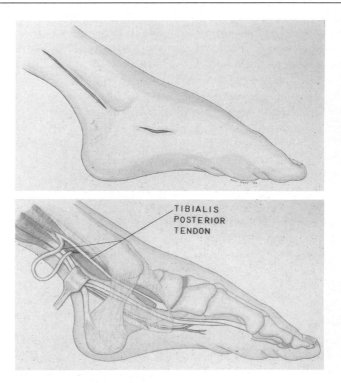

Fig. 2 *Surgical technique of the split posterior tibial-tendon transfer. (Reproduced with permission from Green NE, Griffin PP, Shiavi R: Split posterior tibial-tendon transfer in spastic cerebral palsy.* J Bone Joint Surg *1983;65A:751.)* **Top**, *Medial skin incisions; if a heel-cord lengthening is not performed, the longitudinal 6-cm incision may be placed slightly closer to the tibia, as shown.* **Bottom**, *Surgical technique as described in the text. Care is taken to ensure that both halves of the tendon are approximately the same width.*

The second incision, which is equidistant from the medial malleolus and the posterior aspect of the Achilles tendon, begins at the level of the medial malleolus and continues proximally for 6 cm. The skin and subcutaneous tissues are sharply divided, the tendon of the posterior tibial muscle is identified, and its sheath is split. The freed half of the tendon is delivered into this incision, and the longitudinal split in the tendon is continued proximally to the musculotendinous junction. A heavy nonabsorbable suture is sewn into the stump of the freed half of the tendon, which is tapered distally. The plane directly posterior to the tibia and anterior to the neurovascular structures and the tendons is developed (Fig. 2, *bottom*).

A third incision is made directly posterior and inferior to the lateral malleolus, beginning just proximal to the tip of the malleolus and continuing distally for 2 to 3 cm. The peroneus brevis tendon is identified, and its sheath is split longitudinally. The heavy nonabsorbable suture in the distal stump of the split posterior tibial tendon in the second incision is threaded into a tendon-passer that is used to pass the split portion of the posterior tibial tendon, first directly posterior to the tibia and fibula and anterior to all of the neurovascular and tendinous structures, and then laterally to enter the opened sheath of the peroneus brevis tendon. It is important to adjust the proximal-distal direction of the pull of the tendon so that it passes from posteromedial to lateral. It should be immediately posterior to the tibia and fibula (Fig. 3, *top*).

The distal part of the sheath of the peroneus brevis is opened and the split part of the posterior tibial tendon that already is in the sheath is brought into this and is sutured to the peroneus brevis tendon by weaving it in and out of the tendon. The tension is adjusted so that the hind part of the foot will rest in neutral position once the operation is completed. This adjustment usually can be accomplished by holding the foot in neutral position and pulling hard on the posterior tibial tendon and then reducing the pull slightly. The posterior tibial tendon is then sutured to the peroneus brevis using a 2–0 nonabsorbable suture. The end of the tendon is sutured to the insertion of the peroneus brevis tendon (Fig. 3, *bottom*). The wounds are then closed.

Usually the heel-cord lengthening is performed before the procedure just described; an above knee cast is applied with the knee in extension and the foot in neutral position. The child is allowed to bear weight on the cast as tolerated. Four weeks later the cast is changed, and a below knee walking cast is applied. All immobilization is discontinued 8 weeks postoperatively. If the child is able to actively dorsiflex the ankle to neutral position, then postoperative bracing is not used. If the patient cannot actively dorsiflex the foot to a right angle, a brace should be prescribed to prevent a recurrence of the equinus deformity. If, on the other hand, the anterior tibial muscle functions with a withdrawal action only (associated with active hip and knee flexion), bracing may be used to improve gait. However, the risk of recurrence of the equinus deformity is not as high.

Results

The electromyograms made during gait were used to determine the phasic activity of the posterior tibial muscle (Fig. 4). Normally that muscle is never active during the swing phase of gait.[3] Preoperatively, in all of the patients who underwent a split posterior tibial-tendon transfer, there was continuous activity of the posterior tibial muscle during stance and swing or at least partial phase reversal with swing phase activity.

The results were graded as excellent, good, or unsatisfactory. An excellent result was when the foot was plantigrade, had no postural or fixed deformity, and did not require a brace. These patients, in addition, had heel-toe gait pattern without an increase in hip flexion during the swing phase of gait. There was no varus deformity of the foot during either the swing or stance phase of gait. The patients had good strength of the anterior tibial muscle, and they were able to voluntarily dorsiflex

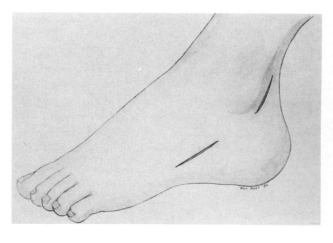

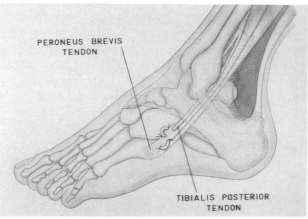

Fig. 3 *Surgical technique of the split posterior tibial tendon transfer. (Reproduced with permission from Green NE, Griffin PP, Shiavi R: Split posterior tibial-tendon transfer in spastic cerebral palsy.* J Bone Joint Surg *1983;65A:752.)* **Top**, *Originally, two separate lateral incisions were made; however, more recently one single incision behind the lateral malleolus has been used successfully. This single incision exposes the peroneus brevis tendon directly posterior and inferior to the lateral malleolus. The split portion of the posterior tibial tendon is passed laterally into this incision. The direction of pull should be oblique from proximal medial to distal lateral. The second lateral incision is also three centimeters long, beginning two centimeters proximal to the insertion of the peroneus brevis tendon. This incision is directly parallel to and is placed directly over the peroneus brevis tendon.* **Bottom**, *The split half of the posterior tibial tendon is delivered into the distal lateral incision. Surgery continues as described in the text.*

the foot at rest without simultaneous flexion of the hip and knee (withdrawal).

A good result was when the foot was plantigrade and had no postural or fixed deformity, but did require night-time bracing to prevent a recurrent equinus deformity as a result of weak dorsiflexors. The gait of

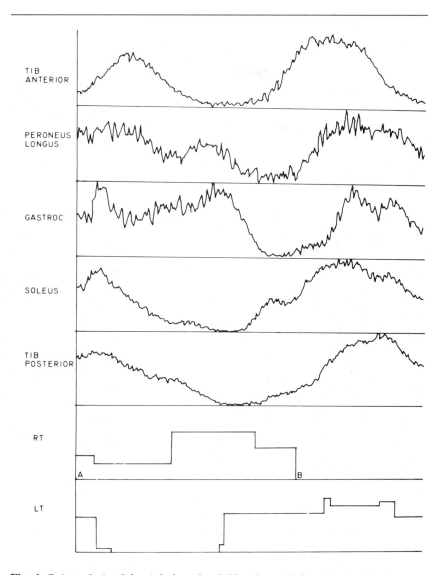

Fig. 4 *Gait analysis of the right leg of a child with a right hemiplegia. This is a computerized analysis of many gait cycles. The upper five lines demonstrate the activity of the five listed muscles. The activity of an individual muscle increases as the tracing moves up from the baseline. This muscle activity is also coordinated with foot placement. Point A is the beginning of the stance phase of gait for the right leg. Point B is the end of stance and the onset of the swing phase. Note that the posterior tibial muscle is active throughout the swing phase of gait. (Reproduced with permission from Green NE, Griffin PP, Shiavi R: Split posterior tibial-tendon transfer in spastic cerebral palsy. J Bone Joint Surg 1983;65A:750.)*

these patients was characterized by exaggerated flexion of the hip and knee in swing phase. Floor contact was made by the entire sole of the foot as a unit. There was no varus deformity of the foot during the swing or stance phase of gait. The foot could be actively dorsiflexed to at least the neutral position of the ankle. This could only be accomplished, however, with simultaneous flexion of the ipsilateral hip and knee (withdrawal).

The result of the procedure was graded as unsatisfactory if there was persistence or recurrence of the varus deformity of the hind part of the foot.

Thirty feet were rated as excellent. Two of these initially had been rated as unsatisfactory. These patients had a fixed varus deformity of the hind part of the foot that was not corrected at the time of the split posterior tibial-tendon transfer. One and one and a half years later, however, these two patients underwent an osteotomy of the calcaneus, and the final results were graded as excellent.

Fifteen feet were rated as good. The varus deformity of the hind part of the foot was corrected in all 15. Because they could not dorsiflex the foot without simultaneous flexion of the hip and knee, these patients all had a so-called steppage gait, although this was less severe than it had been preoperatively. Foot contact was made with the entire sole of the foot at one time. These patients wore a below-the-knee brace at night to prevent a recurrent equinus deformity.

Discussion

Spastic varus and equinovarus deformities are frequently seen in patients with spastic cerebral palsy. The cause of the varus deformity of the hind part of the foot is usually a spastic posterior tibial muscle.[2–4,7,8,11,12] Hoffer and associates[5] postulated that overactivity of the anterior tibial muscle is to blame for the varus deformity of the hind part of the foot in these children. They described the split anterior tibial-tendon transfer that yielded good correction of the varus deformity of the hind part of the foot in their series. It has been my experience, however, that the anterior tibial muscle is weak in most children with a spastic hemiparesis and that, therefore, it is not the offending muscle. In addition, I think the varus deformity of the hind part of the foot is caused by overactivity of the posterior tibial muscle in the face of weak or absent peroneal muscles, whereas a varus or supination deformity of the middle part of the foot is caused by overactivity of the anterior tibial muscle.[2–8,11,13]

Complete tenotomy of the posterior tibial tendon has produced progressive valgus deformity, and anterior rerouting of the posterior tibial tendon has led to progressive calcaneal deformity.[3] Transfer of the posterior tibial tendon anteriorly through the interosseous membrane has been too unpredictable to recommend, even when a gait analysis shows reversal of the normal phase activity.[3,7,8] Lengthening of the posterior tibial tendon has yielded the best results to date in my experience, although recurrence of the deformity has been reported.[11] Simple lengthening of the posterior tibial tendon weakens the posterior tibial muscle, and if both the posterior tibial tendon and the heel cord are lengthened, then plantarflexion strength is significantly reduced. A valgus deformity may result from lengthening of the posterior tibial tendon if the peroneal muscles are spastic and are strong enough to overpower the weakened posterior tibial muscle.

My results show good success in correcting the spastic varus deformity of the hind part of the foot with a split posterior tibial-tendon transfer. In general, the major complication that is encountered with tendon transfers, tenotomy, or muscle release in the spastic child is the development of a deformity opposite to the one under treatment. The split posterior tibial-tendon transfer will consistently correct and prevent the recurrence of a flexible spastic varus deformity of the hind part of the foot, and it has never, in my experience, caused a valgus deformity. When, in addition, the hind part of the foot is in equinus posture, a heel-cord lengthening and a split posterior tibial-tendon transfer will prevent recurrent varus deformity of the hind part of the foot, and the plantarflexion strength of the posterior tibial muscle will not be weakened. Anterior transfer of the posterior tibial tendon combined with a heel-cord lengthening greatly weakens plantarflexion, and, because the spastic posterior tibial tendon has been converted into a dorsiflexor of the foot, a calcaneal deformity may ensue.[2,7,8] Because the plantarflexion strength of the posterior tibial muscle is maintained with the split posterior tibial-tendon transfer, a calcaneal deformity has not been seen as a consequence even when this procedure is combined with a heel-cord lengthening. In addition, recurrence of the varus deformity of the hind part of the foot has not been seen because the peroneus brevis muscle has been reinforced by the transfer of half of the posterior tibial tendon. Another factor in preventing valgus deformity is preservation of the original insertion of the posterior tibial muscle, which continues to function as an inverter of the hind part of the foot.

Conclusions

The split posterior tibial-tendon transfer is a simple procedure that reliably corrects a flexible spastic varus deformity of the hind part of the foot. When this procedure is combined with a lengthening of the Achilles tendon, equinovarus deformity is corrected, and recurrence of the varus deformity is prevented. After split transfer, the posterior tibial muscle cannot function independently as an inverter or as an everter of the hind part of the foot but rather stabilizes the hind part of the foot. A neutral heel without varus or valgus deformity is the result.

References

1. Baker LD, Hill LM: Foot alignment in the cerebral palsy patient. *J Bone Joint Surg* 1964;46A:1–15.
2. Bisla RS, Louis HJ, Albano P: Transfer of tibialis posterior tendon in cerebral palsy. *J Bone Joint Surg* 1976;58A:497–500.
3. Bleck EE: *Orthopaedic Management of Cerebral Palsy*. Philadelphia, WB Saunders, 1979.

4. Gritzka TL, Staheli LT, Duncan WR: Posterior tibial tendon transfer through the interosseous membrane to correct equinovarus deformity in cerebral palsy: An initial experience. *Clin Orthop* 1972;89:201–206.

5. Hoffer MM, Reiswig JA, Garrett AM, et al: The split anterior tibial tendon transfer in the treatment of spastic varus hindfoot of childhood. *Orthop Clin North Am* 1974;5:31–38.

6. Kaufer, H: Split tendon transfers. *Orthop Trans* 1977;1:191.

7. Schneider M, Balon K: Deformity of the foot following anterior transfer of the posterior tibial tendon and lengthening of the Achilles Tendon for spastic equinovarus. *Clin Orthop* 1977;125:113–118.

8. Turner JW, Cooper RR: Anterior transfer of the tibialis posterior through the interosseous membrane. *Clin Orthop* 1972;83:241–244.

9. Watkins MB, Jones JB, Ryder CT Jr, et al: Transplantation of the posterior tibial tendon. *J Bone Joint Surg* 1954;36A:1181–1189.

10. Williams PF: Restoration of muscle balance of the foot by transfer of the tibialis posterior. *J Bone Joint Surg* 1976;58B:217–219.

11. Ruda R, Frost HM: Cerebral palsy: Spastic varus and forefoot adductus, treated by intramuscular posterior tibial tendon lengthening. *Clin Orthop* 1971;79:61–70.

12. Shiavi R, Green N: Ensemble averaging of locomotor electromyographic patterns using interpolation. *Med Biol Eng Comp*, in press.

13. Kling TF Jr, Kaufer H, Hensinger RN: Split posterior tibial-tendon transfers in children with cerebral spastic paralysis and equinovarus deformity. *J Bone Joint Surg* 1985;67A:186–194.

Consensus

Varus Foot in Spastic Diplegia

The varus foot is very uncommon in spastic diplegia, a condition in which there is reasonably symmetric involvement of the lower extremities and minimal involvement of the upper extremities. When the varus foot does occur, it is more common in true hemiplegia or atypical diplegia.

Cause of the Varus Foot

The basic cause of the varus foot is muscle imbalance, with the invertors predominating over the evertors. The primary invertors are the tibialis anterior, tibialis posterior, and triceps surae. The effect of these muscles depends on the position of the subtalar axis, which may vary as a function of foot position, bony deformity, growth, and development. In the normal coupling during stance phase, the peroneal muscles are in synchrony with the triceps surae and tibialis posterior. While in swing phase, the extensor digitorum longus and tibialis anterior are coupled.

Visual Inspection of Gait

As the patient walks, supination and a lack of equinus are observed when the tibialis anterior is involved, and an equinovarus deformity is observed when the tibialis posterior is involved. These observations can be made during both stance and swing phase. The stance phase observation may be confirmed by examination of the child's footwear.

Physical Examination

Passive range-of-motion testing of the tibiotalar joint is done both with the knees straight and flexed to differentiate between soleus and gastrocnemius tightness. The subtalar joint's range of motion is examined with the child seated, and a rapid stretch, in which the forefoot is moved quickly into valgus, is performed with the goal of eliciting a clonic response. If the heel cannot be everted to neutral, the varus may be fixed and not correctable by tendon surgery alone. If varus is confirmed, a standing anteroposterior radiograph and a Harris view are taken to assess alignment and/or bony deformity. Internal tibial torsion can sometimes be seen in conjunction with the true varus foot.

Gait Laboratory Contributions

In many cases of the varus foot, dynamic electromyography (EMG), using fine wire electrodes, provides useful information; however, practical problems with implementation of this method include associated pain, age of the child, cost, and variability of the data. The use of gait analysis to obtain objective data on such parameters as foot pressure distribution, the separation of hindfoot and forefoot kinematics, and the dynamic EMG of various muscle groups, including the peroneals and extensors or digitorum longus, is important for expanding the orthopaedist's knowledge base. Furthermore, evaluating the outcome of surgical procedures requires objective measurements that can also be used in clinical and laboratory investigations. Future refinement of diagnosis and treatment will be enhanced by insights gained from gait laboratory studies. Some of these studies are currently underway, while others are on the research horizons.

Treatment

In treating the varus foot, the following procedures are performed: Achilles tendon lengthening, split anterior tibialis transfer, total tibialis anterior transfer, tibialis posterior lengthening, split posterior tibialis transfer, and total posterior tibial transfer. Depending on the individual patient's condition, the surgeon may choose from the above list individually or in combination. For fixed deformity, calcaneal osteotomy is the procedure most often performed, except in cases of severe deformity.

Section Ten

Goals and Management: Global Perspective

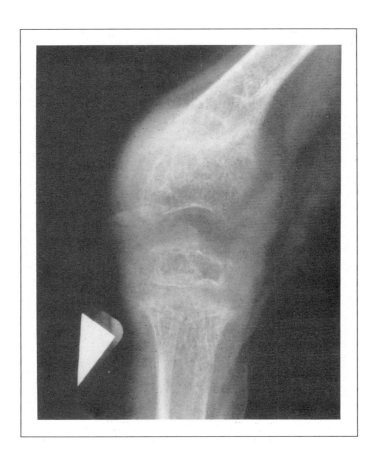

Chapter 34

Orthopaedic Surgeons: What Are We Doing? What Would We Like To Do? What Should We Do?

Michael J. Goldberg, MD
Edward L. Schor, MD

In this symposium, which establishes priorities for those responsible for the treatment of children with spastic diplegia, a trio of philosophical and ethical, but nevertheless pragmatic, questions are presented: What are we doing? What would we like to do? What should we do? A thoughtful answer to these questions must take on a more global perspective.

What Are We Doing?

Using the jargon of the 1990s, as orthopaedic surgeons we are providers of services for our clients (Fig. 1). Our clients are (1) people with cerebral palsy; (2) people with other conditions that have been misdiagnosed as cerebral palsy; and (3) families of people with cerebral palsy.

Cerebral palsy is a nonprogressive motor disorder that originates in the brain and is caused by damage that occurred before or at about the time of birth. Motor disturbance may be apparent in muscle strength, tone, coordination, or in a combination of these. Cerebral palsy varies in severity, and mental retardation or seizures are sometimes associated with the disease.

In addition, our patients are children with conditions that either mimic or are misdiagnosed as cerebral palsy. Spasticity in these patients may have occurred after birth as a result of meningitis or child abuse. There is also an entire group of patients with spastic neuromuscular disease who do not have cerebral palsy, such as those with Rett syndrome. In fact, an analysis of cerebral palsy clinics will reveal a mixture of these patient types. Because so many of our patients are children, we must also include their families as clients.

Providers

As orthopaedic surgeons, we are one of a team of providers, who can generally be placed into one of three groups:

Physicians This group includes orthopaedic surgeons, neurologists,

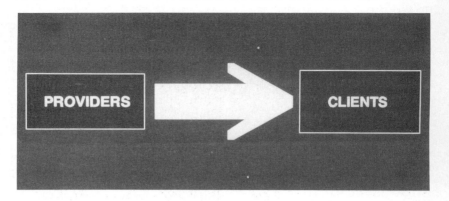

Fig. 1 *A large number of health care professionals are providing services to patients with cerebral palsy and their families.*

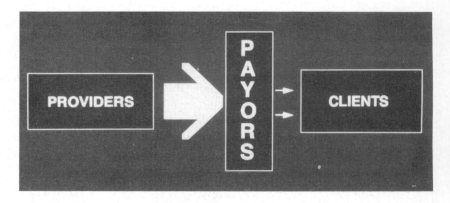

Fig. 2 *The third party payors act as intermediates for providers and clients, serving as a filter for payment of medical services.*

neurosurgeons, physiatrists, pediatricians, radiologists, and, on occasion, ophthalmologists, pediatric surgeons, and otolaryngologists.

Other health-care professionals This group includes physical therapists, nurses, occupational therapists, speech pathologists, and early interventionists as well as social service workers, psychologists, and special educators.

Vendors This group consists of those who supply braces and inserts, customized seating systems, mats and balls, wheelchairs, and other hardware. There are also those who transport patients, pharmacists, computer programmers, and suppliers of software.

The providers require payment for their goods and services, which comes, in large part from third party payors who act as intermediates for providers and clients (Fig. 2). Indeed, the quality and quantity of service that the providers are able to give depends much on the decisions of the third party payors. At times, it appears as if the payors allow some services and disallow others (by refusing to pay for them) with no understanding of what the providers would like to do and should do. But how clearly have we articulated what we would like to do and what we should do?

What Would We Like To Do?

A usual response would be, ''We want to make our patients better,'' or ''We want to assure quality care.'' In fact, we are being held accountable for what we have done (the operations performed, the tests ordered), rather than for what we have accomplished (improved functional performance, enabling a disabled child to become a potential worker and taxpayer). Therefore, we must define what we would like to do, and face the ethical dilemmas that may then arise.

First, we would like to eliminate or at least reduce the number of cases of cerebral palsy. Therefore, we would like to make an investment in basic research, we would like to have a better understanding of the pathobiology of the brain, and we must support and strengthen maternal-fetal medicine programs.

From a narrower viewpoint as orthopaedic surgeons, we want to manage our patients' care to achieve the desired outcomes and to avoid adverse consequences. In addition, we want to do this in a kind and compassionate manner that minimizes suffering.

Let us first analyze the statement, ''Achieving the desired outcomes.'' The questions that immediately come to mind are ''What are they?'', and ''Whose are they?'' The desired outcomes of the child with cerebral palsy are not necessarily the same as the desired outcomes of the parent. The first question often asked by parents of children with cerebral palsy is: ''Will my child walk?''; and then, ''When will my child walk?'' Many cerebral palsy care programs spend inordinate amounts of time, energy, and money trying to achieve this goal. However, is this what adults with cerebral palsy want? Adults with cerebral palsy place communication skills first, independence in performing activities of daily living and self-care second, and mobility or locomotion third.[1] They want to be able to move about easily, without expending a great deal of energy.

In addition to the parent and the child, our society or culture also plays a part in determining the desired outcome. In cerebral palsy, life expectancy is not reduced substantially enough to consider the disease to be transient. Although some children with cerebral palsy reportedly improve,[2] as a rule, cerebral palsy is a lifelong, incurable disease. The child with cerebral palsy eventually becomes the adult with cerebral palsy.[1] Therefore, when establishing priorities for treatment of children with spastic diplegia, we must take our society and culture into account and ask, "Do we make the patient fit the environment, or do we make the environment fit the patient?" When this question is asked, the important considerations are the disease severity and the associated morbidities (mental retardation). The patient has the choice of living independently, living in a sheltered environment, or custodial care. The majority of those with spastic diplegia may be able to live independently; however, the patient's ability to achieve independence is influenced not only by the orthopaedic surgeon and other health care professionals, but by society.

Housing adapted to the needs of the patient, an accessible city, available technology, and an educated populus are important and necessary factors for the patient with cerebral palsy who wishes to live independently. The educational system must be able to assimilate children with cerebral palsy so that they can achieve maximal educational benefit. Society must also be educated so that people with cerebral palsy are integrated into the free marketplace. Some observers have noted that the person with cerebral palsy who lives in a rural area may function better than those who live in urban settings.[3] In rural areas, a person with cerebral palsy often encounters fewer obstructions to travel and is more readily accepted and integrated into the community. Cities, on the other hand, have significant barriers in the schools, public transportation, and other public services. As cities and their systems become dysfunctional, the barriers increase and the handicapped become increasingly disadvantaged.

Thus, our objective is to have goals or outcomes that benefit the patient, the family, and society. This may well prove to be a very uncomfortable triangle. When in conflict, who has priority? The issues that arise are broad. They include those that are comfortable to discuss, such as the timing of orthopaedic surgery as it relates to school, or the type and cost of a wheelchair. They also include those that are a bit uncomfortable to discuss, such as sexuality in the handicapped adolescent and adult; and those that are quite uncomfortable to discuss, such as resources rationing, and the economy of heroic efforts to sustain life.

Once we identify the desired outcomes, we want to achieve them without producing any unwanted or adverse consequences. These adverse consequences may be broadly grouped into five areas (I am sure there are more): (1) anticipated orthopaedic complications; (2) unanticipated medical complications; (3) disruptive education; (4) impact of our care on family; and (5) adverse effects on cost.

Orthopaedic complications are expected, because those are the ones we discuss with all of our patients before surgery. They include such things as wound infection, hardware failure, undercorrection or overcorrection, cast and pressure sores, complications of anesthesia, and complications of blood transfusions, for example.

The medical complications, which I have called unanticipated, include other organ failure, such as worsening of the gastroesophageal reflex, or allowing seizures to get out of control. Another common complication is problems with adequate nutrition. Figures 3 and 4 illustrate a five-year span of multiple surgical procedures on both hips of a

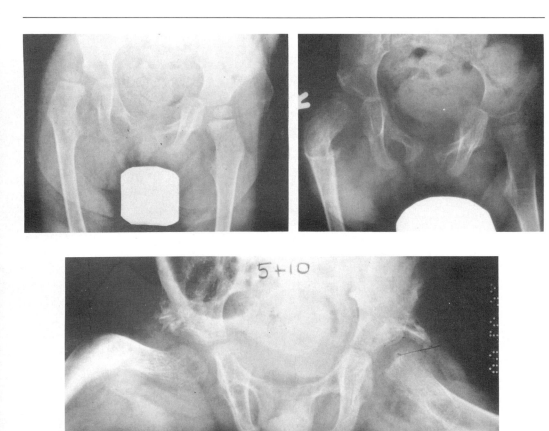

Fig. 3 *Top left: 1985, spastic quadriplegia and subluxation of the right hip of a boy age 2 years 6 months;* **Top right:** *1986, age 3 years 10 months, varus osteotomy of the right hip followed by hardware removal. Early subluxation of the left hip is evident.* **Bottom:** *1988, age 5 years 10 months, bilateral acetabular augmentations. Note progressive varus of right femur.*

2½-year-old boy with spastic quadriplegia, during which time his nutritional requirements were not satisfied and he developed frank nutritional rickets.

The birthday syndrome, so named because each year the child has another orthopaedic procedure, is not compatible with education. Patients with spastic diplegia need to have their education maximized and their ability to communicate refined. In general, this is accomplished better in schools than in hospitals. Therefore, any orthopaedic surgery that contributes to academic failure is undesirable. Many adults with cerebral palsy continue to have difficulty with social and professional integration. The barriers they face are not only those related to

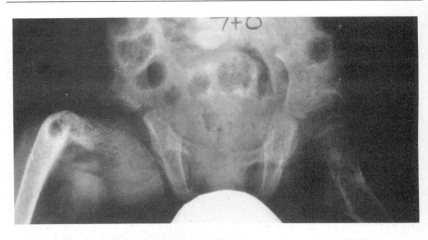

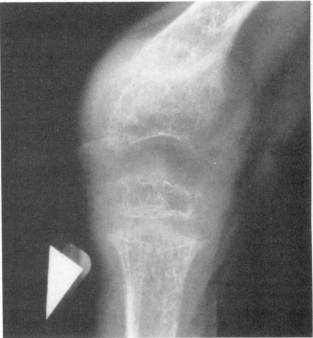

Fig. 4 *Top: 1990, age 7 years. Child clinically is very irritable and visibly undernourished. Progressive varus right femur and generalized osteopenia.* **Bottom:** *1990, age 7 years. The child's knee demonstrates the classic roentgenographic findings of rickets: osteopenia, widened physes, and absent zone of provisional calcification.*

their physical handicap. Many patients with cerebral palsy lack social interactive skills, causing me to question if some of the rigid therapeutic programs involving braces and physical therapy infantilize patients, thereby inhibiting adolescent rebellion and with it the social maturation needed to keep a job in a competitive marketplace. Employment and self-esteem are inextricably linked. Perhaps a better measure of how well teenagers with cerebral palsy are doing is to count how many are becoming pregnant, or how many are abusing alcohol, rather than calculate their stride length or cadence. Until cerebral palsy patients are experiencing the same social problems that trouble unaffected adolescents, we are not accomplishing integration.

One may wonder why patients with polio have more success when entering the workforce. Like cerebral palsy, polio results in significant motor dysfunction necessitating the use of braces and wheelchairs. There are, I am sure, many reasons, but some to consider are: (1) Polio is an infectious disease, whereas the image of cerebral palsy is that of being brain damaged. (2) Patients with polio speak more clearly, while many of the brightest patients with spastic diplegia have distorted speech. (3) Patients with cerebral palsy have been subjected to rigid "programs" of therapy which, I believe, do not promote independence or self-reliance.

The care of children with cerebral palsy often has an adverse impact on the family, both on the relationship of the parents and on the siblings. Everyone in the family must make significant sacrifices.

Another important aspect is cost, which includes utilization of services and dollars. The utilization of services includes physician time, outpatient appointments, and operating room schedules. The utilization of dollars, however, appears to drain resources the fastest. There is evidence indicating that we are heading toward an economy with a limited amount of fixed health-care dollars. Under such circumstances, we will have to weigh the efficacy or appropriateness of therapy, or, whether a treatment works for any one patient (such as a heart transplant for someone with heart failure) against the effectiveness or efficiency of therapy or the value of applying any technique to a large patient population (such as immunization programs). However, what is best for one patient may not be best for a population of patients. For example, compare centoxin, the genetically engineered monoclonal antibody against the gram-negative toxins of septic shock at an estimated $3,800 per dose, with enalapril maleate, a most effective antihypertensive at 60 cents per day.

What Should We Do?

There seem to be important variations in the way children with cerebral palsy (with apparently similar orthopaedic deformities and medical problems) are managed, and differences in their outcomes. Despite our best efforts, we do not know the best way to manage many, if not most, conditions. A system is needed to determine if the way we manage our patients' care is achieving the desired outcomes, and if adverse consequences are being produced in the process. Therefore, we as orthopaedic surgeons need to define the patients being treated and assess their treatment. Although simply stated, it may not be so easy to accomplish; nevertheless, the science and methodology exist.[4-8] I would propose six steps: the first three define the patient; the next three assess treatment.

Diagnostic Criteria

We must establish diagnostic criteria by defining who has cerebral palsy. What essential information is necessary to diagnose this condition? What enables us to make that definitive diagnosis and rule out all other conditions? Is this done by using patient history, physical examination, laboratory data, magnetic resonance images? How?

Severity Indicators

Cerebral palsy varies in severity among children who are affected. What information is most useful in determining how severely the child with cerebral palsy is affected? How can we conclude that one child with cerebral palsy is more severely affected than another? Is it their physical deformity or their functional impairment?[2] Are the number of operations, the amount of physical therapy, and/or the amount of money spent valid measures? What are our severity indicators?

Activity of the Disease

We need to know the activity of cerebral palsy, which is different from the severity. It is easy to think about activity when dealing with disorders such as rheumatoid arthritis, where the erythrocyte sedimentation rate can be an indicator of activity. Nevertheless, some parents say that their child is ''getting worse,'' and some neurologists state that the child will ''outgrow'' cerebral palsy.[2] What clinical data most accurately measure the activity of those with cerebral palsy? Is it patient history, physical examination, or laboratory data?

Therapeutic Options

What are our therapeutic options? For many conditions there exist only a limited number of treatment interventions. Unfortunately, that is not the case with cerebral palsy, where a wide range of treatment modalities are available. These include nonsurgical methods (therapy regimens, pharmacologic treatment, counseling, education), minor procedures (nerve blocks), and major surgery (orthopaedic surgery and neurosurgery). Nevertheless, we need to itemize our options.

Outcomes of Care

We need to determine the outcomes relative to the care that we provide for our cerebral palsy patients. What are the likely outcomes, both desirable and adverse, that could result from the treatment? The goal of medical care is to improve, or at least maintain, the health of our patients, but to know if we are meeting this goal we must critically measure outcomes. Systems are currently being developed that will enable us to measure outcomes,[5] including technical outcomes, the functional health assessment, patient satisfaction, and costs.

The technical outcome includes things measured with rulers and goniometers, such as scoliosis curves and joint range of motion. Functional outcomes include roles and tasks, and physical, emotional, and social functioning. Patient satisfaction includes not only personal satisfaction with the outcome, but also with the process of care. Costs include both the use of existing resources (beds, people) and the costs of providing services (surgery, therapy), as well as balancing individual effectiveness with population efficiency.

Intervening Factors

A number of factors other than the characteristics of the disease might influence the course of cerebral palsy, both its natural history and outcomes. These intervening factors may influence the response to treatment or the cost of care. Examples of intervening factors include sociodemographic factors, other health problems (comorbidities), family and living conditions, access to services, and certain patient/family behaviors, such as compliance with treatment.

Summary

What are we doing? We are providers of health care.

What would we like to do? We would like to manage our patients' care so that desired outcomes may be achieved (whatever they might be) without producing any adverse consequences in the process.

What should we do? We should define the patient with cerebral palsy by establishing diagnostic criteria, severity indicators, and activity of the disease. Then we should assess the patient's treatment by considering therapeutic options, outcomes of care we wish to measure, and any intervening factors that might affect outcomes.

References

1. Bleck EE: Goals, treatment and management, in Bleck EE (ed): *Orthopaedic Management in Cerebral Palsy,* Clinics in Development Medicine. Oxford, MacKeith Press with Blackwell Scientific Publications, 1987, no 99/100, pp 142–212.
2. Nelson KB, Ellenberg JH: Children who "outgrew" cerebral palsy. *Pediatrics* 1982;69:529–536.
3. Bleck EE: Factors affecting independence of the physically disabled. *Dev Med Child Neurol* 1990;32:189–190.
4. Daves AR, Ware JE Jr: Involving consumers in quality of care assessment. *Health Aff* (Millwood) 1988;7:33–48.
5. Goldberg MJ: Measuring outcomes in cerebral palsy. *J Pediatr Orthop* 1991; 11:682–685.
6. Nelson EC, Berwick DM: The measurement of health status in clinical practice. *Med Care* 1989;27(suppl 3):S77–90.
7. Rosenbaum P, Cadman D, Kirpalani H: Pediatrics: Assessing quality of life, in Spilker B (ed): *Quality of Life Assessments in Clinical Trials.* New York, Raven Press, 1990, pp 205–215.
8. Tarlov AR, Ware JE Jr, Greenfield S, et al: The medical outcomes study: An application of methods for monitoring the results of medical care. *JAMA* 1989; 262:925–930.

Chapter 35

Funding for Care of Cerebral Palsy in the United States

Newton C. McCollough III, MD

There is a dearth of information concerning sources of funding for care of children with cerebral palsy in the United States. Much is known about the costs of health care in general, how it is paid for, and the problem of accessing the health-care system by certain of our citizens, notably the poor and the young. A great deal of information is available about the financing of children's health care, especially regarding the financial barriers to universal access of children to the health-care system. Somewhat less is known about the sources of funding for children with chronic disabilities, and very little is known about the funding for care of children with cerebral palsy as a group. It is apparent, however, that the characteristics of health-care financing that affect access to care for the general population, the pediatric population, and the disabled pediatric population also determine the availability of funding for this special group of children. Therefore, any discussion about health-care funding for cerebral palsy must occur within the larger context of the financing available for these larger populations.

National Health-Care Spending and Sources of Payment

National health-care spending has grown from 5.2% of the gross national product in 1960 to over 12% in 1990 (Fig. 1), the highest percentage of any country in the world (Fig. 2). In dollars, this represents a growth from $27.1 billion in 1960 to over $660 billion in 1990 (Fig. 3). In 1987, real health-care spending per capita in the United States was $2,051 compared with $1,515 in Canada, $1,073 in West Germany, $917 in Japan, and $751 in the United Kingdom (Fig. 4). In 1989, the sources of payment for health services in the United States were as follows: private health insurance 33%; out-of-pocket expenditures 21%; federal sources 29%; state and local financing 13%; and other private payments 4% (Fig. 5.). The distribution of health-care financing has changed dramatically since 1965. The proportion of health-care financing provided by federal programs has increased from

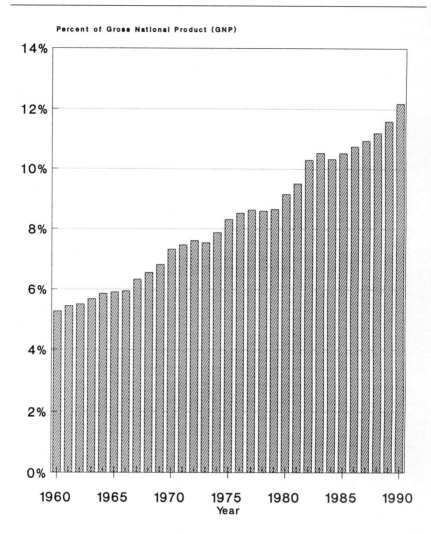

Percent of Gross National Product (GNP)

Fig. 1 *National health expenditures as a share of the gross national product, 1960 to 1990. The 1990 increase in spending marks the sixth consecutive year that health spending grew faster than the overall economy.[1]*

8.3% to 29% and that provided by private insurance has increased from 24% to 33% during the last 25 years. During the same period, out-of-pocket expenses for health care have decreased from 53.4% to 23.5% of total health-care expenditures (Fig. 6).[1]

Despite the fact that the proportion of health-care coverage from both federal and private insurance sources has increased significantly since 1965, it is estimated that more than 37 million Americans still lack insurance coverage.[2] The largest segment of the uninsured population are children under 18 years of age.[3] This is because there has actually been a decline in private health-care coverage of children since 1977,

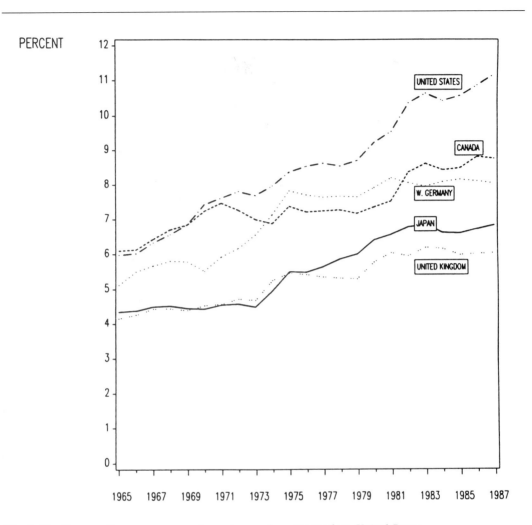

PERCENT

Fig. 2 *Health expenditures as a percentage of gross domestic product, United States and selected countries, 1965–1987.*[1]

when 75% of children were covered. By 1987, only two thirds of the nation's children were covered through their parents' employment-related coverage. This loss occurred almost exclusively among children in two-parent, single-worker homes.[4]

Characteristics of Health-Care Financing for the Nation's Children

The Congressional Research Service has identified the primary sources of health-care coverage for children under 18 in the year 1989.[1] Of the nation's 64 million children under 18 years of age, 72% had

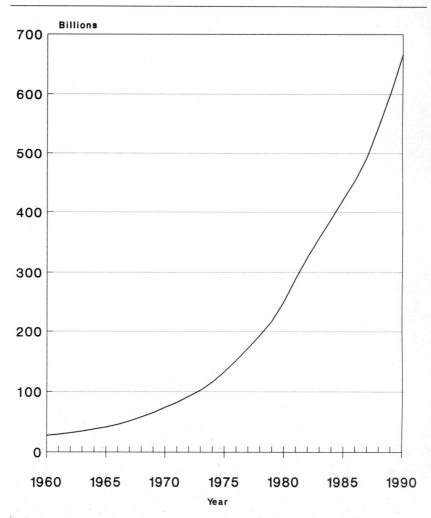

Fig. 3 *National Health Expenditures, 1960 to 1990. Health-care spending grew rapidly in the early 1980s, with annual growth rates exceeding 15% in both 1980 and 1981. Growth rates were more moderate in the mid-1980s, but have accelerated again since 1986. The rate of growth was 10.4% in 1989 and 10.5% in 1990.*[1]

coverage from their parents' job-related insurance; 13% were covered by Medicaid; 2% had "other" health-care coverage; and 13% (8.7 million children) were uninsured (Fig. 7). Chollet[3] has estimated that as many as 12.2 million children, or roughly 19% of the population under 18 years of age, are uninsured or underinsured. Of the total number of uninsured in the United States, 45% are under the age of 24 and 26% are under the age of 18 (Fig. 8).[1]

Americans living below the federal poverty level still represent the largest segment of uninsured, accounting for 12.6 million or 36%.[5] Because children account for the largest segment of all Americans in

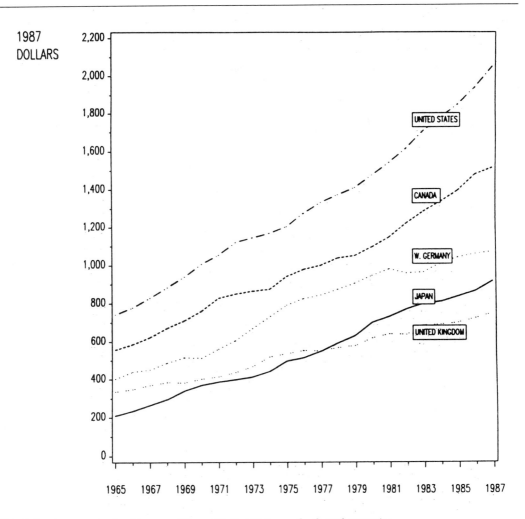

Fig. 4 *Real per capita health expenditures, United States and selected countries, 1965–1987. United States per capita spending rose by 176% during this period, which is comparable to the 167% increase in West Germany and 172% increase in Canada. Japan experienced a considerably higher rate of growth, 339%.*[1]

poverty, the link between income and health insurance coverage for children is particularly significant.

Moreover, the percentage of children with no health insurance increased by 13% between 1983 and 1986,[6] and the percentage of children living in poverty increased by approximately 25% between 1979 and 1987.[7] In 1989, one fifth of all children lived in households with incomes below the federal poverty line ($12,675 for a family of four).[4]

Medicaid has been inadequate to meet the health-care needs of children. The Medicaid program (Title XIX of the Social Security Act) was created in 1965 to provide financial access to health care for low-

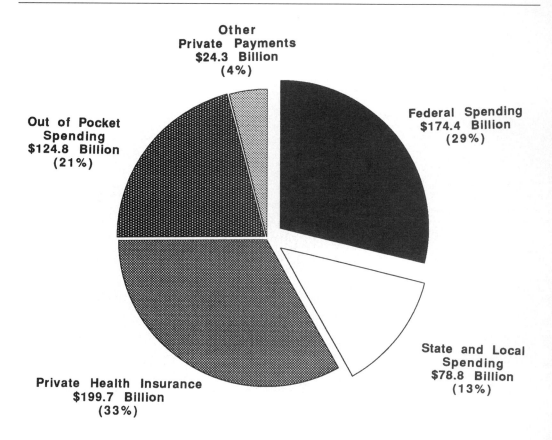

Fig. 5 *National health spending, by type of payer, 1989. Most Federal health spending is for Medicare, but the Federal government also finances health care through Medicaid, the Veterans Administration, the Department of Defense, and the Public Health Service. The largest component of state and local spending is for Medicaid; many state and local governments also finance health services for indigent individuals not eligible for Medicaid.[1]*

income persons. Title XIX mandated a jointly funded federal-state partnership to help eliminate financial barriers to medical care for the poor. The federal government matches state expenditures based on a formula using a state's per capita income. The federal contribution ranges from 50% to 78%; however, each state has a great deal of latitude in setting its own Medicaid policies, resulting in substantial variation in eligibility, benefits, and reimbursement rates.[3] Of the 13 million children under 18 years of age living in poverty, only half are covered by Medicaid.[8]

According to Oberg,[5] "although Medicaid was enacted to finance and improve access to care for the poor, it has developed into the largest public funder of long term care for the elderly. When nursing home care is needed, the elderly spend down to a level of poverty in order to qualify for Supplemental Security Income and Medicaid." Oberg

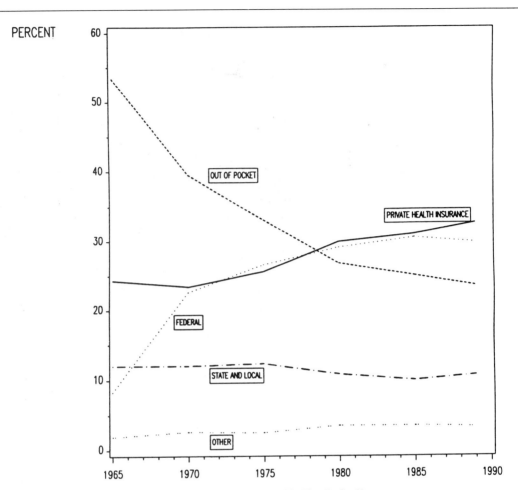

Fig. 6 *Distribution of health spending by payer, 1965–1989. The "other" category includes philanthropy and industrial in-plant spending for health. As can be seen by comparing Figures 5 and 6, percentages vary according to the source of the data.[1]*

examines the trend of Medicaid expenditures since 1972, pointing out a gradual decrease in Medicaid expenditures for Aid to Families with Dependent Children from 18% to 12% of the total by 1987, and a corresponding increase from 53% to 73% of total Medicaid expenditures for Supplemental Security Income recipients by 1987. He further states that the average state Aid to Families with Dependent Children eligibility threshold used for Medicaid fell from 71% of poverty in 1975 to 48% in 1986.

In fact, Benjamin and Newacheck[9] point out that since 1965 the elderly population has gained a progressively greater share of social-welfare spending, while that for children has decreased (Fig. 9). This reversal in social support among these two age groups has occurred during the same period when income levels and relative prosperity have

Persons covered in millions

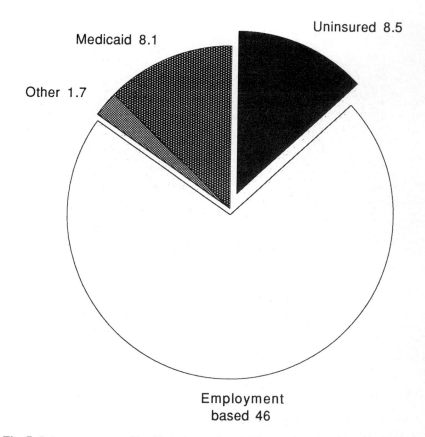

Uninsured 8.5

Medicaid 8.1

Other 1.7

Employment
based 46

Fig. 7 *Primary sources of health coverage for children under age 18, 1989. The rate of uninsurance is twice as high for those under poverty. All poor children will eventually be eligible for Medicaid under the phased-in Omnibus Budget Reconciliation Act 1990 expansions.[1]*

increased for elders and decreased for families with children. Poor and low-income children in two-parent households are more likely to be without health insurance than are poor and low-income children in single-parent households. This reflects the greater accessibility to Medicaid funds by children of single parents.[4]

More recently, federal legislation (Omnibus Budget Reconciliation Act, 1989) has mandated coverage of all pregnant women, as well as all children under six years of age, with family incomes less than 133% of the poverty level.[5]

Persons in millions

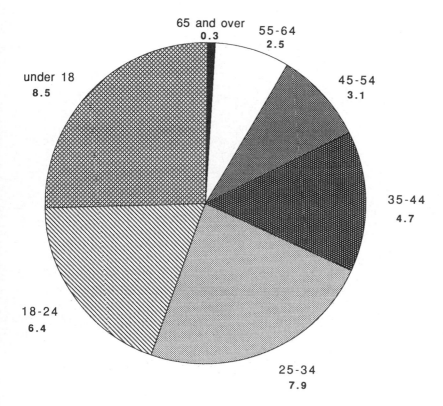

Fig. 8 *Population without health coverage by age, 1989. Older adults make up a much smaller proportion of the uninsured. However, because they are likely to require more health services, they may contribute disproportionately to such problems as uncompensated care in hospitals.[1]*

Health-Care Financing of Children With Chronic Disabilities

Approximately 10%, or 6.4 million children in the United States are affected by chronic health problems. Of these, about half, or 3 million children, have chronic limitations in their activities.[10] Included in this number are the approximately 200,000 children with cerebral palsy.[11]

It has been estimated that 10.3% of disabled children and 19.5% of disabled children in poverty have no health insurance. Further, 40% of all disabled children below the federal poverty line are not covered by Medicaid.[12]

Families of disabled children rely on a variety of sources to cover

449

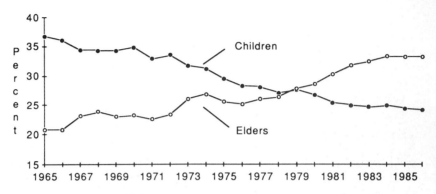

Fig. 9 *Shares of social welfare spending benefiting children and elders, United States, 1965 to 1986. (Reproduced with permission from Benjamin et al.[9])*

health-care bills. According to Newacheck and McMannus (unpublished data, 1989), public insurance covers 25% of disabled children. However, many low-income children are ineligible for Medicaid services because their family incomes are slightly above limits set by the states. In some states, this may be as low as 20% to 30% of the federal poverty level.

Private insurance covered 66% of disabled children in 1984 (P.W. Newacheck, M. McManus, unpublished data, 1989); however, the extent of services a child is entitled to varies greatly. A study of private health insurance coverage of chronically ill children by Fox and Newacheck[13] revealed several deficiencies in coverage of children with chronic disabilities. Many private health-care plans do not provide adequate coverage for physical and occupational therapy, speech therapy, and psychosocial service. For example, only 57% of the plans studied provided coverage for occupational therapy, and only 15% provided coverage for psychiatrists, psychologists, and psychiatric social workers. While a trend toward better coverage for outpatient services and home health care was noted, limits on the number of visits and reimbursement levels are common. There has been a trend for employer-based plans to increase the employee's cost of using covered services by imposing higher coinsurance and deductible requirements.

Of those children under 18 years of age who are insured, 17% do not have major medical insurance to cover special health-care costs, and less than 10% have unlimited coverage. Another factor mitigating against adequate health coverage for disabled children is the frequent requirement that preexisting conditions be excluded. According to Rosenbaum and Johnson,[14] 73% of all employers responding to a major health insurance survey conducted in 1986 indicated that their plans excluded coverage of preexisting conditions.

Federal health-insurance programs, primarily provided via Medicaid, are inadequate to meet the health-care needs of the vast majority of disabled children for reasons noted earlier. Even if a disabled child is fortunate enough to be covered by Medicaid, access to truly comprehensive and coordinated care is virtually nonexistent. For example, some services may be received through public health departments, other services through community health centers, and still other services are provided by urban city or county hospitals. In most instances, none of these institutions communicate with each other. During 1987, 14 states did not cover physical therapy services under the Medicaid program. Occupational therapy was not covered by 23 state Medicaid programs, and 16 states did not cover therapy for speech, hearing, or language disorders.[15]

Many low- and moderate-income families with disabled children turn to the state and federally financed program for Children With Special Health Care Needs, which is designed to provide a range of services to financially and medically eligible disabled children. This program of services is jointly sponsored by federal and state governments and is administered at the state level. The program was created by Title V of the Social Security Act enacted in 1935. The Bureau of Maternal and Child Health is the federal agency that provides these block grants to the states, targeted to medically underserved women and children. The total funding, however, is so low that fewer than half of all states are able to offer comprehensive prenatal programs on a statewide basis.[16] In 1988, approximately $140 million was made available to the state Children With Special Health Care Needs agencies through the federal maternal and child health block grants. During that same fiscal year, the total match by all states amounted to $338.5 million. Combined, these two sources of public funding may only meet as much as 42% of the estimated cost of services needed by the Children With Special Health Care Needs population nationwide (Bureau of Maternal and Child Health, personal communication, 1989).

Shriners Hospitals for Crippled Children makes the largest single private-sector contribution to the care of disabled children on a continuing basis. In 1990, the total Shriners Hospitals for Crippled Children expenditures for orthopaedic hospitals, burn institutes, and research was in excess of $230 million.[17] The 1990 operating budget for the orthopaedic hospitals alone, which care for orthopaedically and neurologically handicapped children, was $162 million excluding research funding. This amount is in excess of the total annual federal expenditure for Children With Special Health Care Needs under Title V. Since the first Shriners Hospital opened in 1922, over $2 billion has been spent by this charity in providing totally free care to disabled children.

Health-Care Financing of Children With Cerebral Palsy

Cerebral palsy is one of the most common causes of chronic childhood disability in the United States. According to Gortmaker and Sappenfeld,[18] the prevalence of cerebral palsy in the United States population is 2.5 per 1,000 population. The only chronic disabling conditions more common than cerebral palsy are asthma, visual impairment, mental retardation, hearing impairment, congenital heart disease, and seizure disorders.[18] It is estimated that between 500,000 and 700,000 persons in the United States are afflicted with cerebral palsy and that 40% of these individuals are under 20 years of age.[11] The incidence of cerebral palsy in newborn children is approximately one per 1,000 live births, which translates into between 3,500 and 4,000 new cases annually in the United States.[11]

Expenses for a child with cerebral palsy, including physician services, speech therapy, medications, special education, and other support services, average $4,490 annually, with 51% paid by the family (United Cerebral Palsy Associations, 1986).

The major sources of funding for the care of patients with cerebral palsy are private health insurance and federally sponsored insurance programs, principally the Medicaid program (Title XIX) and the Children With Special Health Care Needs program (Title V). Deficiencies in coverage by these programs have already been pointed out. No accurate data exist as to the number of cerebral palsy patients who are covered by private insurance and federal programs. However, it is clear that between 13% (8.3 million) and 20% (12.8 million) of all children are uninsured. One must assume that a comparable percentage of children with cerebral palsy are likewise uninsured.

The two major contributors to funding of care for cerebral palsy patients from the private sector are the United Cerebral Palsy Associations and Shriners Hospitals for Crippled Children. Each of these organizations provides substantial resources for the care of children with cerebral palsy.

United Cerebral Palsy Associations is a nationwide network of approximately 180 state and local voluntary agencies (United Cerebral Palsy Associations affiliates), which provide services, conduct public and professional education programs, and support research in cerebral palsy. At the local level, direct services are provided by affiliates to children and adults with cerebral palsy and their families. Services include medical evaluation and treatment, special education, career development, social and recreation programs, parent counseling, and adaptive housing for the disabled.[19] In 1989, United Cerebral Palsy Associations expended $287 million in community services, such as those described above for children and adults with cerebral palsy.[20] Funding of medical care, including therapy services, is limited to the outpatient setting. While United Cerebral Palsy Associations provides a significant amount of uncompensated care, their expenditures are supported to a degree by patient revenues, including third-party payments.

Shriners Hospitals for Crippled Children provide medical, surgical, and comprehensive multidisciplinary allied health care for cerebral palsy patients as inpatients or outpatients in 17 orthopaedic hospitals in the United States. No charge is made to the patient or third party for any service provided in Shriners Hospitals. Of a total of 17,851 admissions to Shriners orthopaedic hospitals in 1990, 2,578 were patients admitted with the diagnosis of cerebral palsy. The average length of stay for these patients admitted for surgery and/or rehabilitation was 10.5 days. The average cost per admission was $7,447. The total expenditures by Shriners Hospitals for Crippled Children for the inpatient care of cerebral palsy patients in 1990 was $19,199,000. Accurate figures are not available for Shriners Hospitals for Crippled Children's contribution to outpatient cerebral palsy care.

Funding for the comprehensive care of patients with cerebral palsy in the United States like funding for the care of other children with chronic disabilities, is inadequate. In addition, the sources of funding and the programs of care for cerebral palsy patients and others with disabilities of childhood are widely disparate and poorly coordinated. The inadequacies of funding for cerebral palsy patients are a part of the larger problem of financing children's health care in the United States. These problems will not be completely solved until a national children's health policy has been developed to integrate and coordinate the public and private resources available.

References

1. Committee on Ways and Means: U.S. House of Representatives: *Health Care Resource Book*. Washington, U.S. Government Printing House, April 16, 1991; Dec 20, 1991.

2. Short PF, Monheit A, Beauregard K: *Uninsured Americans: A 1987 Profile.* Rockville, MD, National Center for Health Services Research and Health Care Technology Assessment, 1988.

3. Chollet D: *Uninsured in the United States: The Nonelderly Population Without Health Insurance, 1986.* Washington, DC, Employee Benefit Research Institute, 1988.

4. Cunningham P, Monheit A: Insuring the children: A decade of change. *Health Affairs* 1990;Winter:76–90.

5. Oberg CN: Medically uninsured children in the United States: A challenge to public policy. *Pediatrics* 1990;85:925–833.

6. Sealing PA: *Profile of Child Health in the United States.* Alexandria, VA, National Association of Children's Hospitals and Related Institutions, 1989, p 19.

7. Children's Defense Fund. *A Vision for American's Future.* Washington, DC, 1989:16. Available Library of Congress 88–063421.

8. Health and Medical Editors: Exclusive healthweek report: Children's health care crisis worsens as millions join ranks of poor and uninsured. *Health Week,* September 10, 1990.

9. Benjamin AE, Newacheck PW: Intergenerational equity and public spending. *Pediatrics* 1991;88:75–83.

10. Gortmaker SL, Sappenfield W: Chronic childhood disorders: Prevalence and impact. *Pediatr Clin North Am* 1984;31:3–18.

11. Sternfeld L: Cerebral palsy. *Health & Medical Horizons.* New York, United Cerebral Palsy Associations, 1991, pp 196–199.

12. Butler JA, Winter WD, Singer JD, et al: Medical care use and expenditure among children and young in the United States: Analysis of a national probability sample. *Pediatrics* 1985;76:495–507.

13. Fox HB, Newacheck PW: Private health insurance of chronically ill children. *Pediatrics* 1990;1:50–57.

14. Rosenbaum S, Johnson K: Providing health care for low-income children: Reconciling child health goals with child health financing realities. *Milbank Mem Fund Q* 1986;64:442–478.
15. Special Report: *Barriers to Care*. Elk Grove Village, IL, American Academy of Pediatrics, 1990.
16. Rosenbaum S, Hughes DC, Johnson K: Maternal and child health services for medically indigent children and pregnant women. *Med Care* 1988;26:315–332.
17. Shriners Hospitals for Crippled Children: *Annual Report*. Tampa, FL, Shriners Hospitals for Crippled Children, 1991.
18. Gortmaker SL, Sappenfeld W: Chronic childhood disorders: Prevalence and impact. *Pediatr Clin North Am* 1984;31:3–18.
19. *Cerebral Palsy Facts and Figures*. New York, United Cerebral Palsy Associations, September, 1989.
20. United Cerebral Palsy Associations: *Live, Learn, Work, Play: Annual Report*. New York, United Cerebral Palsy Associations, 1990.

Chapter 36

Cerebral Palsy in the Rural United States

Walter B. Greene, MD

Because the literature on this subject was unknown to me, a Medline search was initiated. Combining the titles of "cerebral palsy" and "rural" yielded no citations. Also unproductive was a search statement that combined the titles of "child health," "rural," and "developmental disorders." At that point, I became apprehensive that limited data were available regarding children with cerebral palsy who live in rural areas. Further research confirmed that suspicion.

Most of the public health-care dollars for children are dispensed by state governments. Therefore, 50 states are administering in a variety of ways, a multitude of children's health-care programs, none of which are specifically designated for the child with cerebral palsy, nor are they subdivided into rural versus urban populations. Furthermore, geographic data are lacking on children with cerebral palsy whose medical care is financed by private insurance or through other institutions, such as Shriners Hospitals for Crippled Children. Finally, a lack of consensus on what constitutes acceptable care for children with cerebral palsy makes it difficult to determine whether children who live in isolated rural areas are receiving adequate treatment.

Despite these limitations, the assignment remained. I have elected to approach the topic by (1) reviewing the data on the incidence of cerebral palsy in rural areas, (2) examining different aspects of environmental barriers and community acceptance of people with cerebral palsy, (3) evaluating financial considerations and multidisciplinary care for children with cerebral palsy who live in rural areas, and (4) outlining the principles of providing optimal therapy for these children. Finally, two models for providing multidisciplinary care in rural areas will be presented.

Incidence of Cerebral Palsy in Rural Areas

Data on the incidence of cerebral palsy in rural versus urban areas are not available. There is, however, information relevant to other factors associated with cerebral palsy.

Nonmetropolitan women of childbearing age are more likely to be uninsured, and obstetric care is more limited in rural areas.[1] These factors, however, may not significantly affect the incidence of cerebral palsy. Present evidence supports the concept that adverse obstetric factors during delivery cause few cases of cerebral palsy, at least in First and Second World countries.[2-4]

Low birth weight is associated with cerebral palsy,[4] but the data examining this factor in rural versus urban areas of the United States are limited and inconclusive. The 15 states that are predominantly rural ($\geq$ 50% of the state's population residing in nonmetropolitan areas) actually have a lower number of infants with low birth weight.[1] The higher fetal mortality rate that is also observed in these states may partly account for this decreased incidence of low birth weight children. Furthermore, most rural states with a below-average incidence of low birth weight children are Western states that also have large populations of native Americans, an ethnic group that is less likely to bear children of low birth weight. Indeed, a regional study that controlled for the effect of race found rural counties, with one exception, to have a higher rate of infants with low birth weight, very low birth weight, and preterm low birth weight.[5] In the urban counties in this study, infants born of white women had a significantly higher incidence of very low birth weight.

The incidence of cerebral palsy secondary to postneonatal causes is probably higher in rural areas. This is supported by postneonatal mortality rates (deaths occurring between 28 days and one year of life) being higher in nonmetropolitan areas, particularly in black and other nonwhite infants.[1] In a study of children with cerebral palsy living in Saskatoon, the native Indian child is more likely to acquire central nervous system infection.[6] This study supports the concept that postnatal causes of cerebral palsy are higher in the nonwhite rural-based population.

To determine whether the anatomic pattern of cerebral palsy varies in rural versus urban areas, children from North Carolina treated at the Greenville Shriners Hospital for Crippled Children from 1990 were analyzed. For this study, the anatomic patterns were classified as hemiplegia, diplegia, and total body involvement. Total body involvement included those classified by the Shriners Hospital as having quadriplegia, athetosis, athetosis/quadriplegia, and hemiplegia/quadriplegia. The 19 urban North Carolina counties were compared with the 81 rural counties.[7] Of the 212 children with cerebral palsy, 63% of those with hemiplegia (n = 60), 58% of those with diplegia (n = 71), and 58% of those with total body involvement (n = 81) were from rural areas. Therefore, the anatomic pattern of cerebral palsy does not seem to be affected by whether a child comes from a rural or an urban area. Admittedly, these data are limited, but they are the most precise that are currently available. The greater percentage of children from rural areas reflects the proximity of a large number of rural western North Carolina counties to the Greenville Shriners Hospital rather than an actual incidence of cerebral palsy in rural regions of North Carolina.

Environmental Barriers and Community Acceptance of People With Cerebral Palsy in Rural Areas

To define priorities for children with cerebral palsy, it is necessary to understand what is important to them when they become adults. Walking, a focal point for parents of young children with cerebral palsy, is not given the same priority by adults who have cerebral palsy. Bleck[8] reports that adults with cerebral palsy rate walking after communication skills, mobility, and independence in performing activities of daily living. Studies evaluating employment of adults with cerebral palsy also note that independence in mobility and travel is a critical factor.[9–11] Therefore, environmental barriers are a relevant issue for the person with cerebral palsy.

How does the rural environment differ from the urban environment for the child and adult with cerebral palsy? Urban areas, which provide specialized buses and other services for handicapped transportation, may allow better access than small towns, which have no services but similar environmental barriers; ie, curbs, steps, and narrow passageways. However, if rural is defined as living on a farm, then the child with cerebral palsy may contend with fewer environmental barriers. Open spaces and soft ground may provide greater access than cluttered concrete sidewalks.

Unstructured play activities in a farming community may be more accommodating to a child with cerebral palsy, particularly because organized, competitive sports increasingly dominate after-school hours for an urban youngster. The greater necessity of rural children doing chores may also be helpful because even limited motor function can be and usually is accommodated. So what if it takes an 11-year-old child with spastic diplegia longer to weed a garden? This activity naturally integrates the child into family life while providing occupational therapy and a sense of self-esteem.

Environmental barriers in rural areas are sometimes circumvented by nonmedical means. I vividly remember the parents of an eight-year-old child with diplegic cerebral palsy relating how happy and outgoing their child had become since he had been given an all-terrain vehicle. The four-wheeler allowed this child, who lived in a small farming community, to keep up with his friends. Needless to say, I did not deliver my standard, semiscathing lecture concerning the dangers of all-terrain vehicles.

Observations by knowledgeable observers have indicated that in Third World countries, the persons with cerebral palsy who live in rural areas function better than their counterparts who reside in urban centers.[12,13] Bleck,[12] upon observing rural villages in India, noted that unpaved village streets had few obstructions to walking, whereas the city streets had so much congestion that disabled children were largely confined to either their home or school environments. Mainstreaming of disabled children and integration of the disabled into the community occurred by necessity and quite naturally in the villages of India and Nepal.[12,13]

Employment for the person with cerebral palsy may actually be more likely in smaller towns even though specialized mass transit services are unavailable. Ingram and associates[14] found that smaller towns offered better niche employment than cities for the person with cerebral palsy. Perhaps, in rural areas people are more likely to know each other and, therefore, the person with cerebral palsy is accepted as an individual rather than being perceived as an abnormal person with an awkward gait. This is also true of rural areas in other countries where the village serves as an extended family that provides mutual support and acceptance of the disabled person.[12,13]

Financial Aspects of Cerebral Palsy: Rural Versus Urban Areas

All parents of children with a chronic illness such as cerebral palsy, whether living in urban or rural areas, have significant expenses that include the obvious hospitalizations, ongoing therapy, special equipment, and medications, as well as the less obvious need for special schooling, extra transportation, long distance telephone calls, and days out of work.[15] In the United States there are no agencies that completely reimburse families for their out-of-pocket expenses; however, for families with insurance, the financial burdens may be similar whether they live in a metropolitan or nonmetropolitan area. For those who live in rural areas, greater transportation costs may be offset by less frequent therapy sessions.

Is public or governmental support equivalent for uninsured children with cerebral palsy who live in rural areas? I could not find any studies on this question and, therefore, analyzed funding in North Carolina by what is commonly known as the Crippled Children's Services. Crippled Children's Services were started by the federal government in 1935 and were the only significant governmental source providing medical care for low-income children with cerebral palsy and other chronic illnesses until Medicaid was established in the 1960s.[1] In 1981, Congress removed the requirement that each state have a Crippled Children's Service, but in North Carolina, as in most other states, this agency continues to administer monies and sponsor clinics for children with chronic illnesses, albeit under other names and with fewer federal dollars. In North Carolina, this agency now goes by the name of Children's Special Health Services. In the 47 Orthopaedic Clinics sponsored by the Children's Special Health Services of North Carolina, 18% of the children seen during 1990 had a diagnosis of cerebral palsy. Direct expenditures for these children plus their share of the clinic budget in the 1990–1991 fiscal year totalled $1,801,658.52 (J. O'Keefe, personal communication, July 12, 1991).

To determine whether children with cerebral palsy living in rural counties of North Carolina receive an equivalent amount of state monies for health care, I compared expenditures by the Children's Special Health Services during the 1990–1991 fiscal year for the 19 urban coun-

Table 1 Expenditures for children with cerebral palsy*

Expenditure	Dollar Amount	Percent
Inpatient care	$1,267,651	34.8
Outpatient physician fees	78,794	2.6
Occupational & physical therapy	269,551	7.3
Speech therapy	11,423	0.3
Drugs and formula	27,870	0.7
Appliances and supplies	1,976,468	54.3
Total	$3,631,757	100.0

*North Carolina Children's Special Health Services: 1983–1988

ties versus the 81 rural counties. The 81 rural counties accounted for 48% of the state's population and 49% of the expenditures for children with cerebral palsy. Therefore, governmental health care dollars seem to be equally distributed among urban and rural children with cerebral palsy, at least in North Carolina.

The expenditures for children with cerebral palsy by the Children's Special Health Services of North Carolina from 1983 to 1988 are listed in Table 1. Eighty-nine percent of the health-care dollars for children with cerebral palsy are expended on inpatient care and appliances. Reconstructive operations account for most of the inpatient care costs.

Is it possible that children with cerebral palsy from rural areas, who live a long distance from a tertiary center, get appropriate surgical care and adaptive equipment, but are less likely to benefit from a well-coordinated, multidisciplinary team approach started at an early age? With the increased distance and a greater likelihood of being below the poverty level,[1,16] it is certainly conceivable that these children will receive less treatment during early childhood. During this time of rapid growth and muscle imbalance, inadequate early evaluation and treatment might contribute to the development of severe contractures, dislocated hips, and other bony deformities that require extensive surgery. More complex surgery is associated with longer hospitalizations and higher physicians' fees. Therefore, the cost of medical care for the child from a rural area who did not receive appropriate early care could ultimately be equivalent to or higher than the cost for a child living in an urban area.

Evidence supporting the concept that children with cerebral palsy receive less medical management when they live a long distance from tertiary centers was provided by a committee that analyzed treatment of children with developmental disabilities in a six-country area of rural eastern North Carolina.[17] In 1985, only 42% of the children in this region with cerebral palsy who were eligible for public assistance were receiving treatment at any facility, despite the fact that the area had three traditional orthopaedic clinics sponsored by the Children's Special Health Services. These clinics were primarily seeing children with intoeing, out-toeing, knock knees, and flatfeet problems. The child with cerebral palsy was commonly either not being seen by the appropriate specialists or was managed in an isolated fashion by a school physical therapist.

Principles of Providing Optimal Therapy for the Child Who Lives in a Rural Area

Expending time, money, and effort on improving the functional ability of children with cerebral palsy is appropriate and is supported by Walker and associates'[18] study, which showed that the life outcome and satisfaction rating of an individual with multiple handicaps was most strongly related to his/her functional status. On the other hand, it is not possible to cure cerebral palsy or to make these patients function completely normally. Therefore, orthopaedic surgeons, physical therapists, and other health-care professionals working with these children should strive to improve function but, at the same time, have realistic aims and priorities.

The means to provide optimal therapy may be different, but the goals or aims of treatment should be similar whether a child with cerebral palsy lives in an urban or rural setting. Bleck[8] states that next to employment, a prime goal of treatment should be independent living and prevention of institutionalization. Improving function to accomplish these goals not only enhances personal satisfaction of the individual with cerebral palsy, but also is economically beneficial to governments who largely finance this very expensive institutional care.

Scrutton[19] has listed three aims for the physical therapist working with children with cerebral palsy, which are also relevant for any health care professional working with these children.[20] The first aim or goal should be development of an accurate prognosis for locomotive and other problems. Support for this premise is found in Tarran's study,[21] in which she found that parents need early and continuing information about the diagnosis and prognosis of their child. The second aim for managing children with cerebral palsy is identification of problems and determining which problems can either be eliminated or ameliorated. The third aim is to assess a child's home or life situation, then produce a list of practical goals and the means to achieve them, and then discuss this assessment with the parents.

Because cerebral palsy is a multifaceted problem, a multidisciplinary team approach usually provides the most effective means of accomplishing these goals, especially for the child with diplegic or total body involvement. Every person on the team does not necessarily provide ongoing treatment for all children, but they should provide input into the initial evaluation and be available as indicated for subsequent evaluation and therapy. It is of great importance that members of the team communicate their goals to the other members of the team. This provides better understanding of the whole child and, in my experience, is a restraint to impractical treatment. Admittedly, the optimal model for this clinic has not been agreed upon, and local circumstances to some degree will dictate how the clinic will be structured.

The first problem is diagnosis. Primary care providers, whether in rural or urban areas, need to recognize the child with developmental delays and understand the musculoskeletal problems that arise from muscle imbalance at an early age. When the diagnosis of cerebral palsy is established or suspected, the child should be evaluated in a multi-disciplinary clinic where the diagnosis, prognosis, treatment goals, and means to accomplish these should be outlined.

Enhancement of motor development and prevention of contractures, usually by use of physical therapy, are the primary goals of early management.[8] The child who lives in a rural area may ultimately receive surgery and be provided with adaptive equipment, but how can this child receive effective physical therapy? Being treated by a trained pediatric physical therapist three to five times a week is impossible. That frequency of formal physical therapy, however, may not be necessary. Von Wendt and associates[22] analyzed a parent-centered approach to physiotherapy for children living in rural areas of Sweden and found that relatively few parents had difficulties in performing therapy provided that there was adequate contact and support by the physiotherapist. Short and associates[23] observed more effective physical therapy when parents are involved. Siblings can also be effective therapists. Craft and associates[24] found that siblings were effective teachers, role models, and agents of change when they were taught about cerebral palsy and encouraged to do what was feasible to make their brother or sister more independent. Not only did these children with cerebral palsy demonstrate increased range of motion and improvement in motor function, but their siblings were noted to gain an increased sense of self-importance.

Therefore, the young child with cerebral palsy who lives in an isolated rural setting can receive an effective program of repetitive movements and exercise that will enhance motor development. A knowledgeable physical therapist is instrumental in defining the program and instructing parents and siblings, but whether the child and parents should be seen once a week, once a month, or once every six months depends on the child's age, the goals for the child, and the home situation.

Solutions for Multidisciplinary Care in a Rural Area

Many different solutions exist for multidisciplinary management of the child with cerebral palsy who lives in a rural area. I will profile two of these solutions. One comes from a rural, sparsely populated state with a dominating metropolitan area, and the other is a satellite multidisciplinary clinic in a state with a relatively large rural population but no dominating metropolitan center.

Multidisciplinary Care in a Rural, Sparsely Populated State With a Dominating Metropolitan Center: The New Mexico Solution

The population of New Mexico, according to the 1990 census, is 1,515,069. New Mexico ranks 37th in population, but fifth in total area among the 50 states of the United States. Fifty-three percent of the population live in nonmetropolitan areas[1] and about one third of the state's people live in the city of Albuquerque. Carrie Tingley Hospital, a state-supported institution located in Albuquerque, provides medical service for chronic pediatric conditions. Seventy-five percent of the children treated at Carrie Tingley Hospital live outside of Albuquerque. The radius of service for the hospital is approximately 300 miles and reflects the large size of the state. As in other similar children's hospitals, the most common condition seen is cerebral palsy (J. Aceves, personal communication, July 9, 1991; R.B. Winter, personal communication, 1991).

A multidisciplinary team has been assembled to provide care for children with cerebral palsy (J. Aceves, personal communication, July 9, 1991). Included in the cerebral palsy clinic are orthopaedic surgeons, pediatricians, pediatric neurologists, a nurse program coordinator, a physical therapist, an occupational therapist, a speech and language pathologist, a dietician, a dental hygienist, and a parent representative. A new patient clinic is held once a month, at which time the child and family are evaluated by each part of the multidisciplinary team. At the end of the day, an interpretive meeting is held with the family. A written summary of the consultations is given to the family prior to departure. The interpretive session and written report provide the parents with information about the diagnosis and prognosis of their child's condition. The written report provides immediate information to the referring physician, to the school, to local physical therapists, and to the insurance companies. In the following week a separate, more comprehensive medical report is sent to the referring physicians.

A follow-up cerebral palsy clinic is also held once a week. During that clinic all members of the team are available, but the child is seen only by the appropriate specialists. No interpretive meetings are held with the family or with the staff after the follow-up clinics.

Two important members of the team are the clinic coordinator and the parent representative. The nurse coordinator maintains periodic contact with the families to assist them with referrals to other specialists, transportation, and other problems. The parent representative has a child with cerebral palsy and is paid a salary from donated funds. Therefore, the parent representative has the responsibilities of an employee, but the empathy of a parent. The parent representative identifies family-related issues and school placement problems. This person is also a member of Parents Reaching Out Association, a support group and center for information on resources and services.

Satellite clinics are also held by the orthopaedic surgery and pediatric staff but, by necessity, these clinics can neither cover the full state of New Mexico nor provide comprehensive multidisciplinary evaluation and treatment. They are effective in providing follow-up for certain segments of the population and as a preliminary screening for new referrals.

Satellite Multidisciplinary Clinic in a Rural Area: The North Carolina Solution

North Carolina has the second largest nonmetropolitan population in the United States. To provide a multidisciplinary clinic in a rural area located a long distance from tertiary medical centers, the Children's Special Health Services of North Carolina organized one satellite multidisciplinary neuromuscular clinic in March 1987. The success of this clinic has led to the institution of two additional clinics in 1990. Although only minor variations exist, I will restrict description of the satellite neuromuscular clinic to the one started in 1987.

The purpose of the neuromuscular satellite clinic is to evaluate and direct the management of children with neuromuscular disorders in a six-county area. The clinic team consists of a pediatric orthopaedic surgeon accompanied by an orthopaedic surgery resident, two pediatric physical therapists, a developmental pediatrician, public health nurses, a dietician, a social worker, and an adaptive equipment vendor.

The neuromuscular clinic is held monthly in a county health department. A public health nurse from that county serves as the coordinator for the neuromuscular clinic. She is assisted by public health nurses from adjacent counties. The developmental pediatrician and one of the pediatric physical therapists primarily are from a local developmental evaluation center and, therefore, are knowledgeable about the services in the six-county area. They also facilitate communication and assistance from the local pediatricians, neurologists, radiology departments, and physical therapists. The other physical therapist and the social worker are regional coordinators for the Children's Special Health Services. They facilitate communication with state governmental agencies as well as coordinating services within the six-county area. The orthopaedic surgeons come from a tertiary care university center located 150 miles away. To minimize travel time, they are flown in small airplanes maintained by the university and funded by federal support monies. The adaptive equipment vendor also comes from the central portion of the state, but drives to the clinic in a van so that special equipment can be tried or delivered.

New patients are seen by all members of the team. Evaluation and follow-up visits are based on the child's specific problem, but multidisciplinary assessment is strived for on an annual to biannual basis. The patient is kept in a single room, and the different disciplines rotate into the room to see the child. As a result of the close proximity and common purpose of the group, interchange among the disciplines is frequent. In addition, a wrap-up session at the end of the clinic enhances communication.

Local physical therapists working through early childhood intervention programs, home health agencies, or public school systems frequently attend the clinic when one of their patients is present. This direct interchange provides the neuromuscular clinic personnel with a better understanding of the patient's home and school situation, while the treating therapists receive guidelines and practical expectations for treatment. In a similar fashion, public health nurses from the surrounding counties often provide useful information concerning feeding and seizure problems, stresses in the home, and parental understanding of the home therapy program.

Approximately 80% of the patients seen at the satellite neuromuscular clinic have cerebral palsy. Other neuromuscular diseases evaluated include Down syndrome, Duchenne's muscular dystrophy, myelomeningocele, and other types of neuromuscular diseases. Patients with myelomeningocele are seen in conjunction with a myelomeningocele clinic at a tertiary center because the satellite clinic does not provide urologic or neurosurgical treatment.

Eleven clinics were held during the 1990–1991 fiscal year. Fifty new patients were seen and 78 established patients had a total of 154 visits. Therefore, each neuromuscular clinic averaged 4.5 new evaluations and 19 return visits. The relatively large proportion of new patients is related to the transient population stationed at a nearby large military installation.

Discussion

My research suggests that money spent for a child with cerebral palsy in a rural area is equivalent to that spent for a child in an urban area. The availability of multidisciplinary management, however, may be less, particularly for the child who lives a long distance from a tertiary center. That is understandable, especially for families with limited circumstances, as the cost of frequent long trips may be prohibitive.

Transportation barriers must be ameliorated for families with a child needing chronic, comprehensive care. Shriners Hospital for Crippled Children recognizes this need and has provided perhaps the best solution. Members of the Shrine volunteer their time and vehicles to bring needy patients to clinics or pay transportation costs to bring the patient and a parent to the center. The state of New Mexico and Carrie Tingley Hospital have also provided a good solution for their sparsely populated state. Transportation costs of families coming to Carrie Tingley Hospital are paid for by Children's Medical Services (formerly Crippled Children's Program), by Medicaid, or by specifically designated funds. By contrast, in North Carolina, transportation services to tertiary centers are limited. In the best of circumstances, county agencies provide vans that carry patients of all types and ages to tertiary centers. The schedule for the van is variable and sporadic so that the child often cannot be seen in the appropriate comprehensive clinic. More importantly, the counties farthest away from the tertiary centers typically have the most limited resources and, therefore, often provide no transportation services. Difficulties in transportation were the primary reason that the majority of children having neuromuscular disorders and limited resources from a six-county region of eastern North Carolina were either not being served or were being seen in a sporadic and financially burdensome fashion in a tertiary center.

The satellite neuromuscular clinic may be a good solution for rural regions with a relatively large population. These regional neuromuscular clinics provide multidisciplinary care at a more local area and therefore provide services to many children who were not previously treated. That, plus more effective communication with local physicians and physical therapists, have been its relative strengths. The satellite clinic cannot be as comprehensive as a cerebral palsy clinic at a tertiary center; however, except for surgical treatment and orthotic fitting, all services are provided either through the clinic or through local facilities.

In a study of developmentally handicapped children receiving advice from developmental specialists, Cadman and associates[25] found that noncompliance by community care providers was relatively high. Noncompliance by medical personnel was associated with attitudes and beliefs rather than other factors. Therefore, consultants must educate and be clear. Compliance from primary care physicians, local physical therapists, and school systems is particularly important for children who live a long distance from a tertiary center. The written report that accompanies the family when they leave the cerebral palsy clinic at Carrie Tingley Hospital is a good idea. Communication from the satellite neuromuscular clinic has been facilitated by the personnel who work and live in the local region. To gain maximum benefit for patients, specialists in multidisciplinary cerebral palsy clinics must continue to work on this ongoing problem.

Finally, all medical issues being equal, would the typical child with cerebral palsy living in a rural area have advantages over a child growing up in a metropolitan center? This may be true. The reduced environmental barriers have already been mentioned. Rural adolescents are most likely to have both parents at home,[16] a factor that should enhance family support. Family support and self-esteem have been noted as positive factors in people with cerebral palsy who are successfully employed.[11,26] Development of self-esteem may be enhanced by the greater expectation and necessity of all rural children helping with daily chores. By contributing to the family's welfare while participating at their own pace, children with cerebral palsy will achieve maximum function and independence.

References

1. Hughes D, Rosenbaum S: An overview of maternal and infant health services in rural America. *J Rural Health* 1989;5:299–319.
2. Emond A, Golding J, Peckham C: Cerebral palsy in two national cohort studies. *Arch Dis Child* 1989;64:848–852.
3. Naeye RL, Peters EC, Bartholomew M, et al: Origins of cerebral palsy. *AJDC* 1989;143:1154–1161.
4. Stanley FJ: The changing face of cerebral palsy? *Dev Med Child Neurol* 1987; 29:263–265.
5. Moore ML, Buescher PA, Meis PJ, et al: The effect of a preterm birth prevention program in 17 rural and three urban counties in northwest North Carolina. *J Rural Health* 1989;5:361–370.
6. Tervo RC: The native child with cerebral palsy at a children's rehabilitation centre. *Can J Public Health* 1983;74:242–245.
7. Rutledge R, Bell E, Baker CC, et al: A geographic and statistical analysis of the affects of rural and urban residence on trauma deaths in North Carolina. *J Trauma*, in press.
8. Bleck EE: *Orthopaedic Management in Cerebral Palsy*. Philadelphia, JB Lippincott, 1987, chap 6, pp 142–212.

9. Bachman WH: Variables affecting post-school economic adaptation of orthopaedically handicapped and other health impaired students. *Rehab Lit* 1972;3:98–114.

10. Moed M, Litwin D: The employability of the cerebral palsied: A summary of two related studies. *Rehab Lit* 1983;24:266–271.

11. O'Grady RS, Nishimura DM, Kohn JG, et al: Vocational predictions compared with present vocational status of 60 young adults with cerebral palsy. *Dev Med Child Neurol* 1985;27:775–784.

12. Bleck EE: Editorial: Factors affecting independence of the physically disabled. *Dev Med Child Neurol* 1990;32:189–190.

13. Richardson SA: Physical impairment, disability and handicap in rural Nepal. *Dev Med Child Neurol* 1983;25:717–726.

14. Ingram TTS, Jameson S, Errington J, et al: *Living With Cerebral Palsy,* Clinics in Developmental Medicine. London, Wm Heinemann Medical Books Ltd, 1964, no 14.

15. Hobbs N, Perrin JM, Ireys HT, et al: Chronically ill children in America. *Rehab Lit* 1984;45:206–213.

16. McManus MA, Newacheck PW, Weader RA: Metropolitan and nonmetropolitan adolescents: Differences in demographic and health characteristics. *J Rural Health* 1990;6:39–51.

17. Haas K: The minutes of the Neuromuscular Program Committee. Annual Meeting of Neuse Developmental Disabilities Catchment Area Team, Newbern, NC, July 19, 1991.

18. Walker DK, Palfrey JS, Handley-Derry M, et al: Mainstreaming children with handicaps: Implications for pediatricians. *J Dev Behav Pediatr* 1989;10:151–156.

19. Scrutton D: Aim-oriented management, in Scrutton D (ed): *Management of the Motor Disorders of Children With Cerebral Palsy.* Philadelphia, JB Lippincott, 1984, pp 49–58.

20. Bax M: Editorial: Aims and outcomes of therapy for the cerebral-palsied child. *Dev Med Child Neurol* 1986;28:695–696.

21. Tarran EC: Parent's views of medical and social-work services for families with young cerebral-palsied children. *Dev Med Child Neurol* 1981;23:173–182.

22. Von Wendt L, Ekenberg L, Dagis D, et al: A parent-centered approach to physiotherapy for their handicapped children. *Dev Med Child Neurol* 1984;26: 445–448.

23. Short DL, Schkade JK, Herring JA: Parent involvement in physical therapy: A controversial issue. *J Pediatr Orthop* 1989;9:444–446.

24. Craft MJ, Lakin JA, Oppliger Ra, et al: Siblings as change agents for promoting the functional status of children with cerebral palsy. *Dev Med Child Neurol* 1990;32:1049–1057.

25. Cadman D, Shurvell B, Davies P, et al: Compliance in the community with consultant's recommendations for developmentally handicapped children. *Dev Med Child Neurol* 1984;26:40–46.

26. Cohen P, Kohn JG: Follow-up study of patients with cerebral palsy. *West J Med* 1979;130:6–11.

Chapter 37

Risk Factors and Follow-up After Discharge From the Neonatal Intensive Care Unit

Theresa Ricketts, PT
Linda Hanlin, OTR
E. Dennis Lyne, MD

Introduction

Public Law 99-457-Part H[1] provides for a comprehensive, coordinated, multidisciplinary, interagency approach to the delivery of early intervention services to handicapped infants and toddlers, and their families. Close cooperation between hospitals and early intervention providers is essential to the successful implementation of a coherent system of early identification, intervention, referral, and provision of service.[1] Children who have suffered prenatal, perinatal, and/or postnatal complications are most likely to be found in the Neonatal Intensive Care Unit (NICU). The process of identification, intervention, and support should begin in the NICU and build as the child and family move between the medical and educational systems. Because society's ability to fund this type of program is limited, methods of early identification are needed to determine those who are at most risk. A widely accepted general outcome statistic is that the overall handicap rate for infants in the inborn NICU weighing less than 1,500 grams is between 10% and 15%, whereas those in the outborn NICU have a handicap rate of 20% to 25%.

The ability to select a group of neonates who are at highest risk of handicap before their discharge from an NICU allows monitoring of their development throughout infancy, assessment of early intervention techniques, and more efficient use of existing resources.[2] How is this done? Hobel and associates[3] suggest that a screening system be designed that would include intrapartum events in the prediction of the high risk neonate. McCormick,[4] in a study of long-term follow-up, recommends looking at three areas: condition on admission, medical responses to intervention, and sequelae at discharge. An organized, supportive system of follow-up by those professionals who have expertise in this area is indicated. This need is reiterated by Hansen,[5] who states that most parents rely on their pediatricians or primary-care physicians to identify early developmental abnormalities, although a survey by Smith has shown that only 10% of primary-care physicians routinely screen the development of their patients. Studies by Astbury and associates[6] and Blackman and associates[7] support the need for long-term surveillance by specialists. Deficiencies in verbal and perceptual motor skills may not be measurable until a child is closer to five years of age.

It is imperative to develop methods of support and education for families who must make decisions regarding the path of care their child will follow. Forsyth[8] states, "initially most parents feel that their stress is going to end once they go home, but frequently the stress continues after discharge... Parental stress is also known to increase for a week or so before each visit to the follow-up clinic as there is always the fear of hearing something negative about their child's progress."[8]

Our pilot study looked at a variety of risk factors in an NICU population that could serve as indicators of future developmental delay, indicating which children will need specialized services at discharge and will continue to need specialized services during the first three years of life. We also attempted to identify what percentage of children who needed to be followed would be lost to other clinics or elsewhere for unknown reasons. At the request of the Wayne County Interagency Council of Michigan, who funded this project, an "At Risk Scoring System" supplied by the Council was used to identify at risk children (Table 1).

Methods

The "At Risk Scoring System" was developed by the Wayne County Interagency Coordinating Council Subcommittee in an attempt to clarify the eligibility of at-risk infants and toddlers (0 to 3 years) for Public Law 99–457 service. The subcommittee comprised representatives from various infant and toddler programs throughout the county, representatives from medical agencies servicing multihandicapped children, and a representative parent.

After reviewing various risk factors and definitions for developmental delay, the subcommittee concluded that at-risk conditions can be adequately represented by two categories, one including physical/medical conditions and another including psychosocial/environmental conditions. An additional care rating score was to be combined with the risk score; however, this portion was not used in this study.

The authors of the scoring system hypothesized that a score of six or higher would indicate that a child is at risk and in need of early intervention services. This study attempts to assess this scoring system by comparing the risk scores of randomly selected subjects to the follow-up care recommendations of practicing neonatologists.

Sample

Subjects were blindly selected from a computer printout that listed all infants discharged from the NICU over two separate 13-month periods: April 1986 through April 1987 and January 1989 through January 1990. These periods were chosen three years apart so we could compare children needing services at birth to those children requiring services

Table 1 At Risk Category Scoring System

Risk Factors	Risk Score*
Category I Physical/Medical	
Congenital abnormalities, eg, cleft palate, spina bifida, microencephaly, hydrocephaly, etc.	4
Chromosomal anomalies, eg, Down syndrome	4
Genetic disorders, eg, phenylketonuria, sickle cell anemia, etc.	4
Inborn errors of metabolism, eg, Tay-Sacks disease, Hurley disease, etc.	4
Neurologic disorders, eg, neuromuscular disorders, cerebral palsy, seizure disorders, cerebrovascular accident, spinal cord trauma, etc.	4
Respiratory disorders, eg, apnea, asphyxia, bronchopulmonary dysplasia, asthma.	4
Sensory disorders, eg, hearing/vision loss, deafness, blindness.	4
Chronic illness, eg, cancer, cystic fibrosis, diabetes, renal dysfunction	4
Toxic exposure disorder, eg, drug use/abuse resulting in fetal alcohol syndrome/fetal alcohol effect; addiction/withdrawal; parental exposure to medication or teratogen known to cause developmental problems; environmental toxins such as lead, PCB, etc.	4
Severe infectious disease, eg, HIV/AIDS, rubella	4
Parental acute/chronic physical/mental illness, developmental disability/mental retardation.	4
Perinatal complications, eg, birth of a handicapped child, multiple pregnancies, premature/prolonged labor.	3
Prematurity, eg, small for gestational age, birth weight less than 1,500 g.	3
Large for gestational age	3
Atypical or delayed development in one or more areas: cognitive, speech/language, physical, motor, vision, hearing, psychosocial, self-help skills.	3
Failure to thrive, eg, less than tenth percentile in length, weight, and head circumference.	3
Category II Psychosocial/Environmental	
Disturbed infant/mother attachment disorder, eg, infant has persistent feeding, sleeping, eating, nonorganic disorder, withdrawn, unresponsive, inattentive.	4
Teenage parent	4
Child abuse/neglect suspected, reported, family history.	4
Homelessness or inadequate shelter	4
Drug or alcohol dependent parent/caregiver	4
Significant concerns regarding child's competency and well-being	4
Inadequate parenting, eg, unrealistic expectations, inappropriate response to infant's needs, inadequate knowledge of growth and development.	3
Disturbed family interaction due to exposure to negative environment, eg, crime, drugs, violence.	3
Inadequate social support, eg, physical, social, cultural isolation.	2
Parent/child separation due to parental incarceration, divorce, or death.	2
Lack of prenatal care	1
Living at or below federal/state poverty level	1
Inadequate health care or no insurance	1
Parental unemployment	1
Less than 12th grade education	1
History of losses, eg, stillborn, abortion, miscarriage, SIDS	1
Total Score	

*NOTE: A score of 6 or above indicates an at risk condition and need for early intervention services.

at one year and three years after discharge. Any infant admitted to the NICU for any reason was on the list of discharged patients. Twenty percent of the total infant population was selected by choosing every fifth child on the list. This provided 66 subjects from 1986 and 74 subjects from 1989, for a total of 140 subjects. There were no exclusions in this study.

Data Collection

Data collection took place over a three-month period in the summer of 1990. Information was collected from three areas: (1) inpatient medical records (birth and medical history); (2) Developmental Assessment Clinic records (outpatient follow-up documentation); and (3) phone interviews with parents of the subjects.

Birth information gathered from the medical record included maternal age, gestational age, birth weight, sex, perinatal complications, and county the parent resided in. Inpatient treatment parameters examined included diagnosis, length of stay, the need for oxygen and/or ventilation, and discharge recommendations for follow-up.

The Developmental Assessment Clinic attempts to follow children determined to be at risk by the hospital's criteria. The initial visit is two weeks after discharge, to see the neonatologist. Patients return for developmental assessment at six months and 15 months corrected age, and at two, three, and four years chronological age or as otherwise instructed. We looked at compliance with the recommended visits, any additional medical concerns of the neonatologists, and referrals to other clinics and/or ancillary services reported.

Based only on clinical discharge data available in the hospital medical record, the authors assigned risk scores to each child using the At Risk Scoring System designed by the Wayne County Interagency Council. Scores were assigned and accumulated depending on the presence of certain diagnostic and/or environmental factors (Table 1). Each patient's score represents the agreement between two ratings. Any disagreement in scoring was reviewed, and final scores were reached by consensus opinion.

In preparation for phone interviews, introductory letters were sent to parents. Information was given about the prospective study and voluntary participation was requested. An interview form was developed (Form 1) to obtain parental perception of adequacy of their education on discharge from the NICU, nature of developmental follow-up received, and the child's general health and developmental status.

Analysis

Student's t-tests were performed to test the statistical significance of continuous variables. Fisher's exact test or chi-square analysis was done for categorical variables. All p-values were determined using two-tailed tests.

The Receiver Operating Characteristic, which examines sensitivity over all specificities, was used to assess the ability of the risk scores to

Form 1 Patient Interview Form

Chart # _____
Chronological Age _____
Corrected Age _____

1. How old is your child now?
2. While your baby was in the NICU was there any teaching done by health care workers on:
   a. Care your baby might need?
   b. Follow-up visits your baby might need?
   c. Was it helpful to you?
3. Was your baby followed in the Developmental Assessment Clinic?
   a. At what age was their last visit?
   b. Were you scheduled for further visits?
   c. Did you feel these visits were helpful?
4. Since discharged from the NICU did your child have any:
   a. Other medical problems?
   b. Routine health care with another doctor or clinic?
5. How do you feel your child is doing now in comparison to other siblings?
6. At what age did your child;
   LANGUAGE:
   First sounds (baba, dada)
   Initiate and say words
   Say 2–3 word sentences
   Say colors and numbers
   Describe what is happening in a picture
   Say their first and last name
   SOCIAL
   Finger feed
   Drink from a cup
   Remove pants or shirt
   Dress themselves with supervision
   Button their shirt
   FINE MOTOR
   Do they reach for toys and transfer hand to hand
   Bang two objects together or play pat a cake
   Do they pick up objects with thumb and first finger
   Scribble with a crayon
   Will they draw a line
   Will they draw a circle
   Will they draw a + sign
   GROSS MOTOR
   Roll over
   Sit without support
   Cruise around furniture
   Walk alone
   Walk up stairs alone
   How do they go up and down stairs
   Pedal a tricycle or hot wheels
   Balance on one foot
   Catch a bounced ball
7. At any age did you or your child receive special services from a school program, social work program or therapy?
8. Are you or your child still receiving these services? If no, then
   a. Were you ever referred?
   b. How long did you receive services?
   c. Are they now enrolled in a school program?
9. What services do you feel you or your child may have benefitted from? (ie, babysitters, transportation, clinic services nearer to your home?)
10. If you could change anything about your child's care, what would it be?

Table 2 Subject characteristics

Variable Name	No. (%)	Minimum	Maximum	Mean (SD)
Sex:				
Male	77(55.0)			
Female	63(45.0)			
Death:				
Before discharge	8(5.7)			
After discharge	5(3.6)			
Location:				
Detroit	81(57.9)			
Suburban	59(42.1)			
Birth weight (grams)	140	520	5,150	2,596.30(1,066.2)
Gestational age (weeks)	137	22	43	35.35(4.7)
Maternal age (years)	137	14	39	25.88(6.2)
Length of stay (days)	140	1	124	16.61(21.3)

predict follow-up. Sensitivity and specificity were calculated for each subject, based on the risk score being the cut-off point, in order to identify the score resulting in the maximum sum of sensitivity and specificity.

Results

Analyses of the data are presented in three areas: examination of the sample characteristics (Table 2), the At Risk Scoring System, and follow-up care needs. Fifty-five percent of the subjects were male and 45% were female. Five of the infants (3.6%) died before discharge from the NICU, while eight (5.7%) died after discharge. A greater portion, 57.9% were residents of Detroit, and the remaining 42.1% were from the suburban area. Of the parents, 55.7% were contacted for telephone interviews. Other subject variables included birth weight (520 to 5,150 g), gestational age (22 to 43 weeks), maternal age (14 to 39 years), and length of stay in the NICU (1 to 124 days).

Physical/Medical Risk Score

The mean Physical/Medical risk score for the sample was 6.81, with a standard deviation (sd) of 4.4. Comparison of the Physical/Medical risk score by year and by location did not yield significant differences (Tables 3 and 4). Infants who had received some type of follow-up care subsequent to discharge (N = 75) had a mean Physical/Medical risk score of 7.57 (sd 4.79) compared to 5.92 (sd 3.66) for those without follow-up. This difference was statistically significant (p = 0.02). Using the Receiver Operating Characteristic, the highest sum of sensitivity and specificity for the Physical/Medical risk score was 1.49, corresponding to a sensitivity of 0.71 and a specificity of 0.78. Thus, of the subjects followed, 71% had Physical/Medical risk scores of 7 or greater.

Table 3 Risk scores

Variables	N*	Minimum	Maximum	Mean (SD)
Physical/Medical	140	0	26	6.81(4.4)
Psychosocial/Environmental	140	0	9	1.44(2.3)
Sum of risk scores	140	0	31	8.25(4.9)

*Number of patients

Table 4 Risk score comparisons

Variable	Mean (SD)	Mean (SD)	t	p value
By Year:				
	1986 (n = 66)	**1989 (n = 74)**		
Medical score	7.26(5.01)	6.41(3.69)	1.1342	0.2590
Psychosocial score	1.29(2.19)	1.58(2.32)	−0.7659	0.4450
Sum of scores	8.54(5.51)	7.99(4.26)	0.6651	0.5072
By Location:				
	Detroit (n = 81)	**Other (n = 59)**		
Medical score	6.96(4.78)	6.59(3.75)	0.4932	0.6226
Psychosocial score	2.11(2.46)	0.50(1.54)	4.6800	0.0001
Sum of scores	9.07(5.30)	7.12(4.02)	2.4826	0.0142
By Follow-up Status:				
	Follow-up (n = 75)	**No follow-up (n = 65)**		
Medical score	7.57(4.79)	5.92(3.66)	−2.3057	0.0226
Psychosocial score	1.63(2.40)	1.23(2.08)	−1.0350	0.3025
Sum of scores	9.20(5.31)	7.15(4.11)	−2.5658	0.0114

Psychosocial/Environmental Risk Score

The mean Psychosocial/Environmental risk score was 1.44 (sd 2.3). Psychosocial/Environmental risk scores were significantly higher for subjects residing in Detroit (2.11, sd 2.46) than for subjects residing in the suburban areas (0.50, sd 1.54, p = 0.001). Although the Psychosocial/Environmental risk score was higher for subjects receiving some type of follow-up care, the difference was not statistically significant. The Psychosocial/Environmental risk score was less adequate in predicting follow-up. The largest sum was 1.2, with a sensitivity of only 0.28 and a specificity of 0.92. Thus, only 28% of the subjects followed up had an elevated Psychosocial/Environmental risk score (Table 4).

Sum of Risk Scores

The mean for the sum of the risk scores was 8.25 (sd 4.9). The sum of scores did not differ by year, but was significantly higher for Detroit residents (9.1, sd 5.3) when compared to that of subjects residing outside of Detroit (7.1, sd 4.0, p = 0.01). Mean sum of scores also differed by follow-up status. Infants receiving one type of follow-up had a mean sum of 9.2 (sd 5.3), while the mean sum for infants without follow-up was 7.2 (sd 4.1). This difference was statistically significant (p = 0.01). Maximum sum of sensitivity and specificity for the sum of risk scores

Table 5 Comparison of sample characteristics

Variable	N*	Mean (SD)	Mean (SD)	t	p value
By Location:					
		Detroit	**Other**		
Birth weight	140	2,400.91(1,056.11)	2,864.68(1,029.21)	−2.59	0.0105
Gestational age	137	35.03(5.00)	35.78(4.30)	−0.93	0.3552
Maternal age	137	24.10(6.00)	28.22(5.69)	−4.07	<0.0001
Length of stay	140	18.48(23.20)	14.03(18.23)	1.27	0.2064
By Follow-up Status:					
		Follow-up	**No follow-up**		
Birth weight	140	2,340.91(956.42)	2,892.15(1,115.95)	3.15	0.0020
Gestational age	137	34.56(4.07)	36.23(5.22)	2.089	0.0397
Maternal age	137	25.12(6.12)	26.73(6.21)	1.53	0.1293
Length of stay	140	24.17(25.41)	7.88(9.67)	1.22	0.2235

*Number of patients

was 1.4, corresponding to a sensitivity of 0.77 and a specificity of 0.61. This was achieved with a summation risk score of 7. Thus, 77% of the subjects followed had a risk score of 7 or greater (Table 4).

Data were also analyzed to assess the relationship of birth weight, gestational age, maternal age, and length of stay with location and the need for follow-up care (Table 5). The birth weight (p = 0.0105) and maternal age (p = 0.0001) were significantly lower in Detroit versus the suburban areas.

The types of follow-up care received after discharge and up to the time of this study were noted, and 53% of the subjects needed some type of specialized care (Table 6). This follow-up may have consisted of home visiting nurses, home equipment such as oxygen or monitors, therapies, early intervention programs, specialty clinics, or other specialized programs such as parenting classes, federal food programs, and social services. Other significant findings included that families of children with a lower birth weight (p = 0.0020) and a lower gestational age (p = 0.0397) were more likely to seek some type of follow-up care (Table 6). According to the follow-up analysis (Table 6), 39.3% of the total subject population did not fit the criteria for Developmental Assessment Clinic follow-up. Of the 49.3% of the subjects scheduled for clinic visits, 9.3% died and clinic follow-up needs of 2.1% were unknown.

Data gathered on compliance with Developmental Assessment Clinic visits were compiled and comparisons made by year and location (Table 7). Only 9 of the 30 subjects in the 1986 group who were referred to the clinic completed or continued with their Developmental Assessment Clinic follow-up. In the 1989 group of subjects, only 23 of the 39 referred completed or continued with their Developmental Assessment Clinic course. Therefore, within one year, 41.1% of the children referred for follow-up care were lost to this clinic. Within three years, 70% were no longer continuing with follow-up in the Developmental Assessment Clinic.

Table 6 Follow-up characteristics

Variable Name	N(%)*
Follow-up status:	
Yes	75(53.6)
No	65(46.4)
Types of follow-up	
Visiting Nurses Association	63(45.0)
Oxygen/monitors	13(9.3)
Occupational therapy	8(5.7)
Physical therapy	10(7.1)
Speech/language	4(2.9)
Early intervention	10(7.1)
Specialty clinics	15(10.71)
Other	15(10.58)
Developmental Assessment Clinic	
None needed	55(39.3)
Complete/continuing	32(22.9)
Incomplete course	21(15.0)
Never returned	16(11.4)
Expired	13(9.3)
Unknown	3(2.1)

*Number of patients

Table 7 Developmental Assessment Clinic: Characteristics

Characteristic	No. of Patients		
By Year:	**1986**	**1989**	**Total**
None needed	27	28	55
Complete/continuing	9	23	32
Incomplete course	17	4	21
Never returned	4	12	16
Expired	6	7	13
By Location:	**Detroit**	**Suburbs**	**Total**
None needed	28	27	55
Complete/continuing	16	16	32
Incomplete course	15	6	21
Never returned	10	6	16
Expired	10	3	13

Discussion

Public Law 99–457-Part H[1] includes early intervention services for at risk infants. However, as described by DeGraw and associates,[9] this law gives each state a "great deal of latitude in defining developmental delay and determining who will be eligible to receive services." These services are to be supplied, in a state-wide, comprehensive, and coordinated system, to children from birth to 3 years of age and their families. "It is left to each state's discretion to include other groups of children who are at risk of developmental delay, such as those with biological risk factors, including prematurity, low birth weight, or perinatal risk factors, and those at environmental risk—biologically normal infants whose early life experiences, including maternal and family care, health care, nutrition, and patterns of physical and social stimulation, are sufficiently limited that there may be a high probability of developmental delay."[9]

This pilot study stated that a variety of risk factors in a NICU population would serve as indicators of future developmental delay. A second component of this study attempted to identify children that needed follow-up services at discharge as well as identify whether these children continued with follow-up services or were lost to our medical system. The At Risk Scoring System supplied by the Wayne County Interagency Council was used to establish indicators of the at risk population. Recommendations for meeting the needs of the at risk infants/ toddlers and their families, which were based on the findings of this study, generally fell into three categories: (1) a system to indicate risk factors; (2) a system for meeting communication needs between families, medical, and educational personnel; and (3) coordination of care extending beyond the initial hospital experience.

The At Risk Scoring System was beneficial in finding the children who needed follow-up care. After using the scoring system, we felt that this tool needed a more in-depth description of the multiple factors that put a child at risk. Some of the literature reviewed supported not only factors concerning the neonate, but also many maternal and socioeconomic factors.[3,4,6,7,9] Though this system did provide a broad base of multiple risk factors, the instructions issued were not detailed, resulting in a dilemma caused by imprecise terminology and difficulty with scoring. A portion of this system, the care rating score, was discarded because its implementation was not clearly defined. In both the Physical/Medical and the Psychosocial/Environmental scales, questions were raised regarding definitions of categories. The consistency of scoring as well as the knowledge base of the nonhealth-care professional using this system may vary. Finally, once they have been identified, what steps should be taken for the at risk infant and family?

This study pointed out some problems involving follow-up care. Within one year (1989), 58.9% of children had not continued with the follow-up visits. At three years after discharge, (1986), only 30% had continued or completed their recommended Developmental Assessment Clinic course. During the telephone interviews, a variety of responses were received regarding follow-up visits. Several of the parents did not remember or understand the need for the follow-up visits. One parent responded that her family physician did not see the need for continued visits. Another parent stated that insurance coverage for developmental assessments was not available to her, illustrating the need for communication between medical personnel and families, as well as the need for coordination of care. A case manager system would initially empower parents with information and assistance that would enable them to make the educated decisions regarding the recommendations of the medical staff. This type of program may prevent a loss of children from medical and developmental care.

A major limitation of the study is the possibility of reviewer bias. Discharge recommendations for follow-up were present in the medical chart and, therefore, were not always unknown to the reviewer. We feel, however, that the criteria on which the risk scores are based are objective and that the resulting bias to our results, if any, is minimal. Nevertheless, these risk scales should be evaluated in other populations in which the reviewers are blinded to the discharge recommendations.

References

1. Gilkeson L, Hilliard AS, Schrag E, et al: Point of view: Commenting on P.L. 99–457. *Zero to Three* 1987;7:13–17.
2. Allen MC, Capute A: Neonatal neurodevelopmental examinations as a predictor of neuromotor outcomes in premature infants. *Pediatrics* 1989;83: 498–505.
3. Hobel CJ, Hyvarinen MA, Okada DM, et al: Prenatal and intrapartum high-risk screening. *Am J Obstet Gynecol* 1973;117:1–9.
4. McCormick MC: Long term follow-up of infants discharged from neonatal intensive care units. *JAMA* 1989;261:1767–1772.
5. Hansen R: Developmental screening: Child and environment. *J Calif Perinatal Assoc* 1983;3:27–30.
6. Astbury J, Orgill AA, Bajuk B, et al: Neurodevelopmental outcome, growth and health of extremely low-birthweight surivors: How soon can we tell? *Dev Med Child Neurol* 1990;32:582–589.
7. Blackman JA, Lindgren SD, Herman A, et al: Long-term surveillance of high-risk children. *Am J Dis Child* 1987;141:1293–1299.
8. Forsyth SC: Physical and occupational therapy in the neonatal intensive care unit. *NDT* 1984;7:13–20.
9. DeGraw C, Edell D, Ellers B, et al: Public Law 99–457: New opportunities to serve young children with special needs. *J Pediatr* 1988;113:971–974.

Chapter 38

Priorities for Treatment of Children With Spastic Diplegia

Andre J. Kaelin, MD

Spastic diplegia is characterized by a central, nonprogressive neurologic lesion occurring early in life. The clinical manifestations express themselves relative to the psychomotor development of the child. There is no cure for the underlying lesion, but preventive measures may decrease the number of new patients, and treatments directed toward the motor dysfunction are able to improve the functional status of affected individuals.

The physiopathology and pathology of spasticity, as well as conservative and surgical treatments, have already been widely discussed in this symposium. I prefer to discuss the organization of public health systems in different European countries because government organizations are mainly responsible for preventive programs and full-range care of spastic patients.

Each country of Europe has its own historic, socioeconomic, and cultural past. This diversity is evident in the different ways of organizing treatment programs for patients with spastic diplegia. Medical school, postgraduate, and specialty programs are very different in each country, and the continental scientific societies found in the United States are rare in Europe. For example, the European Pediatric Orthopaedic Society has been in existence just 10 years, and the European Orthopaedic Society will be founded in 1993. Exchanges between European pediatricians, neurologists, rehabilitators, and orthopaedists are uncommon and based on personal contacts.

For the past 50 years, Western European countries have had the privilege of individualized care, with the patient's family being able to choose the type of treatment, institution, and doctors. Eastern countries developed nationwide institutionalized programs without the alternative choice of a private medical system.

When dealing with health problems, southern Europe, which has a stronger universal tradition, is more individualist and fatalist than northern Europe, which stresses social change.

The socioeconomic condition of each country and its importance to the quality of medical care are difficult to evaluate, but studying perinatal and infant mortality rates is a way to compare health systems.

Countries, Health Systems, and Care

The health-care systems in France, Germany, Austria, Holland, and Great Britain are highly organized. Patients are fully insured by these systems, which cover the perinatal period, medical treatment, physical therapy, orthoses, adapted school programs, and professional integration. Performance of health-care systems depends more or less on the financial status of the country. For example, Belgium and Italy have problems with organization, and Spain is benefitting from a period of economic growth. In countries such as Italy, Spain, and Great Britain, where the public-health system is saturated with patients, 20% to 40% of the population are insured by private companies. Diplegic patients are usually not eligible for private insurance because of the length and the cost of their treatment.

The Swiss system relies on private insurance for preventive measures and on state aid and their social security system for treatment and educational and professional integration of patients with congenital diseases.

If we compare the internal growth income with the cost of health care, it is possible to determine the accessibility of medical care. If the computed index of growth income/health-care cost is high, accessibility of the general population to medical care is good. The majority of the developed countries have an index of 20 to 22. The United States has an index of 10, which means that expensive and high-quality medical care is not available to everyone. On the other hand, Japan and Switzerland have a higher index (Tables 1 through 3).

According to public-health data, life expectancy is longer in Japan and Switzerland than in the United States, and the infant mortality rate is also lower (Tables 4 and 5). These data are important because prenatal care and birth monitoring should be applied to all pregnant women in order to decrease the number of "at risk" babies. Only social programs can provide care and educate pregnant women.

An efficient network of government-supported health service encourages early screening and neurologic assessment of low birth weight and premature babies in order to provide appropriate care as soon as possible. The full range of treatment itself should continue, under the control of multidisciplinary teams including orthopaedists, neurologists, pediatricians, physical therapists, occupational therapists, orthotists, logopedists, psychologists, and specialized teachers. Government support is mandatory in the organization of such programs.

For example, France's program is very well organized. From the beginning of this century, large rehabilitation hospitals were developed, initially to treat patients with tuberculosis and polio. Immunization and antibiotics eradicated those diseases, and now these institutions are devoted mainly to the treatment of functional impairments resulting from spasticity and neurologic diseases. Despite medical treatment,

Table 1 Gross national product by inhabitants (1989)*

Country	Amount (United States Currency)
Switzerland	33,941
Sweden	27,281
West Germany	24,070
Japan	23,973
United States	21,607
France	21,055
Austria	20,906
Belgium	19,528
Italy	18,729
Holland	18,708
Great Britain	16,912

*Union de Banques Suisses, La Suisse en chiffres, 1991.

Table 2 Yearly health cost by inhabitants 1987*

Country	Amount (United States Currency)
United States	2,051
Sweden	1,233
Switzerland	1,225
France	1,105
Germany	1,093
Holland	1,041
Austria	982
Japan	915
Belgium	879
Italy	841
Great Britain	759

*Evenement du Jeudi. Paris, 1991;345:85.

Table 3 Accessibility index: Gross national product/yearly health cost

Country	Index
Switzerland	27
Japan	26
Sweden	22
Belgium	22
Great Britain	22
Italy	22
Germany	22
Austria	21
Holland	18
United States	10

psychologic support, and professional help, adults disabled by spastic diplegia and their families complain of the difficulty of integrating into a normal social, family, and professional life.

Table 4 Infant mortality in 1987

Country	Deaths/1,000 live births
Japan	5
Sweden	5.7
Switzerland	6.8
France	7.4
Belgium	8
Germany	8.3
United States	10.1
Portugal	27

(Data from Schneider H: Regionalisation in obstetrics: Functions of a perinatal center. *Bulletin de perinatologie* 1991;15:9–12.)

Table 5 Life expectancy 1986*

Male	Years	Female	Years
Japan	74.4	Switzerland	81
Switzerland	74	France	80.7
Italy	72.6	Japan	80.5
France	72.5	Italy	79.1
Germany	72.4	United States	78.3
United States	71.3	Germany	78.1
Portugal	70.7	Portugal	77.6

**Evenement du Jeudi* 1991;345:77.

Swiss Organization

In Switzerland, the different cantons or states each handle their own health-care system. Depending on urbanization, the number of citizens per medical doctor varies from 254 citizens per doctor in canton Basel to 1,224 citizens per doctor in canton Appenzell. Access to full-range care for spastic patients varies in the same way. In Switzerland, five university hospitals provide optimal full-range care, and the social security system supports the cost of all treatment, education, and vocational training for all spastic patients.

Each center has its own organization. In Basel, spastic children are treated by an orthopaedic surgeon whose specialty is neuro-orthopaedics. In Zurich, the pediatric rehabilitation department is in charge. In Bern, a neuropediatrician handles coordination of care, and in Geneva a team of pediatric neurologists and orthopaedists organizes the multidisciplinary care for spastic patients.

Orthopaedic research teams are mainly active in Basel under the direction of Professor Jurg Baumann; his research program covers all the treatment fields: gait analysis, surgical correction, rehabilitation, and orthosis. In the orthopaedic clinic of Geneva, Professor Taillard developed with Yves Blanc an electromyocinesigraphic model for gait assessment.

In Switzerland, the organization of care for spastic patients is based on a social insurance system, that pays all medical and educational costs, including hospitalization, physiotherapy, orthoses, special schools, and transport fees from home to school, as well as professional training and architectural modifications for the home.

The system is effective and heavily administered. Medical doctors and an ad hoc commission of the social security system are responsible for distribution of funds.

Global Care in Geneva: Urban Areas

In Geneva, the number of new diplegic patients decreased more than 40% in the last ten years because of the prenatal examination program. Pregnancy monitoring consists of monthly clinical examinations and blood tests performed during the first eight months of pregnancy, then every two weeks until delivery. Two ultrasonographic examinations are recommended, at 18 and 32 weeks of gestation. Amniocentesis or chorionic villous sampling are not performed routinely.

Between 1985 and 1989, prenatal transport of high risk cases to a hospital providing neonatology and pediatric intensive care units has doubled. High risk and low birth weight babies are screened for brain lesions by a specialized pediatrician. As soon as a cerebral lesion is suspected, the neuropediatrician and the orthopaedist are consulted. A neuroreeducation program begins as early as possible in order to provide stimulation and to comparatively assess development. Neuroreeducation is executed by specialized physical therapists trained in the Bobath method.

If the diagnosis is confirmed, a nurse supports the family at home, helping the parents to cope with the disease and to enhance personal contacts. Rehabilitation aims at developing the intact functions and preventing secondary disorders. Orthoses and surgery are used when spontaneous progress slows down or stops.

Kindergarten and primary public schools provide a wide spectrum of possible integration, from a normal school setting to classes in the Children's Hospital, which provides an intensive therapy program. Coordinated medical and surgical care is provided by a team of physicians and surgeons located in the same building. Periodic functional and ergonometric assessments, as well as psychologic and intelligence tests, will help the team to choose the best school system and, then, the best professional training. The mean level of education of diplegic patients is comparable to that of normal teenagers and young adults. However, social and professional integration remain far from complete. Even patients who have a college-level education find it difficult to compete in the workforce. Fewer than 50% of these patients eventually marry.

Failure to integrate adult spastic patients represents the biggest problem now faced by orthopaedic surgeons. Media campaigns try to present a positive image of handicapped patients. Prenatal and postnatal screening programs, treatment methods, and educational measures can be considered successful only if there is real potential for a normal adult life.

Chapter 39

Goals and Management in Scandinavia

Jørgen Reimers, MD

In Scandinavia it is possible to specialize in orthopaedic surgery without any special examination or training in pediatric orthopaedics. Most surgeons' knowledge about treatment of cerebral palsy is, therefore, quite accidental. All treatment is given free of charge.

Sweden

For a population of 8.3 million, Sweden has 44 clinics for children, as well as general clinics whose staffs include a pediatric neurologist and the local orthopaedic surgeon, who does the simple surgery. There are also two or three experts in cerebral palsy surgery who travel to these clinics to see difficult cases; these experts do the more involved surgery at the University Hospitals.

Finland

In this nation of 4.7 million, cerebral palsy surgery is performed by two orthopaedic and two pediatric surgeons. Five orthopaedic and some pediatric surgeons have extensive experience with cerebral palsy, but most orthopaedic surgeons in Finland have neither training nor interest in cerebral palsy surgery.

Norway and Iceland

I have no information from these countries. However, I know that in Norway, most children with cerebral palsy are treated by one orthopaedist.

Denmark, Including Greenland and the Faroe Islands

For a population of 5.2 million, there were five experienced pediatric orthopaedic surgeons, who took care of the treatment in cerebral palsy.

However, ten years ago, the special orthopaedic hospitals belonging to the Home and Society for Crippled Children were incorporated into the public hospitals, and the earlier emphasis at these institutions on care for the handicapped changed in favor of surgery for arthrosis. I am now the only orthopaedic surgeon with extensive experience in treatment of cerebral palsy working at the only department in Denmark for pediatric orthopaedics. Our waiting list for nonacute cerebral palsy is more than 1.5 years.

Of course, many children are treated at different clinics by pediatric neurologists and therapists and are also seen by an orthopaedic surgeon. But, perhaps because deterioration of the untreated child with cerebral palsy is gradual, many parents seem to be satisfied with treatment that does not include surgical corrections.

There are, in principle, two sorts of surgeons. One says, ''If you ask for it, it is of course possible to operate, but you must realize that the muscles will then become weaker!'' The other says, ''We must operate upon the muscles and tendons to weaken the muscles. Then the spasticity and the deforming force of the muscles will decrease!'' What answer would a surgeon who has not learned about cerebral palsy surgery give to the parents?

We have some special schools for handicapped children, but most children with cerebral palsy attend special classes in normal schools.

Chapter 40

Cerebral Palsy Treatment in Moscow Children's Hospital No. 18

Evgeny G. Sologubov, MD

Moscow Children's Hospital No. 18 is a 420-bed children's ortho-paedic and rehabilitation hospital. There are ten departments within the hospital: nine focus on children with cerebral palsy and one, which contains 60 beds, treats children with spinal injuries. There are 30 beds for newborns, 120 beds for children up to 3 years of age, 90 beds for children 3 to 7 years of age, and 120 beds for older children. Within this group of beds for children with cerebral palsy, 120 are for surgical treatment. In 1990, more than 3,000 patients were treated at the hospital; approximately half of these were from Moscow and the remainder were from other Soviet Republics. The average inpatient stay is one week.

There are a variety of different disciplines within the hospital. There is a research department that studies the pathophysiology of cerebral palsy. Medical departments include neurology, orthopaedic surgery, neurosurgery, urology, and radiology. In addition, there are physio-therapists, teachers, and other specialists (Fig. 1). There also is an independent school for 180 pupils. In addition to the inpatient service, there is an outpatient service in which over 25,000 patients are seen yearly. Sixty-three percent of the outpatients are from Moscow and the remainder from other Republics.

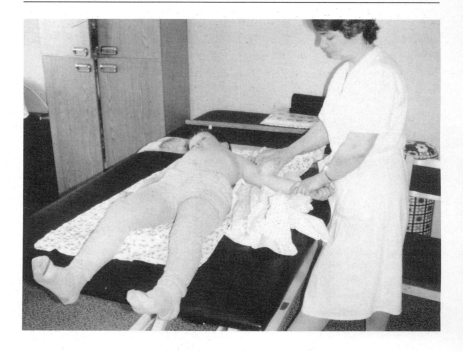

Fig. 1 *Patient with cerebral palsy receiving ice massage therapy.*

Consensus

The papers in this section concern themselves with health care delivery for cerebral palsy patients in the United States and throughout the world. The discussion in this section concerns itself with cerebral palsy of all varieties, not just spastic diplegia.

What Are We Doing, What Should We Be Doing, and Where Are We Going?

As orthopaedic surgeons, we are only one of the health-care providers for these children. We would like to be able to eliminate or reduce the number of new cases and to provide care that achieves the desired outcomes without producing adverse consequences. Some of the initial steps in achieving this would be: (1) establish diagnostic criteria; (2) establish risk factors; (3) establish severity indicators; (4) quantitate the severity of cerebral palsy; (5) determine the therapeutic options; (6) design outcome studies that provide us with the necessary information about our treatment methods; and (7) find treatment factors that affect the natural history and outcomes.

Funding

Funding for cerebral palsy in the United States comes from private health insurance, governmental agencies, and private benefactors. While the number of uninsured children is unknown, it may approach 13% to 19%. Perhaps up to 10% of other children with other chronic illnesses have no insurance. Forty percent of disabled children who come from families below the federal poverty line are not covered by Medicaid. Shriners Hospitals are the largest single provider of care for children with cerebral palsy. The United Cerebral Palsy (UCP) Association is also a major contributor to funding of care for cerebral palsy patients. The UCP is a nationwide network of state and local agencies that provide a significant amount of compensated care; however, their expenditures are also supported to a great extent by patient revenue, including third party payors. Medicaid, which was enacted to finance and improve access to care for the poor has developed into the largest public provider for long-term care for the elderly.

Rural Care

The delivery of rural care varies from state to state. There are several different models. In some, like North Carolina, satellite clinics are available for provision of this care. In others, such as new Mexico, a large central clinic is probably the best solution.

Urban Health Care for the Cerebral Palsied Child

As the centers of many large cities continue to disintegrate, the health-care facilities and ability to use public facilities decrease precipitously for the disabled person. The primary concern in the disintegration process is the disruption of the family, which forms the cornerstone of adequate health care. There is also a loss of essential services including transportation and of functional partners such as schools, municipal recreation programs, government systems, etc. Very often the disintegrating urban society places the care of the disabled child in its lowest priority level. All this adds up to a lack of access to health care, and also a lack of follow-up for those identified as high risk from neonatal intensive care units. This affects directly the government-mandated public law for free, early intervention services.

The key to establishing priorities in this dysfunctional environment include the following: (1) the average citizen, who remains surprisingly strong and caring for children; (2) the establishment of priorities for children and mothers in the public domain; (3) partnership with such viable organizations as churches, which tend to be extremely helpful, especially in the educational areas; (4) the emphasis on a positive attitude because, in most cases, the positives outweigh the negatives; and (5) the creation of a networking system that emphasizes whatever positive is remaining in the structures. The true key is love and concern, for the child and for those less able to care for themselves.

European Systems of Delivery of Care

In the Scandinavian countries, the number of specialists may be limited and the waiting lists may be up to one and one half years. Many patients attend special schools, but others are in regular schools. All care is free including physical therapy. In Switzerland, care is provided by the cantons, which are similar to our states. Private insurance pays for preventative measures; state organizations and social security systems pay for the treatment, education, and vocational training of persons with congenital diseases. In Russia, one example was the Moscow Children's Psychoneurological Clinical Hospital. This 420-bed hospital has a clinic and an independent school. It is a full-service hospital with a variety of specialists involved in the care of handicapped children as well as the therapists needed to treat this abnormality.

Index